BOOKS BY THE SAME AUTHOR

1. Advanced Public Administration
2. Public Administration: Theory and Practice
3. Public Financial Administration
4. Public Health Policy and Administration
5. Public Personnel Administration: Theory and Practice
6. Administration and Management of NGOs: Text and Case Studies
7. Panchayati Raj in India: Theory and Practice
8. Urban Development and Management
9. Management Techniques: Principles and Practices
10. Encyclopaedia of Disaster Management (Set in 3 Vols.)
11. Management of Hospitals: Hospital Administration in the 21st Century (Set in 4 Vols.)
12. Hospital Core Services
13. Hospital Managerial Services
14. Hospital Preventive and Promotive Services
15. Hospital Supportive Services
16. Health Care System and Management (Set in 4 Vols.)
17. Health Care Management and Administration
18. Primary Health Care Management
19. Health Care Organisation and Structure
20. Health Care, Policies and Programmes
21. Nursing Services: Management and Administration
22. Distance Education in 21st Century
23. Encyclopaedia of Higher Education in 21st Century
24. Human Values and Education
25. Stress Management
26. Population Policy and Family Welfare Administration
27. International Administration
28. International Civil Service : Principles, Practice and Prospects
29. Social Welfare Administration (2 Volumes)
30. Family Planning Programme and Beyond
31. Education Policy and Administration
32. Human Resource Development in 21st Century
33. Disaster Management
34. Slum Improvement through Participatory Urban Based Community Structures
35. Development Planning and Administration
36. Public Health Administration
37. Hospital Administration: Theory and Practice
38. Principles, Problems and Prospects of Co-operative Administration
39. Personnel Administration in Co-operatives
40. Public Personnel Administration and Management
41. Right to Information and Good Governance
42. Health Education: Theory and Practice
43. School Health Education
44. Good Governance: An Integral Approach
45. Disaster Administration and Management

IN PRESS

46. Education of Lifestyle and Lifetime Diseases
47. Health Education of Communicable and Non-Communicable Disease
48. Health Education Administration : From International Level to Village Level
49. Education for Healthy Urban Cities
50. Environment and Value Education
51. Women Health Education
52. Rural Health Education

ENVIRONMENTAL HEALTH AND VALUE EDUCATION

DR. S.L. GOEL
Vice-President, Executive Council,
Indian Institute of Public Administration, New Delhi
Professor of Public Administration (Retd.)
DCS, Panjab University, Chandigarh
Emeritus Fellow, University Grants Commission
Director, State Bank of India (Local Board), Chandigarh
Director, National Horticulture Board, Ministry of Horticulture,
Government of India, New Delhi
Formerly Member UGC, Member Distance Education Council
and Member All India Board of Management, AICTE

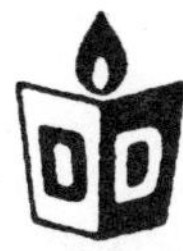

DEEP & DEEP PUBLICATIONS PVT. LTD.
F-159, Rajouri Garden, New Delhi-110027

ENVIRONMENTAL HEALTH AND VALUE EDUCATION

ISBN 978-81-8450-117-9

Typeset by S.S. COMPOSERS,
3190, Mohindra Park, Shakur Basti, Delhi-110034.

Printed in India at MAYUR ENTERPRISES,
WZ Plot No. 3, Gujjar Market, Tihar Village, New Delhi-110018.

Published by DEEP & DEEP PUBLICATIONS PVT. LTD.,
F-159, Rajouri Garden, New Delhi-110027.
Phones: 25435369, 25440916
E-mail: ddpbooks@yahoo.co.in • ddpubs@gmail.com
Showroom:
2/13, Ansari Road, Daryaganj, New Delhi-110002 • Telefax: 23245122

Contents

Preface

Health affects and is affected by other factors. Environment is basic to health promotion. Tord Kjellstrom in his Article, Health Hazards of the Environment: Measuring the Harm in *World Health,* June 1988 rightly feels that whenever a dramatic out-break of "pollution disease" occurs, the attention of the world focuses on a severe "symptom" rather than the "diseases" itself. The dramatic out-breaks with a mass media appeal only occur under special circumstances. But the daily exposure of millions to pollution which causes severe health effects goes unnoticed and unreported. The underlying causes tend to be the same; hazardous chemicals or other agents used or produced by industrial or agricultural technologies that have at the same time brought prosperity and development at least to some parts of the community.

Towns like Minamata in Japan and Bhopal in India have unwillingly become notorious reminders of the side-effects of industrialization, but the suffering of the victims of pollution disease in those towns must spur us to intensified efforts to prevent pollution disease wherever it occurs.

A number of major disease out-breaks caused by environmental hazards have occurred. The examples given overleaf have become prominent partly because of the high numbers of people affected in a local area and partly because of the very dramatic suffering of the community, but also because of the often extensive and detailed health effect studies subsequently carried out. Each dramatic outbreak has triggered epidemiological and other studies, which provide details about the extent of the exposed population, the numbers initially affected, those with severe long-term health effects, and the prevalence of less severe consequences. These measurements of the health effects of pollution are essential as they will pin down the exact causes and will provide the detailed information required to take effective preventive action.

There is a need to educate the people about environmental health programme. These may includes:

- Emphasizing it is the people's programme not the authorities.
- Working with people, not against them.
- Building self-confidence, not destroying it.
- Supporting and helping, not coercing people.
- Concentrating on positive not negative approaches.

- Working with all sectors, not just a few.
- Cooperating with organizations, not "taking them on."
- Drawing on community resources, not funding everything.
- Encouraging participation not passivity.

Values are essential to keep good health. Values provide the essential parameters which are essential for positive health.

For a harmonious and a better quality of life in the twenty-first century, what is required is a new national as well as global socio-political agenda for the establishment of a new social order with a sound foundation of physical culture, mental culture and soul culture, and working hand-in-hand to produce the enlightened, educated and complete man of genuine culture. This enjoins integration of physical sciences with the science of spirit or spiritualism. If materialism is a quest for a better quality of outer life, spiritualism is the quest that begins with the ascent of man and society towards humanism and pursuit of eternal human values that will guarantee the advancement of contemporary civilization and the glory of man and society. The integration of the two is imperative for the betterment of mankind by putting an end to the prevailing disequilibrium, disharmony and disorder in the human life at all levels from home to the global village. It would elevate man to his higher spiritual status as he would be fully aware of the divinity in himself as well as in all creatures—of the fatherhood of God, the fellowship of humanity and the brotherhood of man. Whenever and wherever spiritual qualities are lacking in man, there is nothing to prevent the society from falling into decay.

Ethical and moral values are the basis of good life as ethical culture indeed ennobles human life. Ethics, religion and spirituality have become synonymous terms in common parlance as they co-exist in the development of moral culture and righteous and virtuous life. Moral living starts through dedication to ideal principles, maxims and human values. A righteous and virtuous life and a clear conscience provide the backbone of spiritual as well as a humane material progress of the civilized man and his society.

Rabindranath Tagore beautifully sums up the essence of values "Perfection has its two aspects in man, which to some extent be separated, the perfection in being and perfection in doing. It can be imagined that through some training or compulsion, good works may possibly be extorted from a man who personally may not be good . . . where the questions not that of utility but of moral perfection, we hold it important that the individual be true to his goodness. His outer good work may continue to produce good results, but the inner perfection of his personality has its immense value, which for him is spiritual freedom and for humanity is an endless asset through we may not know it, for goodness represents the detachment of spirit from the exclusiveness of our egoism, in goodness we identify ourselves with the universal humanity. . . . In order to realize his unity with the universal, the individual man must live his perfect life which alone gives the freedom to transcend it." Rabindranath Tagore (The Religion of Man) XIV, 120-21.

N.K. Ambasht, Ajit Singh in their article "Education of Learners in Life Coping Skills: An Emerging Need" in *Journal of Value Education*, Vol. 2, July 2001 observe: "The present scenario in the country demands immediate significant interventions to help students to withstand/overcome stresses, strains and frustration, depression, etc. One of the significant interventions is to train the students to acquire life coping skills and develop desirable attitudes. This has to be a deliberate and planned effort. Graded curricular inputs have to be made from early years of education to the higher and processional level of education."

According to Sathya Sai Baba, "Education must instill the fundamental human values—Truth, Right Conduct, Peace, Love and Non-violence and these should constitute the life and breath of students. Development of these correspond to the five domains of human personality—intellectual, physical, emotional, psychic and spiritual—leading to holistic and integrated development. The five human values are the pillars on which stands the entire approach.

In this book, having ten chapters, an effort has been made to promote the emphasis on environment and value education to promote good health. It is hoped that those who are interested in the promotion of health would find this book useful.

Chandigarh S.L. GOEL

CHAPTER I

HEALTH EDUCATION

"The aim of health education is to help people achieve health by their own actions and efforts. Health education begins therefore with the interest of people in improving their condition of living, and aims at developing a sense of responsibility for their own health betterment as individuals and as members of families, communities or governments."

—*World Health Organization*

Health Education

"Health education aims at promoting the greater possible fulfilment of inherited powers of the body and the mind and the happy adjustment of individuals to society. It is the educational approach to health problems and as such is concerned with practical measures for the promotion of health and the control and treatment of disease."

—*WHO*

It has been rightly said that healthy mind is in healthy body. Therefore, students in higher education must be made aware of the significance and meaning of health and how to achieve good health. For this health education must be imparted to students otherwise the unhealthy practices like smoking, drinking, taking of drugs, etc. would make the life of youth miserable. Therefore there is a need to include in the syllabus of colleges and universities a chapter on health education through which they can improve their lives for better health as well as help the society in the promotion of good health. This can also check the spread of violence caused by the influence of unhealthy practices like drinking, etc. Let us now understand the significance, and meaning of health as well the need and scope of health education for students in higher education.

SIGNIFICANCE OF HEALTH

Good Health is a prerequisite to human productivity and the "development" process. It is essential to economic and technological development. A healthy community is the infrastructure upon which to build an economically viable society. The progress of society greatly depends on the quality of its people. Unhealthy people can hardly be expected to make any valid contribution towards developmental programmes. Health is man's greatest possession, for it lays a solid foundation for his happiness. Charaka, the renowned Ayurvedic physician is known to have said: "Health was vital for ethical, artistic, material and spiritual development of man."

Buddha has said that of all the gains, the gains of health are the highest and the best. Health is not only basic to leading a happy life for an individual but it is also necessary for all productive activities in the society. Who would deny that a soldier who is not keeping good health cannot be expected to defend the frontiers of his country even when he is provided with the latest sophisticated weapons? Similarly, who would deny that an unhealthy farmer with the best possible technological know-how would not succeed in producing the best that can be expected of him? Obviously what is true of an unhealthy soldier or an unhealthy farmer is also true of other categories of workers. Thus, no industry can expect the optimum output if it does not employ healthy workers or does not make and provide adequate facilities for proper maintenance of their health. Undoubtedly, professional efficiency, good health and productivity are inter-related. Yet, health cannot be bestowed upon people if they themselves do not make any effort to maintain a proper balance between their external and internal environments.

Whatever one may say, a disease stricken society can hardly hope to extricate itself from the clutches of poverty and ignorance that keep it backward and underdeveloped in many areas of life. A nation can become truly healthy only when it succeeds in overcoming also these deficiencies stemming from cultural, social, economic and other causes. A nation that is ill-fed can hardly afford to exhibit efficiency in any field. In fact, an epidemic or endemic disease in any part of the world can pose a potential danger to all mankind and even a challenge to modern science. The planning commission has stressed the vital importance of public health in the enrichment of community life. It has been stated:

"Health is fundamental to the national progress in any sphere. In terms of resources for economic development, nothing can be considered of higher importance than the health of the people which is a measure of their energy and capacity as well as of the potential man-hours for productive work in relation to the total number of persons maintained by the nation. For the efficiency of industry and of agriculture, the health of the worker is an essential consideration."

In this address to 31st Session of WHO Regional Committee for South-East Asia held at Ulan Botor, Mongolia (22-28 Aug., 1978), Dr. Nyam-Osor, Minister of Public Health, Mongolia read a passage from a poem by Dashdorjiin Natragdorj, which glorifies "Health." It is being reproduced below.[1]

"Happiness, happiness, happiness
It maybe of different origin on this earth
But the happiness of being healthy
Is the real happiness."

Thus, there can be no two opinions that health is basic to national progress and in terms of resources for economic development nothing could be of greater significance than the health of the people. To quote Herophilas, C., 300 B.C.—

"When health is absent
Wisdom cannot reveal itself
Art cannot manifest
Strength cannot fight,
Wealth becomes useless
And Intelligence cannot be applied."

As such good health must be a primary objective of national development programmes. It is a precursor to improving the quality of life for a major portion of mankind.

MEANING OF HEALTH (See Chart 1.1)

Health is viewed differently by different people all over the world. The World Health Organisation defined health as "a state of complete physical, mental, and social well-being and not merely an absence of disease or infirmity."[2]

Thus, good health is a synthesis of physical, mental and social well-being. As stated in the First Five Year Plan—

"Health is a positive state of well-being in which harmonious development of mental and physical capacities of the individuals lead to the enjoyment of a rich and full life. . . . It implies adjustment of the individuals to his total environment—physical and social."

Some people even define it as a condition under which an individual is able to mobilise all his resources—intellectual, emotional and physical—for optimum living. Thus, health is not static; on the contrary, it fluctuates on a scale which ranges between optimum health as defined by WHO to complete lack of health.

Dr E. Berthet, Secretary-General of the International Union for Health Education, Paris, defines health as follows:

"We no longer ought to define health only in terms of sickness, but rather in relation to the harmonious development of every individual's personality. After all, it represents a balanced measure of a person's total potentials whether biological, psychological and social; and to the notion of individual health we should add the concepts of family and community health."[3]

The Health Charter should serve as a spring board to renewed activities, for the health and happiness of humanity.[4] It is beautifully expressed in the Vedic benediction:

May all humanity be happy

CHART 1.1

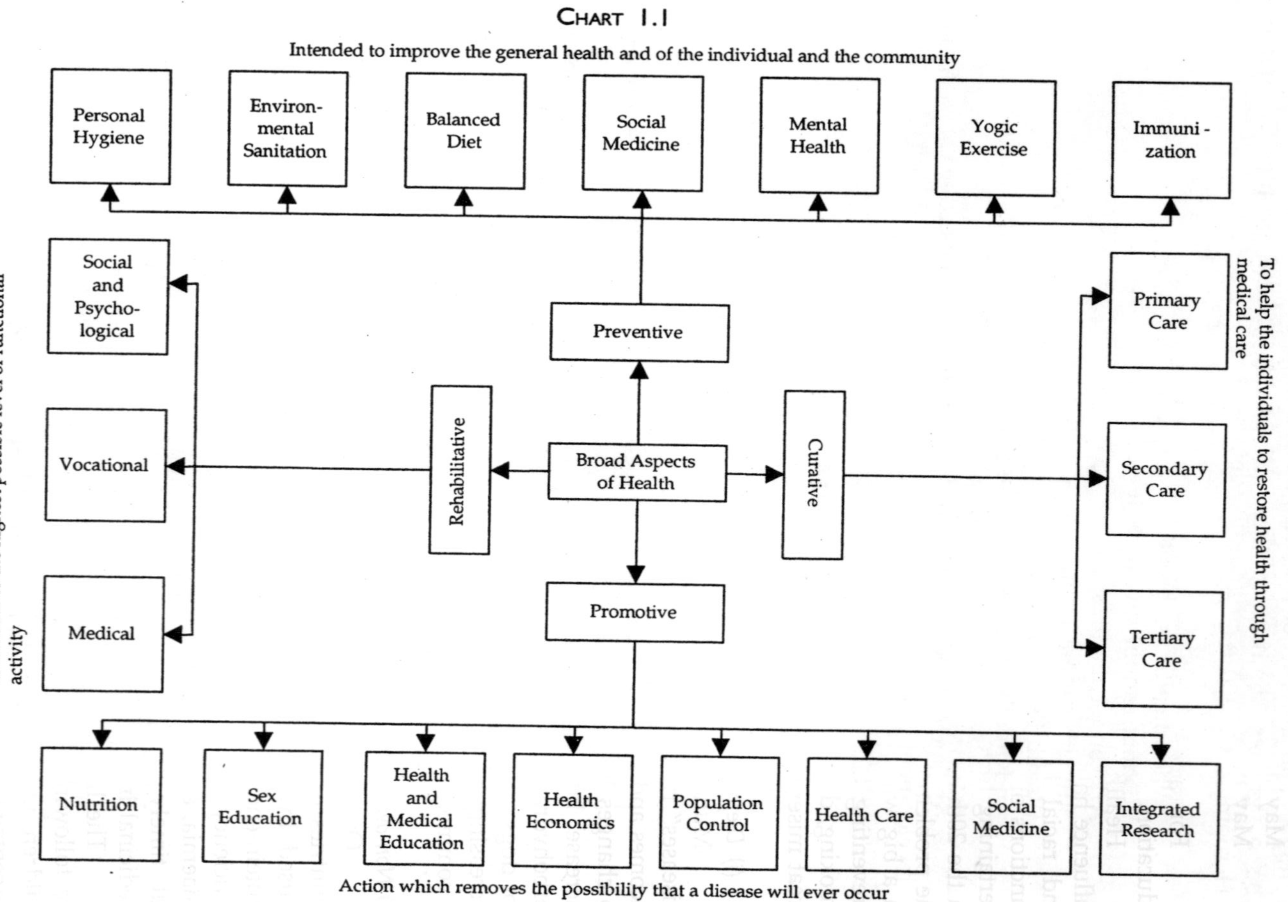
Intended to improve the general health and of the individual and the community
Personal Hygiene
Environ- mental Sanitation
Balanced Diet
Social Medicine
Mental Health
Yogic Exercise
Immuni - zation
Social and Psycho- logical
Vocational
Medical
The combined and co- ordinated use of medical, social, educational measures for training and re-training the individual to the highest possible level of functional activity
Preventive
Rehabilitative
Broad Aspects of Health
Curative
Promotive
To help the individuals to restore health through medical care
Primary Care
Secondary Care
Tertiary Care
Nutrition
Sex Education
Health and Medical Education
Health Economics
Population Control
Health Care
Social Medicine
Integrated Research
Action which removes the possibility that a disease will ever occur

May all be without disease
May all witness auspicious sights
May none have to undergo suffering

For achieving this, we have to understand the role of health education.

Health Education is the sum of experiences which favourably influence habits, attitudes and knowledge relating to individual, community and racial health. Health Education has been an integral part of the functions of health personnel since time immemorial to educate the people pertaining to factors which influence their health. We have been engaged in the 20th century in finding out new technology and medicines to tackle the problems of health. That is why super specialty hospitals have come up in a big way. However, we have ignored the role of health education in preventing killer diseases resulting from faulty life- style, use of alcohol, smoking, drugs, etc. Let us analyse these health hazards which are causing great misery to individual, families and society.

(I) *(i) Dietary Lifestyles*

Muhammad Al-Khrateeb[5] in his Article "New Lifestyles' New Diseases" rightly remarks that Recent Social development—such as bigger incomes and greater availability of a wide variety of commodities—have led to changes in lifestyles that threaten health. Coronary diseases are on the increase because of changes in diets; people are eating more fats, carbohydrates and animal proteins; fast-food restaurants offer ham-burgers, hot dogs and fried chicken; the intake of salt from canned food is rapidly increasing; access to transport facilities reduce physical exercise; and stress is common in their daily life.

(ii) Non-availability of balanced Diet

On the other hand, there is a large population in the developing countries especially India which is suffering from a number of diseases caused by malnutrition and under-nutrition. Some of the diseases are protein-energy malnutrition-related diseases e.g., low birth weights, Iodine deficiency disorders, Vitamin A deficiency disorder, iron deficiency, Anaemia, etc. These diseases do not require super specialists' interventions but timely Primary healthcare and education of mother and simple medicinal interventions.

The International Conference on Nutrition (ICN) in 1992 enunciated the following goals: (1) reduce severe and moderate malnutrition among children under five years of age by half of the 1990 levels, (2) increase the percentage of newborns having an adequate birth weight (2500 grams or more) to 90%, (3) reduce to less than 10% and possibly eliminate iodine deficiency disorders, (4) eliminate Vitamin A deficiency and its consequences including blindness, and (5) reduce iron deficiency anaemia.

Drawing up an integrated national strategy for the prevention of non-communicable diseases is both advisable and economically justifiable. But prevention of such diseases cannot be achieved through the efforts of health officials alone. Health education has to be made accessible to the entire population and non-health institutions and various mass media should be mobilized to this end. Research data yielded by national as well as international studies show that early intervention can make the prevention of diseases possible.[6]

(2) Use of Excessive Alcohol, Smoking and Drugs

World Health, July-August, 1995 has published figures about prevalence of alcohol, tobacco and drugs which are quite alarming.[7] In developed countries, typically 70-90% of adults consume alcohol. Studies in a number of industrialized countries suggest that 5-10% of drinkers are dependent on alcohol.

For several diseases, including cancers of the mouth, Oesophagus and pharynx, as well as for many forms of injury including motor vehicle accidents, industrial accidents, drowning, falls, suicide and homicide, the contribution of alcohol is well known, the risk increasing steadily with the amount consumed.

World-wide, there are about 1100 million smokers with 800 million in developing countries and 300 million in developed countries. About 6000 million cigarettes are smoked every year. In developed countries, about 41% of men and 21% of women regularly smoke cigarettes. In developing countries, about 50% of men but only about 8% of women smoke.

Tobacco causes about 3 million deaths a year now, with about one-third of them in developing countries. If current smoking trends persist, tobacco is likely to kill approximately 10 million people a year in 30-40 years time, with about 70% of them in developing countries.

If current smoking trends persist, about 500 million people currently alive (about 9% of the world's population) will eventually be killed by tobacco, and half of them will be in middle age when they die, losing about 20-25 years of life. In many developing countries heroin and cocaine use is becoming more common and increasingly problematic. In several countries heroin use is increasingly replacing traditional patterns of substance use including opium smoking. In many developing countries drug injecting is becoming increasingly common, and in these countries injecting often means the sharing of injecting equipment, with the risk of HIV, hepatitis and other infections.

One crude estimate suggests that, world-wide, between 160,000 and 210,000 deaths every year are associated with drug injecting. Norman Sartorius in his Article, "Putting a Higher Value on Health" in *World Health,* June 1986 has cautioned about the negative effects of the use of these horrible drinks in excess. To quote:[8]

"The abuse of psychoactive substances including alcohol, tobacco and narcotic and psychotropic drugs cause enormous damage to the health and productivity of nations. It undermines the quality of life of individuals and their families, and threatens the welfare of communities. The health consequences of abuse are also grave, and range from violence and delinquency to liver cirrhosis, brain damage and lung cancer."

Dr. H. Mahler, Former Director General of World Health Organisation in his Article, "Smoking or Health: The Choice is Yours" rightly stated. "Smoking increases the risk of lung cancer, heart disease and respiratory infections of all kinds. In fact, many of the diseases associated with smoking have become current only in the last few generations, when the habit of smoking factory made cigarettes became widespread."

The latest report of South-East Asia Region on Health situation in 1994-97 has clearly brought out the consequences of the use of these substances. A major problem with the use of alcohol is its impact on the health and well-being of the family. A study carried out in India in 1996 reported that drinking families from lower income groups spend from 15% to 45% of their income on alcohol. A high proportion of hospital beds are occupied by the physically and mentally damaged victims of alcohol dependence. Many beds occupied by accidents-affected patients are because of alcohol.

The causal relationship between tobacco use and diseases such as cancers, cardiovascular diseases, and chronic respiratory disorders is increasingly being studied in most countries of the Region. In India the number of avoidable cases of chronic heart and obstructive lung diseases has been estimated at 12 million per year. Cancer incidence data reveal that almost 50% and 25% of cancers in men and women respectively are related to tobacco use. The incidence of oral cancer caused by chewing tobacco is estimated to be one of the world's highest, at about one-third of all cancer cases. Annually, tobacco-related conditions are reported to cause 635,000 deaths in India.[9]

The basic question is how to tackle these non-communicable diseases? How to motivate the people using these substances not to do so? What can be done by health experts? The only answer to these questions is the need of strengthening Health Education intensively. Muhammad Al-Khateeb[10] suggests that drawing upon integrated national strategy for the prevention of non-communicable diseases is both advisable and economically justifiable. But prevention of such diseases cannot be achieved through the efforts of health officials alone. Health education has to be made accessible to the entire population, and non-health institutions and various mass media should be mobilised to this end. Research data yielded by national as well as international studies show that early intervention can make the prevention of disease possible.

Achieving 'Health for All' requires much more than just setting up a health centre in every district and providing a high standard of medical care within easy reach of everyone. A key element in the primary healthcare approach to Health for All is health education, which seeks to bring about a change in behaviour patterns by making essential health information available to all people in a simple, direct and effective manner. It is hoped that people will thus be motivated to evaluate their habits and practices, and will modify them according to the requirements of health protection and promotion.

Behavioural change, however, is too complex a process to be initiated simply by providing a set of facts. The motivation to break a habit must be much stronger than the force of habits or the pleasure derived from a certain practice. The spiritual dimension can be highly influential in this process of behavioural change.[11]

In spite of overwhelming evidence linking tobacco consumption and various diseases, including cancer, the consumption of cigarettes in nearly all countries of the world is increasing. The rise in tobacco consumption is especially seen among women and the youth. Non-smoking campaigns over the past years have been less than successful. This is mainly because of the aggressive advertisements and counter-attacks by the tobacco industry and the fact that nicotine is addictive. Moreover, most governments are reluctant to take a strong stand on this issue considering that tobacco is a source of revenue and of foreign exchange.

The need for heightened global advocacy for tobacco control has been stressed by Dr. Gro Harlem Brundtland, WHO Director-General, in her statement to the Fifty-first World Health Assembly in May 1998. To quote her:

"I am a doctor, I believe in science and evidence. . . . Tobacco is a killer, Tobacco should not be advertised, subsidized or glamorized."

Of late there is a move to ban Tobacco companies from sponsoring Sports events in India leading to a major debate as to whether it would be at the cost of the Sports activity and so on.

MEANING, NATURE AND SCOPE OF HEALTH EDUCATION

The most important aim of Health Education is to alter behaviour which may have directly or indirectly influenced occurrence of spread of diseases in a given cultural setting. A culturally relevant health education programme can be planned Only after understanding the behaviour in all its manifestations. One of the best definitions of Health Education was offered by Wood in 1926: "Health Education is the sum of experiences which favourably influences habits, attitudes and knowledge relating to individual, community, and racial health:"[12]

Different authorities have differently viewed the aims of health education. According to one source:[13]

"The aim of health education is to help people achieve health by their own actions and efforts. Health education begins therefore with the interest of people in improving their condition of living, and aims at developing a sense of responsibility for their own health betterment as individuals and as members of families, communities or government."[14]

Another source highlights that, "Health education aims at promoting the greater possible fulfilment of inherited powers of the body and the mind and the happy adjustment of individual to society. It is the educational approach to health problem and as such is concerned with practical measures for the promotion of health and the control and treatment of disease."

Unfortunately, the experts and development planners have failed to improve the lives of the people as they do not understand properly the science to communicate effectively with each other or with the people they are trying to help. Most of the people in authority today, who are guiding the people in this field, have not realised the urgency of such education and the benefit it can generate; consequently governments have not taken any substantial steps in this direction.

Health education does not mean merely removal of ignorance. On the contrary, it involves four important things:

(i) It provides a person with appropriate knowledge to enjoy decent health and also the knowledge about the occurrence and spread of disease thus enabling him to adopt relevant preventive measures;
(ii) It creates in him an interest in his own health and well-being;
(iii) It even creates in him an interest for the health of other members of his family as well as of those living in his surrounding; and
(iv) It creates in him a desire to support health education programmes in his area.

Besides, Health Education should make the people understand the benefits that they can derive from modern medicine. K.S. Sanjive, Professor of Medicine has said:

"It will not be an exaggeration to say that the paramount step in the effort to take modern medicine to every coener of the country and every citizen is health education. Health education in its widest sense of getting every one to understand what modern medicine can do to diminish disease and death and to be properly motivated to utilise this knowledge in their daily lives, requires the simple quality of sincerity more than highly specialised techniques."[15]

Neglect of health education is one of the main reasons why scientific medicine is not taking root in the country and people are steeped in ignorance and superstition.

ESSENTIALS OF HEALTH EDUCATION

Health education would be possible only if the health educator and the receiver are in constant dialogue with each other. It is not wholly correct that the purpose of health education is to manipulate the receiver. What might be more appropriate is a circular diagram in which the parties to the "Communication Contract" as it is sometimes called, function dually as senders and receivers. This model would avoid the possibilities of misinterpretation. We know that even well-planned campaigns can end in failures if there is no proper monitoring or feed-back to make sure that the wrong effect is not being created by the communicator, however innocently.

In a democratic society, the dynamic power which impels governments to action is the voice and enlightenment of the people. People can only pressurise their executive or legislative machinery to undertake suitable health measures when they themselves are aware of the means of warding off disease and promotion of positive health. This knowledge (Health Education) is therefore a pre-condition and prerequisite to creating the demand for health and setting the pace of implementation of environmental sanitation and the total health policy.

FUNCTIONS OF HEALTH EDUCATION PROGRAMME (See Chart 1.2)

No health education programme can function in isolation. A health education programme has to be an integral part of various other development programmes. Functionally, a health education programme should aim at bringing about the following change as shown in Chart 1.3.

(1) A Change in Knowledge

The most important need which health education programme can serve is to provide appropriate knowledge about health and diseases to the people. This knowledge should be provided in such a way that the recipients do not find it hard to accept it. How to provide this knowledge in an acceptable way? This is the first challenge faced by a health educator. Meaningful responses are relatively easier to learn than the meaningless ones. The health educator can do a lot better by making his demands on the response of receivers which are meaningful. For instance, the health educator who gives a big lecture to the mother on the value of practising family planning without indicating its benefits to her as an individual would be showing inadequate understanding of this principle, for she has to look into her own benefits first. Vigorous efforts would be required to proliferate suggestions that are realistic and meaningful.

(2) A Change in Attitude

A change in attitude is possible only when the new knowledge that is offered is acceptable to the recipients. Its utility should also be well known to them. Normally, provision of appropriate knowledge should lead to formation of positive attitudes not only towards a person's own health but also towards the health of other members of the community.

(3) A Change in Behaviour

Once positive attitudes are formed, these must reflect in the behaviour of the recipients. They should not only become mindful of their past behaviour but should also avoid doing things which can in any way influence occurrence or spread of diseases.

CHART 1.2

Feedback
Message
Sender
Receiver
Sender
Receiver
Message
Feedback

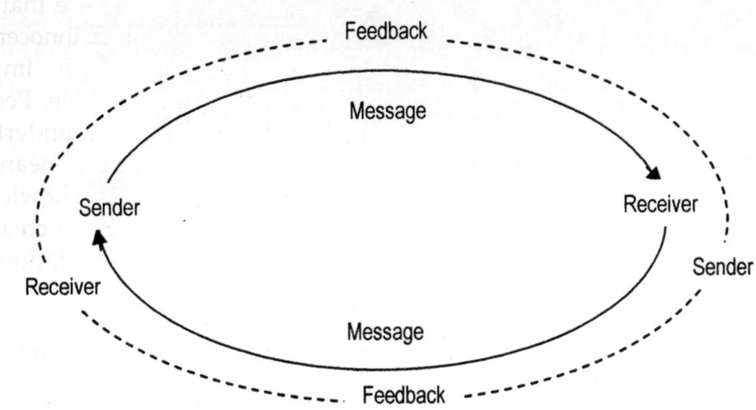

CHART 1.3

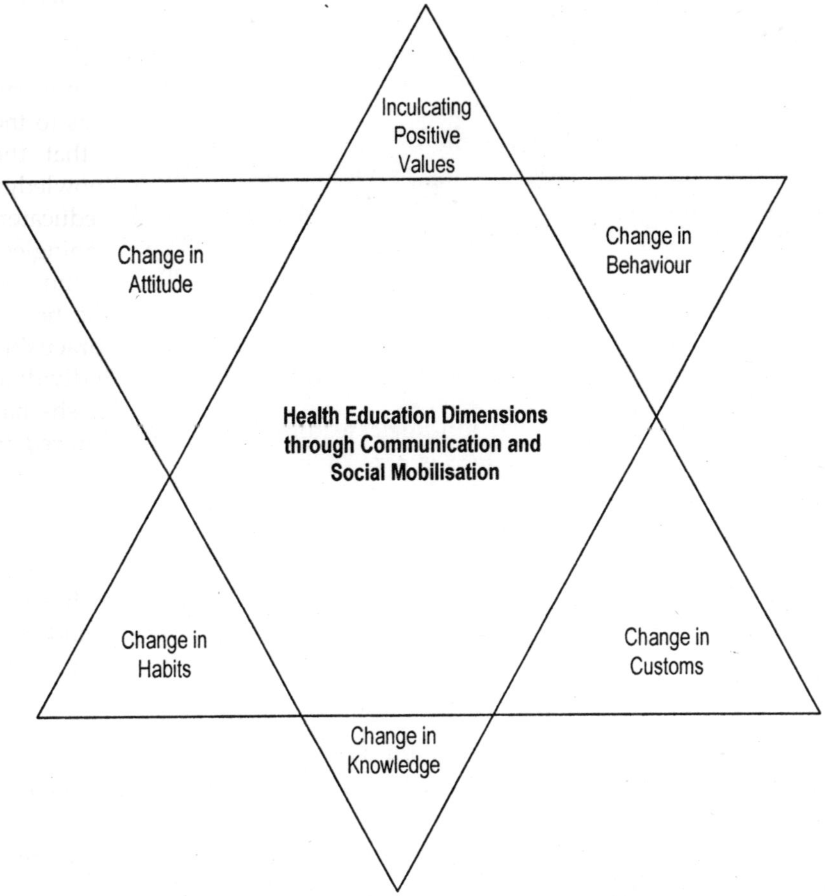

Inculcating
Positive
Values
Change in
Attitude
Change in
Behaviour
Health Education Dimensions
through Communication and
Social Mobilisation
Change in
Habits
Change in
Customs
Change in
Knowledge

(4) A Change in Habit

The change in the behaviour of the recipients must lead to habit formation. A habit can be formed only when the behaviour becomes repetitive. If proper habits are formed, not only the individuals concerned but the whole community will be benefited. Habit formation, however, is a slow process and it has been well said, that 'habits die hard'.

The persuasive communicator or health educator should be interested both in the long range effects of his messages and in their initial effects. As a matter of fact, he should be interested in turning the learned responses into habitual ones. What are the other principles that guide the establishment of a response? First, the probability of response will increase with the increase in the number of rewarded repetitions. As long as the stimulus with reinforcement following each correct response is not adequately repeated, it will not become a habitual response. Many messages are short-lived because of lack of reinforcement and are likely to become extinct. Second, in order to establish habit patterns, it would be necessary to have a shorter interval between response and reward. Third, habit formation is easier when stimuli are presented in isolation. A nutrition message when unaccompanied by another message such as sanitation message facilitates habit formation. Fourthly, timely increase in reinforcement will further strengthen habit formation. Fifth, receiver's original level of motivation will also influence her habit formation. The mother having a better level of motivation from the beginning will find habit formation much easier. Sixth, providing timely information about receiver performance, would lead to further improvement in performance. Providing selective information to a mother on the positive aspects of her performance will also improve her performance. Thus, communication of health ideas can yield the desired result if the above principles are followed religiously.

(5) A Change in Customs

Acquisition of positive attitudes leading to appropriate habit formation must sooner or later, evolve into customs. Only when a substantial number of people in a given cultural setting start behaving in a customary manner, one can say that behaviour has become a part of their customs.

Don Palmer in his article, "Social Health: A True Story, Culture and Tradition as Medicine" in the *Daily Tribune* dated 26th January 2000, rightly stresses the need of health education. Modern urban life, devoid of the goodness of social health, can be particularly tough for young indigenous inhabitants of developed countries. Some kill themselves, while many more drift into drugs, alcohol and crime. Now a prison programme is helping in rehabilitation of aboriginal offenders by reintroducing them to their cultural traditions."

It needs to be re-emphasised that health education is a slow process and that it proceeds gradually—a part of the process may get established without any problem but additional efforts may be required to complete the whole process. This process may be directed towards the following important programmes: (See Chart 1.4)

(a) Personal hygiene.
(b) Knowledge of modern medicine, i.e., use of health services.
(c) Nutrition.
(d) Mental health.
(e) Prevention of communicable diseases.
(f) Care of children.
(g) Environmental sanitation.
(h) Human physiology.
(i) Lifestyle diseases.
(j) Education about alcohol and drugs.

Health education must be imparted keeping in mind latest developments in the field of health. Life is changing fast and the individuals must be educated in the new technology—its role and limitations. Mr. V. Tatochenko, a member of the WHO Expert Panel on Maternal and Child Health in his Article on "Education for Health" said, "Rapid changes in lifestyles and the evolution of views on health and disease call for new departures in health education. A quick glance of health education material of even one generation ago will show how fast it tends to get out of date. Medical facts, it has been estimated, get outdated within a decade or so. Effective health education, therefore, requires a continuous stream of knowledge, development of the people's ability to absorb it, and decisions taken on the basis of a constantly changing body of information.[16]

METHODS OF HEALTH EDUCATION

Health organisations are set-up to promote positive health. A good health organisation must establish environmental linkages, i.e. points of interactions with the environment. These can be classified into four categories: enabling, functional, normative and diffused. The enabling linkage ensures and protects the organisational authority to operate, its access to resources and its power to achieve results. Functional linkage is to link the programme with the task environment. Normative linkages try to modify the behaviour of the people into the existing value system of the society. Diffused linkages imply reaching the clients through public relation (health education).

Sociologists have categorised diffusion process which leads to a widespread acceptance of the programme into five critical stages: awareness (the individuals first introduction to a new idea or practice), interest (the stage at which he actively seeks further information and background data), evaluation (the stage of assessment on critical grounds), trial (a limited

CHART 1.4

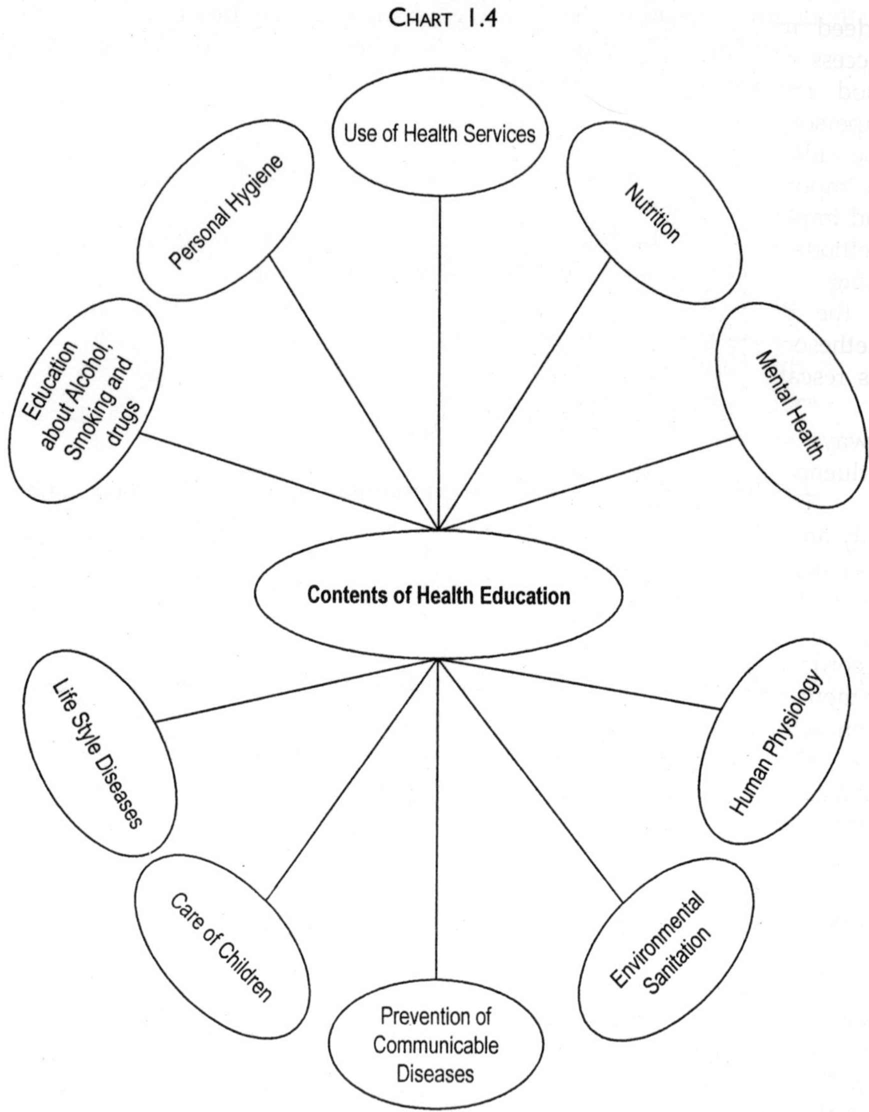

phase of experiment), and finally acceptance or adoption. These processes have been occurring for centuries. The need of the present day health administration is to accelerate adoption of the health programmes and to control diffusion process in a short span of time to achieve effective implementation of health programmes.

Changes in knowledge, attitudes, behaviour, habits and customs can be brought about by 'personal' as well as 'impersonal' methods of health education. These methods have certain advantages and disadvantages. While personal methods involve face-to-face interaction, the impersonal methods do not require such a close personal contact. Personal methods are indeed more convincing and generally more successful. However, the success of personal methods greatly depends on the establishment of a good rapport between the health educator and his recipients. The impersonal methods are relatively simpler and even less time-consuming. The radio, the newspapers, the posters, and the pamphlets, etc. can all play an important role in imparting health education. Experience with personal and impersonal methods of health education have revealed that if both the methods are used simultaneously one can obtain better results than simply using one or the other method. The most important aspect in the adoption of the programme is the use of inter-personal relationships. Alastair Metheson, Deputy Director of UNICEF's division remarks on the basis of his research that:

"To get people to act in way that conform to new values almost always requires that mass communications to be reinforced by personal intluence."[17]

Thus, we see that communication, i.e. dissemination of information is only an important element in health education. The adoption or acceptance may not take place simply by communicating health information. A study conducted by United States Public Health Services has revealed that, "Unfortunately knowledge alone does not motivate a person to act in accordance with it. He may well know the correct answers to questions without really believing and accepting such information as the basis for his own action."

Dr. Gisela Gastrin, a Finnish physician mentions in his article, "How Education Helps"; "People can be motivated to adjust their outlook towards health and disease, but before this can happen their negative attitudes have to be countered with factual information. Education needs to be a part of a comprehensive programme in which responsibilities involving the health authorities and others are clearly delineated and resources allocated."[18]

For effective health education, people's involvement is essential. Eric R. Ram[19] in his article, "Information is Power" in *World Health*, rightly says that making people aware of their rights and responsibilities helps them to determine their own health priorities and take part in solving their own health problems, a step so essential in the process of empowerment of the people. We have to employ all credible channels of communication, including the traditional methods of story-telling and drama, in order to reach all people. Films, radio and television whenever available can be useful, but we have to recognize their limitations; they are useful in creating awareness among people in their communities, but to bring about a real change in health practices, people have to decide for themselves and take responsibility for their own health.

It was mentioned by Dr. E. Berthat in his article, "A New Role for Teachers" that besides information and motivation, action is indispensable. He said that "Information and motivation are not enough; it remains for governments to ensure that a good health infrastructure is available to all the people. Health education has to convince the men and women who are responsible for taking decisions that health is a basic raw-material for their country's eventual social and economic development."[20]

A health educator, as a persuasive communicator can make the best possible use of the personal methods of health education. But he has to see that the messages which he is delivering get mentally registered with his recipients. Actually, he can present his message and then wait until he gets the requisite response from his recipients. D.F. Skinner has distinguished between two types of approaches to the learning situation, as 'operant behaviour' and 'respondent behaviour'. The two situations have also been described as involving instrumental learning and conditional learning. In 'instrumental learning situations', which involves 'operant behaviour', the health educator will present his message and then wait for the receiver to make a correct response. When the receiver makes this response, the health educator will attempt to fix the response by the appropriate award or reinforcement. On the other hand, in 'conditioned learning situation' which involves 'respondent behaviour', the health educator presents his message in such a way that he elicits the response that he wants from his recipients and thus the stimulus that originally served to elicit the response becomes the reinforcing or rewarding element in conditioning. Undoubtedly, conditioning is much more efficient than instrumental learning. It is, however, necessary for the health educator to be aware of both kinds of situations since the condition for using 'respondent behaviour' may not be present in the persuasive situation. The health educator has to be aware that the recipients of his messages differ in the ways in which they learn a given response. They may give different responses essentially in the same situation because of certain specific reasons.

TRAINING OF PERSONNEL FOR HEALTH EDUCATION

We can divide the personnel for health education in two categories, i.e., Health Workers like teachers, social workers, physicians, nurses, etc., and Specialists, i.e., the persons specially trained for this function.

Objectives of training for Health Workers are:

(1) To create an awareness and understanding of the health education aspects of health work and of the principles and procedures to be considered in achieving these purposes.

(2) To foster an interest in health education in all health personnel;

(3) To teach the right way to communicate with individuals families, community groups, and the general public;

(4) To stress the importance of team work for the realisation of effective health education; and

(5) To strengthen the aspects of health education in the curriculum of medical education.

The main objectives of training health education Specialists are:

(a) To establish professional standards to secure public confidence. It is essential that such specialists possess an ethical code and technical competence which govern their behaviour and standards of performance.
(b) To prepare specialists to encompass health education planning, organisation, coordination, dissemination, training, studies and research.

The health education Specialist should acquire through his basic education and post-graduate training the following qualities:

(a) A high degree of competence involving a thorough understanding of the importance and implication of cultural, economic and social influences in relation to health.
(b) Special competence in planning, organisation, administration, evaluation, etc., of health education aspects of health programmes.
(c) The ability to give technical leadership in planning .and conduct of health education, training for health workers and workers in closely related fields (content, methods, planning, etc.).
(d) Skill in giving technical guidance and consultation on planning, preparation, pre-testing, production, and use of visual materials.
(e) The ability to assume technical leadership in cooperation with others in planning and execution of studies, and research on major health education problems.
(f) Thorough knowledge of educational principles and methods involved in planning and arranging of seminars, conferences, meetings, courses, teaching units, etc.
(g) They should acquire latest information from research in teaching and learning relevant to health education.

CONCLUSION

Without evaluating the impact of health education programmes on the bulk of the people, one cannot possibly identify positive as well as negative aspects of the programme. An objective evaluation of the health education programme alone can help one improve the guidelines for future action. 'Cost-benefit' analysis should be an integral part of this evaluation, so that one may assess how available resources have been utilized. Through objective evaluation; one may also be able to curtail mass production of ritualistic health education material as produced by various health education bureaus. The amount thus saved can be effectively utilised for a more purposeful and meaningful health education programme.

Health education is the most difficult task as habits, usages and customs are deeply entrenched. But health administration would fail in its purpose if it could not produce social change through health education. That is why it has been said that "it is easier to destroy mountains than to change our customs."[21] Professional training helps the health experts to deal with the health changes effectively. Their pharmacopoeia in both fields must be strong in order to translate the findings of biological investigations into social application. So over and above each technical act; there is a corresponding education function which doubles the value of the act, increases its efficiency and endows it with real human and social value. G. Borkar in his book, "Health in Independent India" writes that all progress in public health depends ultimately on the willing assent and cooperation of the people and their active participation in measures intended for individual and community health protection, considering how much of illness is the result of ignorance of simple hygienic laws or indifference to their application. In practice, no single measure is productive of greater returns to outlay than health education.[22] Thus, health education can influence the lives of people for many generations. WHO conducted an interview of a Mongolian Feldsher. He stated that "conducting continuous health education is my first duty, prevention is our basic principle. Every effort is made to raise the health knowledge of the people. Child care, correct feeding and vaccinations are among the most important topics for health education."[23]

Notes and References

1. WHO, SEARO, S.E.A./RC/31, p. 59.
2. Govt. of India, First Five Year Plan, p. 88.
3. WHO, *World Health*, May 1979, p. 23.
4. Govt. of India, First Five Year Plan, p. 511.
5. Muhammad Al-Khateeb, "New Lifestyles, New Disease" in *World Health*, July 1989, p. 23.
6. *Ibid.*
7. WHO: *World Health*, July-August, 1995, p. 16; *World Health* June, 1986, p. 2.
8. *World Health*, Feb.-March, 1980.
9. WHO: SEARO: Health Situation in the South-East Asia Region, 1994-97, New Delhi, 1999, pp. 149-51.
10. *World Health*, July 1989, p. 23.
11. Abdulmoneirn Aly: Health Education Through Religion, in *World Health*, July 1989, p. 27.
12. John J. Hanlon, Principles of Public Health Administration, St. Louis, 1960, p. 402.
13. WHO, Technical Report Series. No. 89, p. 4.
14. WHO, *Ibid.*, No. 156, p. 3.
15. K.S. Sanjive, Planning India's Health, Orient Longman, New Delhi, 1971, p. 64.
16. WHO, *World Health*, Feb.-March 1979, p. 24.
17. UNICEF, UNICEF News, "Communication: A Tool for Development", issue 84/1975/12, p. 18.

18. WHO, *World Health,* Nov. 1975, p. 14.
19. *World Health,* Jan.-Feb. 1989, p. 9.
20. *World Health,* May 1979, p. 25
21. Bosnian proverb.
22. WHO Technical Report Series, 1954.
23. Borkar, Health in Independent India, p. 217.

CHAPTER 2

ENVIRONMENTAL EDUCATION

> Over the years, together with a spreading of environment consciousness, there has been a change in the traditionally-held perception that there is a trade-off between environmental quality and economic growth as people have come to believe that the two are necessarily complementary. The current focus on environment is not new—environmental considerations have been an integral part of the Indian culture. The need for conservation and sustainable use of natural resources has been expressed in Indian scriptures, more than three thousand years old and is reflected in the constitutional, legislative and policy framework as also in the international commitments of the country.
>
> —*T.R. Baalu*
>
> Union Minister of Environment and Forests

Environmental Education*

Oh, Mother Earth !
Your hills, snowclad mountains, forests,
In all shapes and formations
Bring happiness to us.
I bow you
With all my might, I shall save
Your cultivable, fertile and nourishing black and red
Soils which are strong and resistant,
And protected by our ancestors,
From getting weak by destruction and degradation.
—(*Atharva Veda,* Kand-123, Sukti-I, Mantra-11)

We have to make our youth in colleges and universities conscious about environment so that they can protect it and spread the message further to save humanity. Therefore, environment education must form an important aspect of curriculum both at under-graduate and post-graduate level whether one offering any group of subjects.

A GOOD ENVIRONMENT IS THE KEY TO HEALTH AND DEVELOPMENT (See Chart 2.1)

Environment has been defined by Webster's New Collegiate Dictionary as "the aggregate of all the external conditions and influences affecting the life and development of an organism."

Shri T.N. Chaturvedi in his Editorial to *IJPA,* July-Sept. 1989 (Special Number on Environment and Administration) rightly sees the intimate relationship between human beings and nature since times immemorial. To

* See Appendix 2.1: Core Module Syllabus for Environmental Studies.

CHART 2.1

Environmental Education

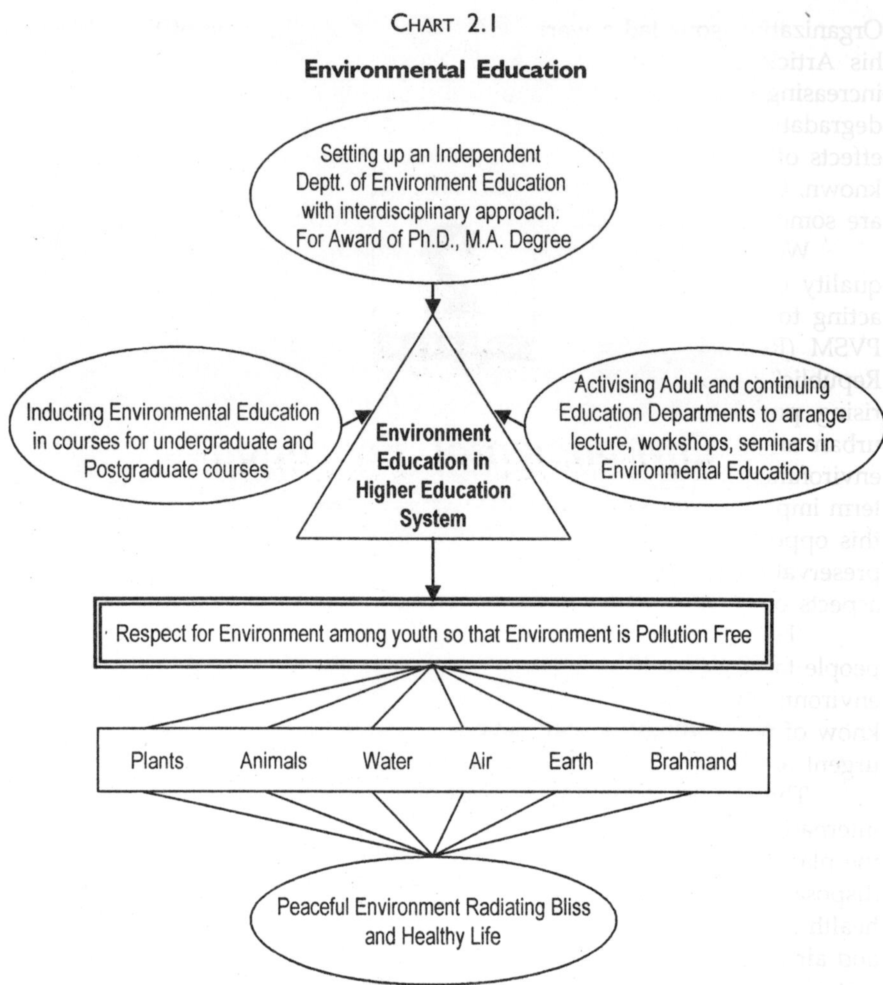

quote: "Man, since his origin, has lived in harmony with Nature through the ages, holding Nature in awe and reverence. The Vedas, folklore and scriptures of different religions, faiths and beliefs also speak of the need for harmony with the universe, which is the habitat not only of men but also of all animals, birds, insects, plants and vegetation. The mutually supportive role of all living things is often mentioned as a crucial factor for a balanced social and harmonious existence. The ecological balance is inherent in the very process of creation. Everywhere, the seers, poets and thinkers, through the ages, have referred to the need for living in harmony with environment. In fact, the Taitariyopanishad looks at the relationship between man and his environment in its totality and stresses complete harmony and interdependence between them in order to attain real prosperity."

Dr. Hiroshi Nakajima, Director-General of World Health

Organization, sounded a warning alarm about degradation of this planet in his Article, "A Wounded Planet."[1] He rightly visualises that it is now increasingly evident that more and more diseases stem from the degradation caused by man to his own environment. The potential harmful effects of industrial development on our global ecosystem are now better known. Ozone layer depletion, acid rain, climate change, chemical pollution are some examples of the man-made wounds to our planet.

We are at a turning point; warnings of the damage to our health and quality of life are growing louder. An increasing number of people are acting to stop the degradation of our environment. Lt. Gen. I.F.R. Jacob, PVSM (Retd.) Govemor, Punjab in his message, "Fifty years of Indian Republic" in the *Daily Tribune* (26th January, 2000), remarked that with our rising population the civil services and environment, especially in the urban areas, are under great stress and strain. The degradation of our environment has to be arrested immediately otherwise it would have long-term impact on the quality of life of future generations. We should also take this opportunity to educate our children regarding the importance of the preservation of our environment. Dr. Wilfried Kreisel[2] also elaborates the aspects of environment which affect health of mankind.

"How can we make environmental health a more potent force to serve people faced with growing threats to their health? How can our improving environmental health technology be better used to foster positive health? I know of no country-developing or industrialised in which this issue is not urgent and important. I know of many countries in which it is critical."

The remarkably wide range of environmental concerns include the international problems of acid rain, the greenhouse effect, and depletion of the planet's ozone layer. It includes national concerns with medical wastes disposal, radioactive and toxic wastes control, transportation accidents, health aspects of urbanisation and traffic, occupational health and safety, and air and water pollution. It also includes local concerns over inadequate water supplies and sanitation facilities, water quality, clean air, solid wastes management, and finding a balance between the economic incentives of development and a decent quality of life. In the report on Our Common Future, the World Commission on Environment and Development (sometimes called the Brundtland Commission) pointed out that the situation is getting increasingly critical.

EDUCATION, AWARENESS AND INFORMATION

Priority is accorded by the Ministry of Environment and Forests to promote environmental education, create environmental awareness among various age-groups and to disseminate information through Environmental Information System (ENVIS) network to all concerned. Special emphasis is given to non-formal environmental education through seminars/symposia/workshops, training programmes, eco-camps, audio-visual shows, etc. The Ministry has been organising a National Environment Awareness

Campaign (NEAC) since July 1980. As a part of this campaign, 19 November to 18 December every year is observed as the National Environment Month. The main themes for the 1997-98 campaign were Pollution Prevention and Control, and Conservation and Plantation of Trees for Environmental Protection. A large number of organisations have been granted financial assistance by the Ministry to organise various activities for creating environmental awareness. The Ministry also provides financial support for setting up eco-clubs at schools and for production of films on environment.

A new scheme, Paryavaran Vahini, was launched in 1992-93 to create environmental awareness and to ensure active public participation by involving the local people in activities relating to environmental protection. Paryavaran Vahinis are proposed to be constituted in 194 selected districts all over the country which have a high incidence of pollution and density of tribal and forest population. The Vahinis also play a watch-dog role by reporting instance of environmental pollution, deforestation, poaching, etc. They function under the charge of District Collectors, with the active cooperation of the State/Union Territory governments. This scheme is entirely financed by the Ministry of Environment and Forests.

K.B. Powar in his article, "Environmental issues and Universities"[3] in Environment Challenges and the Universities, AIU, New Delhi, states that the universities have an important role to play in generating public awareness, protecting the environment and promoting sustainable development. As John Berry succinctly puts it: (J. Berry, 1993, Canadian Universities: "Responding to the Challenges of 90's ACU, BULL, Curr. Doc., pp. 2-8)" . . . universities are the best source of expertise to conduct the necessary research and guide the development of policy framework.

They are also the training ground for the next generation of society's leaders who need to be educated, regardless of their discipline, with a broad and sensitive understanding of the issues." This is particularly true for India where the universities are charged with the responsibility of undertaking teaching, research and extension activities. The role of universities was discussed at a conference on 'University Action for Sustainable Development' held at Dalhousie University, Halifax, Canada in December 1991, and which was attended by 33 Vice-Chancellors and Presidents, from 10 countries. The declaration issued at the end of the conference emphasizes that "universities and their graduates must be significant actors if (human) demands (upon the planets) are to be shaped into sustainable and equitable forms necessary for a wholesome future environment." The Halifax declaration IAU (UNU) AUCC/DV 1991 Universities and Sustainable Development: The Halifax Declaration, Doc..No. 104 (June 1992, pp. 18-19) asked the universities to:

- "Ensure that the voice of the university is clear and uncompromising in its ongoing commitment to the principle

and practice of sustainable development within the university, and at the local, national and global levels.
- Utilize the intellectual resources of the university to encourage a better understanding on the part of society of the inter-related physical, biological and social dangers facing the planet Earth.
- Emphasize the ethical obligation of the present generation to overcome those current malpractices of resource utilization and those widespread circumstances of intolerable human disparity which lie at the root of environmental unsustainability.
- Establish whatever programmes are necessary within the university to generate the capability and the capacity necessary to develop appropriate environmental technologies and practices as well as to diminish environmental illiteracy and enhance ethical awareness on the part of faculty, students, and the public at large.
- Cooperate with one another and with all segments of society in the pursuit of practical, effective revision and reversals of those current practices which contribute to environmental degradation, to South-North disparities and to inter-generational inequity.
- Employ all channels open to the university to communicate these undertakings to UNCED, to governments and to the public at large."

S.C. Gupta rightly defines Environment Education:[4] "In the university system, research, teaching and extension are the three major components with differences in emphasis at different levels. The emphasis on teaching will naturally be more confined to undergraduate programmes whereas teaching and research together will be emphasized at the postgraduate level. The extension component, it is needless to say, need to be continuously provided from undergraduate to postgraduate level. The introduction of the environmental education component will be possible through (a) institutions of degrees or diplomas in Environment Science, (b) introduction of the environmental education component in the existing structure for different disciplines at undergraduate and postgraduate levels, and (c) through provision of research/doctoral programmes of inter-disciplinary nature in relation to problems of environment.

International Union of Conservation of nature and nature Resource defined Environmental Education as:

"The process of recognizing values and clarifying concepts in order to develop skills and attitudes necessary to understand and appreciate the inter-relatedness among man, his culture and his biophysical surroundings. Environmental Education also entails practice in decision making and self-formulation of a code of behaviour about issues concerning environmental quality. Tbilisi Conference (1977) held at Gorgia under the auspices of UNESCO and UNEP mentioned the following as the contents of

Environment Education:

- To consider the environment in its totality natural and built, Technological and social (economic, political, cultural, historical, aesthetic and moral).
- To be a continuous, life long processes, beginning at the pre-school level and continuing through all formal and in-formal stages.
- To be interdisciplinary in its approach, drawing on the specific content of each discipline in making possible a holistic and balanced perspective.
- Examine major environmental issues from the local, national, regional, and international points of view so that students receive insight into environmental conditions in other geographical areas.
- Explicitly consider environmental aspects in plans for development and growth.
- Emphasize the complexity of environmental problem and thus the need to develop critical thinking, problem-solving attitude and skills.
- Promote the value and necessity of local, national and international cooperation in the prevention and solution of the environmental problems.
- Utilize diverse learning environments and a broad array of educational approaches to teaching/learning about and from the environment with due stress on practical activities and first hand experience.

In environment education in universities and colleges, emphasis is laid only on plants, animals, air, water, etc. These are being taught from scientific point of view. The need is more of management to see that all the education given is applied and acted upon. Management can help in communication, co-ordination and control to make a unified impact. Hence, management of environment is most essential. We must be stress our efforts to uplift environmental education by integrating through management to improve the quality of all our educational programmes as at present, it is lopsided.

Thus, there is a need of understanding the concept of ecology as explained in our Ancient Sanskrit Literature, so that we may lead life with right focus and perspective in the present times. The Ancient Sanskrit Literature gives us the genuine principles to adjust with our environment and lead a spiritual life full of bliss. Few countries have the natural resources that we in India have. That is, why India was known as golden sparrow. But, then, again, few countries have as little consciousness and respect for our resources as we in India have. Therefore, environmentalists and government must help build a resource consciousness that will lead to conservation and balance of our rich ecological heritage.

The Vedic Rishis had forewarned the need to protect the environment. They mentioned the need of performing the daily Yajnas for protecting the ecology. Dharmasastras prohibited men from disturbing the bio-diversity and eco-system as it is against the tenets of religion and it is considered a sinful activity (Papakarama). In the epic age, man and environment lived in harmonious relationship. The Rgveda considered the oldest manuscript dealing with relationship of environment and human beings, but Atharveda has dealt meticulously about various aspects of environment and showed more concern forecology. Even the Aryans of the Vedic period were aware of the flora and fauna and ecology.

Many other hymns were also written which wanted people to maintain equilibrium of Bhuloka, Suryaloka and Antariksalokas, i.e. earth and other astronomical objects. As stated in various ancient Sanskrit literature, e.g. Gita, Vedas, Manuscript, mind of human beings is always restless, the more it gets the more it wants, resulting into a vicious circle of greed and temptations without any need. People soon cutting trees, do excessive mining, kill animals causing polluted environment. Vedic Rishis had always stressed the planting of trees (Dyaurvana girayovrkṣ-akesah) and avoiding cutting of trees (ma kakambiramudvrho Vanaspatisastrtrvikimnasa R.V. 6.48.17).

Atharvaveda's love for earth is outstanding (Prithvisukta) as mother earth bestowed love on all the creatures living on it. We should not unnecessarily dig the earth as laid down in 35th Mantra of Bhumi Sukta (Yat me Bhume Visvanabhi tadepi Sohatu ma te marma vimrgvadi ma te hrdeyamapinam).

Puranaic mythology believes in worshipping nature, thereby, bringing harmony in eco-system. Even the Great Rishis like Vyasa, Valmiki and others wrote scriptures of eternal values under the trees and the beautiful surroundings. They, with the help of their disciples, maintained beautiful links with environment. All the Rishis even taught the values of good relationship with the eco-system to their disciples, who included many would be kings. Thus, the kings were well versed with the importance of the eco-system.

Ayurveda laid great stress on eco-system as it provided the flora and fauna which was used as medicine for the health of human beings. The names of Charaka and Susruta are noteworthy as they identified the nature and properties of herbs, plants, etc. which were useful to human beings.

Sanskrit writers like Kalidas in their various works dwelled upon the proximity of nature and human beings. The description given by Sanskrit writers is so enchanting that one feels united with nature. Even English writers like Wordsworth appreciated flowers and the beauty of nature.

Our environment is a blessing for us, as it provides basic necessities of life. More and more research on the flora and fauna of the environment will lead to new knowledge for the benefit of human beings. Destroying environment is like cutting the branch of a tree on which one is sitting. Environment must be made better and better based on the sermons contained in our ancient Sanskrit Literature.

Gandhi had conviction of plain living and high thinking. When a man wants to multiply his daily wants, he falls from the ideal. Man's happiness really lies in contentment. Discontentment makes a man slave to his desires. And there is no slave equal to that of the desire. "The less you possess, the less you want, the better you are. Once Gandhi said, "the secret of happy life lies in renunciation. Renunciation is life. Indulgence spells death.

Kautilya in his Arthasastra was firm about preservation of forests, reservoirs, etc. and maintenance of cleanliness in the habitations. He further added that fines should be levied whenever roads are made filthy. Variety of large trees were grown and an officer had to judiciously inspect tree-care and killing of birds and animals was banned.

Nisha Singh in an article, "Environment Education: A Forgotten Commitment "in *University News* clearly define that Environmental Education (EE) emerges to be a comprehensive life long education, responsive to changes in a rapidly changing world. It emphasise on the interdependence of man, society and nature. It attempts to focus on the highly complex relation between development and natural systems. "Environmental education is a process aimed at developing a world population that is aware of and concerned about the total environment and its associated problems and which has the knowledge, attitudes, motivations, commitments and skills to work individually and collectively towards the solution of current problems as well as the prevention of new ones." International Union for the Conservation of Natural Resources defines Environmental Education to be a process of recognising values and clarifying concepts in order to develop skill and attitudes necessary to understand and appreciate the interrelatedness among man, his culture and his biological surroundings.

The Environmental Education proposes to develop in an individual a sense of responsibility and commitment to preserve environment for a better tomorrow. Environmental education includes three broad aspects, i.e. education for the environment, education through the environment and education about the environment.

The first, the foremost and a highly relevant aspect today is the development of attitudes, skills and evaluation abilities for the proper use and the development of environment, i.e. educating for the environment. Where the environment is used as a vehicle for gathering concepts, knowledge and skills related to specific academic disciplines it is the education through the environment; and acquiring an understanding of the total environment constitutes education about the environment. A conceptual model of curriculum based on the goals of Environmental Education was proposed by UNESCO. The goals being:

(i) to foster clear awareness and concern about economic, social, political and ecological interdependence in urban and rural areas;

(ii) to provide every person with opportunities to acquire the knowledge, values, attitudes, commitment and skills needed to protect and improve the environment; and

(iii) to create new patterns of behaviour of individuals, groups and society as a whole towards the environment. This model illustrates how scope can be integrated through grade levels and across appropriate disciplines.

The term environment in Sanskrit literature encompasses broader areas than the definitions given in the context of various commissions and conferences in India, abroad and United Nations System. Most of these definitions are limited to deal with the problems of developed countries and even their solutions pertain to them. In developing countries like India, Environment includes all and its boundary is unlimited. Sanskrit literature reveals that our ancestors never looked upon forests as well as domestic and wild life animals and human beings and Environment, as just a cluster, but they deemed it as a total Biological live landscape with perfect rythum and harmony. Eminent scientist like Einstein strongly believed in nature's inherent harmony. His concern throughout was to find a unified foundation of physics. According to our Seers and Sages as well as Einstein's observations were that "nature is like a vibrating Veena" with perfect rhythum with live waves. They were also aware of the vital functions of non-living entities such as clouds which move and break down, rivers grow, air gains strengths and speed, etc.[5] We cannot forsee a situation where environment can be seen in the context of individual countries. It has to be seen globally and solutions for it are to be seen globally. Even president Roosevelt dwelt upon this idea when he remarked that poverty anywhere is a danger to prosperity.

Sanskrit literature has always been perceiving the problem in toto and its solution also in toto. To quote Sanskrit verse:

सर्वे भवन्तु सुखिनः सर्वे सन्तु निरामयाः ।
सर्वे भद्राणि पश्यन्तु मा कश्चित् दुःख भाग्भवेत् ।।

(Vedic Benediction)

(May All Humanity Be Happy
May all be without disease
May all witness auspicious sights
May none have to undergo suffering)

Man is a discovering specie. Economic man has always had to be concerned with his environment. Until recently, environment was seen as a boundless cornucopia, to be enjoyed, plundered and rearranged for profit. Today, many thoughtful people see it as a limited resource. The relationship between modern man and his environment is a major and a growing problem. The very survival of man as a specie depends upon intelligent and moral human action with respect to these problems.[6]

Environment and development are closely inter-linked. Development cannot subsist on a deteriorating environmental base. Implicit in this is that development cannot take place without exploiting the environment, but harmony between the two is a pre-requisite for the safeguard and preservation of all life on Earth. Development in the absence of emphasis on effective environment, ironically has resulted into pollution of air, water and soil, which in turn has invited the resurgence of a number of life threatening diseases like Cancer, Asthma, Jaundice, Malaria, Dengue, Gastroenteritis, Plague, Tuberculosis, Respiratory illness, Mental disorder, etc. This situation is arising perhaps due to our orientation in deep seated ideologies of production and consumption.[7]

According to the UN Report, "Sustainability means meeting the needs of present generation without compromising the abilities and opportunities of future generation. It thus, implies both intergenerational and intra-generational equity. Sustainability is an important dimension of human development. Human development is a process of enlarging people's choices. But such enhancement must be for both present and future generations without sacrificing one for the other." Thus, sustainable development is a technique of eating the portion of bread and butter by the present generation in such a way that it must last long so as to enable the future generations to enjoy over it.[8]

Bahuguna follows the way and is showing it to all of us. The way is R'ta. Our saints discovered it through communion with nature. The native people can teach us R'ta through their reverence for nature.[9]

Our earth is an infinitely insignificant part of the cosmos. Life is only a recent and insignificant development on earth. Man is only one amongst millions of species—plants as well as animals, past and present, confined to only the outer surface of the earth of a few inches out of 8,000 miles of earth's interior and a few feet above in the atmosphere. We are exposed to space hazards. Some 65 millions years ago a heavenly body crashed down on our planet leading to existinction of many life species including Dinosaurs. In 1908 a comet or a meteor with a mass between 1,00,000 to 10,00,000 tonnes exploded over central Siberia. The impact was 1500 times more powerful than the bomb dropped in Hiroshima and destroyed an area of woodland 40 kms. by 50 kms large.

Man is also, like-wise, participating in many social circles—concentric circles—family, village, block, district, state, country, continent and the global society at large. Life exists between a small temperature band. A few degree higher temperature resulting from changes in solar radiation or any other reason will burn up life and few degrees lower will freeze all life to death. A few degrees rise in maximum temperature will melt all polar ice resulting in sub-merging of all landmass and the terrestrial life forms. Any minor change in the composition of the atmosphere—because of cosmic developments—crashing of a space object on the earth or resulting from human civilization, burning of hydrocarbons—resulting in green house effect, rising temperature, melting of polar ice and flooding and sub-mergence of land masses, exhaustion of mineral resources, ozone hole, environmental degradation, disappearance of flora and fauna with unspecified effects on human life, appearance of diseases as deadly or deadlier than AIDS, cancer, etc. can extinguish human life. In the light of cosmic level scales and possible variations in cosmic parameters—within the very narrow limits of which alone human life is possible—there is every reason to believe that human life hangs by a slender thread.

We are standing at such a cross, that there is no scope of looking back, but to act swiftly with a courage of conviction, to control the rising curves of population graphs. The old frame of 20th century is already spreading its weak and withered look over the paths on which the man has treaded during the last millennium. The beseeching old look are now reverently assessing our past unresponsive attitudes which limited the man's actualism only to the sensual and lustful desires which consequently kept on loading this planet with sustained effects of pollution on every bit of life-prone existence.[10]

Ever since the dawn of civilization, man has been constantly engaged in the pursuit of unraveling the mystery of nature with a view to arriving at the fundamental values of life. Today, the world is in a state of turmoil, the causes of which seem to be beyond man's comprehension and capabilities. Paradoxically enough, man seems to be lost in the world of plenitude. His soul is starved in the midst of unbounded materialistic pleasures and comforts that science and technology of today have placed at his disposal. Now man everywhere is be deviled by complex and complicated moral, cultural and social issues. The harder he strives to extricate himself out of the web of these problems, the more he is caught and involved in it. Underneath the morass of conflicting values lies man's quest for the real meaning of life and the destiny to which it leads.

With all the scientific and technological revolutions that humanity has achieved so far, we have not risen above the level of satisfying the bare physical needs of man. Science does not help us to discuss the fundamental moral and spiritual values of life or how to live and here we see that the advancement of science hassled to mankind's lopsided growth and development.

R.Venkataraman, former President of India, in his article, "Need for Ecological Balance" in *Bhavan's Journal* (April 15, 2002) states that Modern civilisation has brought in its trail many ill effects caused by our failure to respect and preserve the balance of ecological factors in the human environment. More often than not, we have in our decision-making allowed economic and material considerations to outweigh human and spiritual ones. Much of this has happened in the developing nations because we have attempted to develop along western models forgetting that the west is already suffering from the consequences of indiscriminate use of modern technology. It is this failure to understand the western experience of development that has all too often faces to adopt policies that are economically disastrous. There has been haphazard growth of our large cities where inhabitants are condemned to psychological and social effects of overcrowding; slums have come up in the periphery, where the poor live without basic civic amenities; crime has increased; family as a cohesive unit and as apart of small community is breaking up and the individual lacks security and a sense of belonging. In the rural areas the very sources of livelihood of the people are being threatened. There is the pollution of lakes, of rivers and the sea. . . . In fact, man has not understood nature and its secrets and will realise it only after destroying its boundaries.

CRISIS IN MANAGING ENVIRONMENT

Ever since the United Nations Conference on Human Environment held at Stockholm in 1972 proclaimed the right of the people to a clean environment, the Government of India as well as the state governments have initiated a number of measures to control the various types of pollution. However, the disastrous consequences of a technological civilization which has disturbed the delicate balance of various ecological factors are yet to be fully realized by the humans. Until recently nature was able to absorb the pollutants added to it and again provide a clean environment on the planet. But today an advanced industrial society and greedy humanity is polluting the environment at a rate faster than the nature's capacity to remedy the same. The United Nations has given a timely call to halt the suicidal tendency of the humanity to destroy the very planet which has been sustaining its existence.[11]

Dr. Zbigniew Bankowski, spells out the code of ethics to protect the environment. It would be unrealistic, however, to suppose that the damage that has been done, and still continues to be done, can be arrested and undone in the short-term. Rather, long-term global policies must be envisaged and, if they are to be successful, they will require changes in our perceptions of man in nature. If our global physical environment is not to be further degraded, we must change our conceptual environment, our ways of thinking and behaving. Perhaps the worst environmental pollution is pollution of the mind, and the greatest need is for well thought out principles of environmental ethics.

All spheres of human conduct private and public, are subject to ethical principles or rules. When governments or other corporate bodies despoil the environment in the name of development or political dominance or national security, when government adopt *laissez faire* policies that permit the exploitation of nature for narrow, short-term gains, they contravene the basic ethical principle of the greatest good for the greatest number of people. It is necessary to approach the problem in a holistic manner by linking sanitation with religion, culture, health, agriculture, environment and production of energy. The basic attitude that needs to be formed is to link it with Bhakti. It has to be stressed that cleanliness is godliness and unless cleanliness becomes a part of our lives, we cannot be true devotees of God.[12]

As early as in 1972, the United Nations Declaration on Human Environment warned: We see around us growing evidence of man-made harm in many regions of the earth; dangerous levels of pollution in water, air, earth and living beings; major and undersirable disturbances to the ecological balance of the biosphere, destruction and depletion of irreplaceable resources; and gross deficiencies harmful to the physical, mental and social health of men, in the man-made environment, particularly in the living and working environment.

The Tribune editorial Sept. 6, 2002, "Who cares for the earth: has rightly hit on the policies of the developed world, To quote: The environmental health of the planet did not improve after the path-breaking earth summit at Stockholm in 1972. It did not change in spite of the decibel level being raised at Rio in 1992 to a point that ensured the whispered reservations of the rich could be heard across the globe. The message from Johannesburg that hosted the latest round of the World Summit on Sustainable Development is not encouraging either. It is the same old story of the poor being allowed a forum from which they can share with the rest of the world their concerns about environment-related issues. However, in the end it is the will of the rich that prevails. The fact that President George W. Bush did not deem it necessary to be present on the occasion conveyed in clear terms what the USA—the biggest polluter—thought about such summits. At Rio Ms. Meneka Gandhi had stolen the thunder by insisting that for a safe and fair world order it was necessary to adopt the principle that made the polluter pay for messing around with the fragile ecology of the planet. She received applause, but at the end of the day countries like the USA continued to add to the rising pollution levels without any sense of remorse. The Earth Summit 10 years ago at Rio de Janerio grandly resolved to save all nature, from the humblest algae to the majestic elephant. It agreed that the planets delicate climate urgently needed protection before global warming rises to dangerous levels. What has been the contribution of the developed community at Rio? They asked the smaller nations to comply with the strict provisions while they busied themselves in buying unused greenhouse emission permits from countries that in any case do not produce even a fraction of the permissible level.

In addition, the multinational corporations are responsible for environmental degradation. The multinational corporations and their role in raising the pollution level is not a secret. Union Carbide was responsible for the Bhopal tragedy and the USA did not allow the law to get hold of the guilty for trial in India. In the UK a company by the name of British Nuclear Fuels Ltd. dumped approximately 182 kg of plutonium into the Irish sea over the past 50 years. Lobsters from the polluted region and near the Norwegian coast have been tested positive of high levels of radioactive contamination. Should anyone be allowed to play in these waters? What about eating the contaminated seafood? World leaders need to do an honest introspection for saving the planet from certain disaster. They must realize that every living being shares the same earth. If the lungs develop cancer, the rest of the body cannot survive by removing the lungs.

Environment is common for all the countries as well as inter-connected as polluted environment can move freely through diffusion as already explained in the introduction. A global effort based on the wisdom contained in Sanskrit literature and new knowledge generated through science and technological research should be employed to combat the menace of environmental degradation. The developed world should not remain isolated as the impact of endangered environment would rècoil on them. All the affluence of the developed world would be of no use if the total environment is not smoothing.

Churamani states that just as waves merge into sea and become one, so developed and developing countries should think of ocean, i.e. collective approach and not isolated approach. Life is nothing but a wave in the vast sea. Each wave is having a feeling of individuality and it does not consider itself the part and parcel of the sea or the sea itself but considers itself separate from the vast sea. The feeling of separation has caused its existence in the universe. The drama of action and reaction of wave motion always continues in the sea. None can judge how many water waves are taking birth and how many are dying. The waves are of different strengths and their strengths and their existence is also of different time periods.[13]

Therefore, there is a need of redefining the environmental issues so that a peaceful solution can be found to make it fit for all the people of the world to live. We should also associate rural and urban Governments in protecting the environment as these institutions understand the problem and can provide operational solution. Today, we are thinking and tackling Physical environment but the major problem resides in the realm of mental, social, spiritual and astronomical objects. So a complete solution by all the countries is essential. We must consult Sanskrit Literature for solution beyond Physical environment, i.e. in the sphere of Metaphysical.

Bernard Lovell, and Al Gore also emphasize Ethical basis which is the core view of Ancient Indian Sanskrit Literature. "The vital question is whether the framework of society in which science is perused can develop the ethical basis and moral purpose necessary to ensure that in our future progress we overcome the forces leading to decay and destruction.[14]

To me, as a student of Sanskrit, environment includes study of all human beings in their physical, social, psychological and spiritual needs and relationships as well, their environment in terms of water, air, plants, animals and heavenly bodies. Ancient Sanskrit literature considers environment cosmic in sweep and it includes transcendental and psychic categories besides physical and natural.

It is realized that industrialization is essential if an economy is to develop. But the transformation of natural resources for industrialization is accompanied by serious environmental degradation. When this transformation of nature by man, instead of showing a symbiotic relationship between man and nature, shows a man centric effort to conquer nature and ultimately overpower it, the economy that is aimed to be built by man to protect himself and prosper, is itself stressed. This gives the background of one's understanding on industrial ecology. If mankind is to live over generations, the eco-system, which feeds them, has to be sustained and there comes the question of controlling man's exercise of power over nature.[15]

Most of the environmental problems of the present day are essentially man-made. The role of man is therefore important because it is his attitude and values which shape the environment. In developed countries mad race after materialism puts too much pressure on environment. The materialistic attitude of man multiplies the human needs and ultimately leads towards resources exploitation, without considering the future consequential disharmony with the environment. Man has to evolve a balanced way of thinking, acting and feeling towards the environment. So human ethics, attitude, values, decision making analysis of ecological, economic, social and technical aspects come under the scope of environmental education.[16]

Education, including formal education, public awareness and training should be recognized as a process by which human beings and societies can reach their fullest potential. Education is critical for promoting sustainable development and improving the capacity of the people to address environment and development issues. While basic education provides the underpinning for any environmental and development education, the latter needs to be incorporated as an essential part of learning. Both formal and non-formal education are indispensable to changing people's attitudes so that they have the capacity to assess and address their sustainable development concerns. It is also critical for achieving environmental and ethical awareness, values and attitudes, skills and behaviour consisted with sustainable development and for effective public participation in decision-making. To be effective, environment and development education should deal with the dynamics of both the physical/biological and socio-economic environment and human (which may include spiritual) development, should be integrated in all disciplines, and should employ formal and non-formal methods and effective means of communication.[17]

Unfortunately, knowledge of environment hygiene and awareness of pollution hazards are seriously lacking amongst even our enlightened citizens. The Stockholm Conference of Human Environment in 1972 heralded the efforts, both national and international to "establish programmes of environment education, interdisciplinary in approach, in school and out of school en-compassing all levels of education and directed towards the general public in particular the ordinary citizens living in rural and urban area, youth and adult alike, with a view to educating him as to simple steps he might take, within his means to manage and control his environment."

Archana Aggrawal in an article, "Education for Environmental Awareness" in *University News,* Oct. 21, 1996 states that the need of the hour is to prepare suitable strategies of Environmental Education for saving our environment. Environment education denotes a study of environment and its dynamics: environmental degradation and its various forms, factors degrading environment and its impact on man's life. In particular, it includes the following major areas:

(i) Detailed study of environment alongwith all the pertinent facts and forces that pollute environment;
(ii) Study of the impact of environmental pollution and changes on the life of man;
(iii) Use of education as a motivational force and as a promotional agency for right understanding of environment and its degradation, for controlling environmental degradation and for prospering environment. What is it? How is it destroying the earth? Why is environmental balance necessary? How can we save it?
(iv) To evolve pollution control ideas, devices and measures and to adopt them to deal with environmental degradation and its consequences and to improve the environment through education and training of every citizen including training of teachers and the personnel needed for promoting environmental education.

Article 51A of the Constitution of India states:

"It shall be the duty of every citizen of India to *protect and improve the natural environment including forests, lakes, rivers and wild life and* to *have compassion for the living creatures."*

New Education Policy of 1986 has also emphasized this: "There is a paramount need to create a consciousness of the environment. It must permeate all the ages and all sections of society.

'Environmental Sciences' should be introduced at undergraduate and postgraduate level. Several new courses at both the levels should be introduced in science, engineering, commerce and arts such as, Environment and Development, Agriculture and Environment, Chemical Aspects of Air Pollution, Waste Water Treatment, Industry and Environment, Production through Waste Material, etc. Production of electricity from the waste is now becoming popular. This solves the problem of disposal of waste as well as providing fuel for electricity generation. Project work at postgraduate level that usually forms part of these courses can provide good opportunities for useful investigations related to environment. Areas can be identified which need more attention. Projects as a survey of environmental awareness among people; a study of environmental awareness among teachers; effect of pollution on health, etc. can be undertaken. Moreover, Searches exploring the condition of environment, factors polluting environment, effectiveness of various measures used in different industries for controlling pollution and their after-effects should get full attention. Co-curricular activities like scouting, NCC: NSS are part of school curriculum. Volunteers can make attempts to promote environmental awareness through several activities like plays, songs, talking with peoples, tree plantation, maintenance of healthy environment, etc.

It is of great significance that judiciary is also taking keen interest in protection of environment. To create this awareness, to feel by oneself about the critical importance of environment, environment education is a must as it can create positive attitude among the minds of people. Since 1972, the syllabus at the primary and secondary and Higher Education levels is becoming gradually environment conscious. In particular at school level, environment is included in geography, physical science and life science, though no uniformity exists in their coverage or level. However, in 1992, the Supreme Court heard a public interest litigation case on the urgent need to impart environmental education for all the students from the primary to the university level and gave directions to the government that environment should be made a compulsory subject for all the students—the future citizens of the country—to enable them to protect the public health, prevent pollution and save all forms of life as envisaged under Article 51A(g) of the constitution. This will give a boost to frame a standard syllabus on environment education for the future generation and we can hope that they will be saved from the confusion and unawareness of the people in the present generation. In Delhi, old vehicles of above 20 years were banned. It is very difficult to discuss all. Concerned over the lack of awareness among people about the protection of environment, the Supreme Court fined 10 states Rs. 15,000 each for failing to respond to its notices seeking information whether they had included environmental studies in the school and college curricula as direction by it on 21st Sept., 2003.

Taking strong exception to the states of Assam, Arunachal Pradesh, Bihar, Goa, Jammu and Kashmir, Jharkhand, Madhya Pradesh, Maharastra and West Bengal not responding to the court's notices, a Bench comprising Mr. Justice N. Santosh Hedge and Mr. Justice B.P. Singh said the fine should be deposited by them within four weeks.

The court warned that if they failed to deposit the fine within the stipulated period, the Chief Secretary of each state would be held responsible.

The court was hearing a public interest litigation (PIL) by Magsaysay Award winner environmentalist-lawyer M.C. Mehta highlighting the issue of non-compliance of the 1991 court order by the states in which a series of directions were given about maintaining the ecological balance and launching of a sustained campaign on protection of environment.

The court had specifically said every state was required to make the environmental studies at school and college levels compulsory and issue directions to the education boards and the universities in this regards.

The court had made it mandatory for the states to include environmental studies in the school and college course from the 1992-93 academic session.

The University Grants Commission (UGC) was also directed by the court to prescribe the course for environmental studies at the graduation and the post-graduation level.

"Eco Clubs in colleges" have been set-up in order to widen the base of the green brigade in the country, the Ministry of Environment has directed states and the union territories to set-up National Green Corps (NGC) also in colleges and increase the number of the eco-clubs in schools. Dr. Satnam Singh Ladhar of the Punjab State Council for Science and Technology said that the clubs were set-up throughout the country in 2001 under a scheme which was evolved by the Ministry of Environment. At that time the ministry had proposed to set-up 100 clubs in each district. "Every state has been directed by the Ministry to set-up 50 eco-clubs in colleges.

UGC in its document six months module syllabus for environment studies for undergraduate courses stressed the need for environmental education to quote the document. The importance of environmental science and environmental studies can not be disputed. The need for sustainable development is a key to the future of mankind. Continuing problems of pollution, loss afforest, solid waste disposal, degradation of environment, issues like economic productivity and national security, Global warming, the depletion of ozone layer and loss of biodiversity have made everyone aware of environmental issues. The United Nations Conference on Environment and Development held in Rio de Janeiro in 1992 and World Summit on Sustainable Development at Johannesburg in 2002 have drawn the attention of people around the globe to the deteriorating condition of our environment. It is clear that no citizen of the earth can afford to be ignorant of environment issues.

Accordingly, the matter was considered by UGC and it was decided that a six months' compulsory core module course in environmental studies maybe prepared and compulsorily implemented in all the Universities/ Colleges of India.

CONCLUSION

The experts committee appointed by the UGC has looked in to all the pertinent questions, issues and other relevant matters. This was followed by framing of the core module syllabus for environmental studies for undergraduate courses of all branches of Higher Education. We are deeply conscious that there are bound to be gaps between the ideal and real. Genuine endeavourers required to minimize the gaps by intellectual and material inputs. The success of this course will depend on the initiative and drive of the teachers and the receptive students. (See Appendix 2.1)

The ultimate purpose of Environment education should be to ensure the following as mentioned in Sukal Yajarved 36-71 and the Chart 2.2.

ओउम् द्यौ शान्ति ।
अन्तरिक्ष शान्ति ।
पृथिवी: शान्ति ।
आप: शान्ति ।
औषधय: शान्ति ।
वनस्पतय: शान्ति ।
विश्वे देवा शान्ति ।
ब्रहा शान्ति ।
शान्तिरेव शान्ति ।
सा मा शान्तिरेधि ॥

शुक्ल-यजुर्वेद 36-17

CHART 2.1

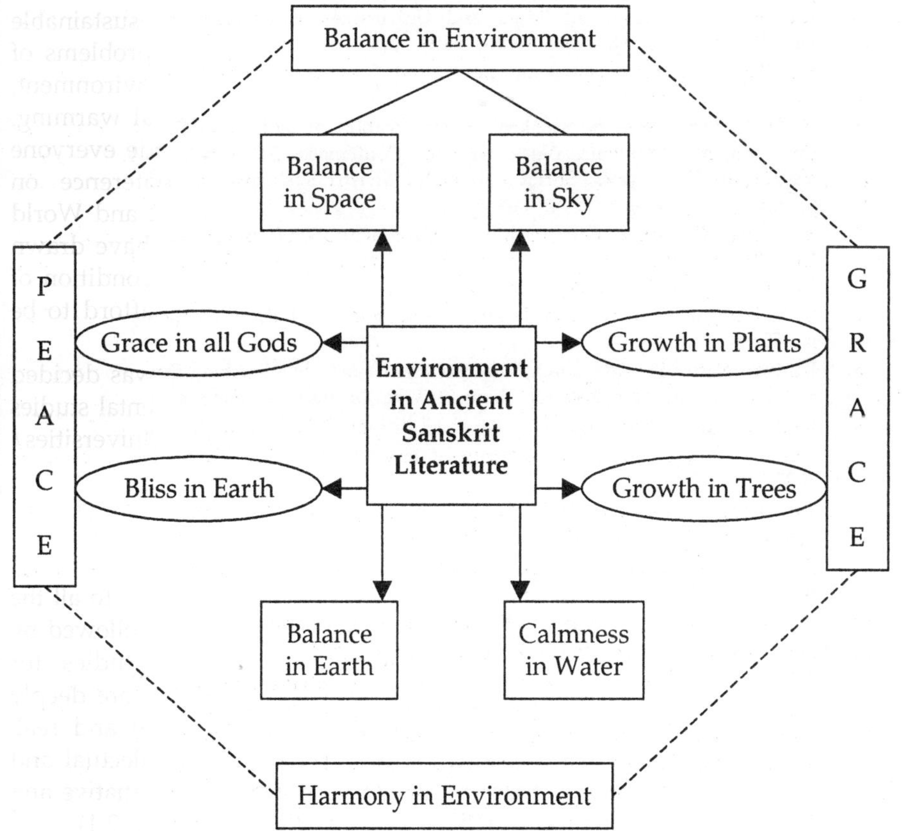

Let there be balance in the space !
Let there be balance in the sky !
Let there be peace on the earth !
Let there be calmness in waters !
Let there be growth in plants !
Let there be growth in the trees !
Let there be grace in all Gods !
Let there be bliss in the Brahman !
Let there be balance in everything !
Let there be peace and peace !
Let such peace be with everyone of us !

Notes and References

1. Hiroshi Nakajima, "A Wounded Planet", in *World Health*, January-February 1990, p. 3.
2. Dr. Wilfried Krielsel, "Environment Health in 1990's in *World Health*, January-February 1990, p. 5.
3. K.B. Pawar, Environment Issues and Universities, in *Environment Challenge and the Universities*, AIU, New Delhi, 1994, pp. 2-3.
4. S.C. Gupta, Environmental Studies, Need For Planning and Co-ordination, in *Ibid.*, p. 12.
5. A.N. Yellappa, Role of Sanskrit in Preservation of Wild Life Bio-Diversity and Environment", Souvenir, World Sanskrit Conference, 5-9 April, 2001, Ed., Prof. Vachaspati Upadhyaya, Shri Lal Bahadur Shastri Rashtriya Sanskrit Vidyapeeth, p. 183.
6. S. Murty, Economic Growth and Environment: Some issues in Environmental Challenges of the 21st Century ed. S. Radha and Amar Singh Sankhyan, New Delhi, Deep & Deep, 2002, p. 44.
7. O.P. Monga, Ecology, Development and Society: Future Challenges, in *Ibid.*, p. 75.
8. Baidya Nath Prasad Singh, Environment and Sustainable Development: A suitable Strategy Needed for their Striking Balance, in *Ibid.*, p. 72.
9. Raghbir Singh Pirta, The Himalayaṣ, Tehri and Bahuguna, Ibid p. 277.
10. Gurcharn Singh, Pollution to Purity of Environment, New Delhi, Deep & Deep, 2005, p. 113.
11. S.P. Ranga Rao, and M.S. Prakasa Sastry, "Control of Water Pollution in Andhra Pradesh" in *IJPA*, July-Sept. 1999, p. 548.
12. Zbigniew Bankowski, "A code of Ethics" in *World Health*, January-Feb. 1990, p. 18.
13. Parmod Churamani, Way to Mental Freedom, Chapter 5.
14. Lean, Geoffrey, Rich World Poor World, p. 332.
15. S.S. Narata Rao and Pratibha Narata, Industrialization and Environment: Agenda for the 21st century in Environmental challenges of the 21st century, Editors S. Radha and Amar Singh Sankkyan, 2002, p. 124.
16. Maba Kumar Patnaik and P. Sasi Bhushan Rao, Environment Education for 21st century in Environment Management and Audit, Editors, P. Pasi Bhushan Rao and P. Mohana Rao, Deep & Deep, New Delhi, 2000, p. 206.
17. Agenda 21, UNCED, Rio-de Janerio, Brazil, June 3-14, 1992, Chapter 36.

Appendix 2.1

CORE MODULE SYLLABUS FOR ENVIRONMENTAL STUDIES FOR UNDER GRADUATE COURSES OF ALL BRANCHES OF HIGHER EDUCATION

Unit 1: The Multidisciplinary Nature of Environmental Studies

Definition, scope and importance (2 lectures)

Need for public awareness.

Unit 2: Natural Resources

Renewable and Non-renewable Resources

- Natural resources and associated problems.
- Forest resources: Use and over-exploitation, deforestation, case studies, timber extraction, mining, dams and their effects on forests and tribal people.
- Water resources: Use and over-utilization of surface and ground water, floods, drought, conflicts over water, dams, benefits and problems.
- Mineral resources: Use an exploitation, environmental effects of extracting and using mineral resources, case studies.
- Food resources: World food problems, changes caused by agriculture and overgrazing, effects of modern agriculture, fertilizer-pesticide problems, water logging, salinity, case studies.
- Energy resources: Growing energy needs, renewable and non-renewable energy sources, use of alternate energy sources, case studies.
- Land resources: Land as a resource, land degradation, man induced landslides, soil erosion and desertification.
- Role of an individual in conservation of natural resources.
- Equitable use of resources for sustainable lifestyles. (8 lectures)

Unit 3: Ecosystems

- Concept of an ecosystem.
- Structure and function of an ecosystem.
- Producers, consumers and decomposers.
- Energy flow in the ecosystem.
- Ecological succession.
- Food chains, food webs and ecological pyramids.

- Introduction, types, characteristic features, structure and function of the following ecosystem:
  (a) Forest ecosystem,
  (b) Grassland ecosystem,
  (c) Desert ecosystem.
- Aquatic ecosystems (ponds, streams, lakes, rivers, oceans, estuaries) (6 lectures)

Unit 4: Biodiversity and its Conservation

- Introduction—Definition: genetic, species and ecosystem diversity.
- Biogeographical classification of India.
- Value of biodiversity: consumptive use, productive use, social, ethical, aesthetic and option values.
- Biodiversity at global, National and local levels.
- India as a mega-diversity nation.
- Hot-spots of biodiversity.
- Threats to biodiversity: habitat loss, poaching of wildlife, manwildlife conflicts.
- Endangered and endemic species of India.
- Conservation of biodiversity: In-situ and Ex-situ conservation of biodiversity. (8 lectures)

Unit 5: Environmental Pollution

Definition

- Causes, effects and control measures of:
  (a) Air pollution
  (b) Water pollution
  (c) Soil pollution
  (d) Marine pollution
  (e) Noise pollution
  (f) Thermal pollution
  (g) Nuclear hazards
- Solid waste Management: Causes, effects and control measures of urban and industrial wastes.
- Role of an individual in prevention of pollution.
- Pollution case studies.
- Disaster management: floods, earthquake, cyclone and landslides. (8 lectures)

Unit 6: Social Issues and the Environment

- From Unsustainable to Sustainable development.

- Urban problems related to energy.
- Water conservation, rain water harvesting, watershed management.
- Resettlement and rahabilitation of people; its problems and concerns. Case studies.
- Environmental ethics: Issues and possible solutions.
- Climate change, global warming, acid rain, ozone layer depletion, nuclear accidents and holocaust. Case studies.
- Wasteland reclamation.
- Consumerism and waste products.
- Environment Protection Act.
- Air (Prevention and Control of Pollution) Act.
- Water (Prevention and Control of Pollution) Act.
- Wildlife Protection Act.
- Forest Conservation Act.
- Issues involved in enforcement of environmental legislation.
- Public awareness. (7 lectures)

Unit 7: Human Population and the Environment

- Population growth, variation among nations.
- Population explosion—Family Welfare Programme.
- Environment and human health.
- Human Rights.
- Value Education.
- HIV/AIDS.
- Women and Child Welfare.
- Role of Information Technology in Environment and human health.
- Case Studies. (6 lectures)

Unit 8: Field Work

- Visit to a local area to document environmental assets—river; forest/grassland; hill; mountain.
- Visit to a local polluted site—Urban/Rural/Industrial/Agricultural.
- Study of common plants, insects, birds.
- Study of simple ecosystems-pond, river, hill slopes, etc.

(Field work equal to 5 lecture hours)

SIX MONTHS' COMPULSORY CORE MODULE COURSE IN ENVIRONMENTAL STUDIES: FOR UNDERGRADUATES

Teaching Methodologies

The Core Module Syllabus for Environmental Studies includes

classroom teaching and Field Work. The syllabus is divided into eight units covering 50 lectures. The first seven units will cover 45 lectures which are classroom based to enhance knowledge skills and attitude to environment. Unit eight is based on field activities which will be covered in five lecture hours and would provide students first hand knowledge on various local environmental aspects. Field experience is one of the most effective learning tools for environmental concerns. This moves out of the scope of the text book mode of teaching into the realm of real learning in the field, where the teacher merely acts as a catalyst to interpret what the student observes or discovers in his/her own environment. Field studies are as essential as class work and form an irreplaceable synergistic tool in the entire learning process.

Course material provided by UGC for classroom teaching and field activities be utilized.

The universities/colleges can also draw upon expertise of outside resource persons for teaching purposes.

Environmental Core Module shall be integrated into the teaching programmes of all undergraduate courses.

Annual System

The duration of the course will be 50 lectures. The exam will be conducted along with the Annual Examination.

Semester System

The Environment course of 50 lectures will be conducted in the second semester and the examinations shall be conducted at the end of the second semester.

Credit System

The core course will be awarded 4 credits.

Exam Pattern

In case of awarding the marks, the question paper should carry 100 marks. The structure of the question paper being:

Part-A: Short answer pattern.	25 marks
Part-B: Essay type with inbuilt choice.	50 marks
Part-C: Field Work.	25 marks

Source: UGC, Six months' Module Syllabus for Environmental Studies for Undergraduate Courses, New Delhi, 2003, pp. 7-8.

CHAPTER 3

HEALTH AND ENVIRONMENTAL EDUCATION

> Economic growth, without being specifically attuned to human needs and human realization is not worth very much. Once more you hear everywhere people speaking about unclear energy, oil energy, solar energy, wind energy, and everybody seems to be overlooking the fact that without human energy, there would be no kind of progress either socially or economically.
>
> —*Dr. Mahler*

Health and Environmental Education

Environment Protection is Everybody's Mission to help Build a Healthy, Wealthy and Prosperous Nation.

—*D.C. Naik*

Health of the people and environment are directly linked. In the new millennium, health and environment are becoming of serious concern as they affect each other and the total process of socio-economic development. It has been beautifully said that Health is Wealth. Healthy people would work in all directions—agriculture, animal husbandry, etc. radiating happiness which is vital for a stimulating environment. Healthy individuals would interact among themselves in a positive way. These positive interactions would make a positive environment. That is why it has been stated that Healthy Human beings rather than capital is key to healthy environment development. If all of us make use of environmental resources to meet our basic needs and not engaged in exploitation to satisfy our greed and lust, then both the environment and the people would remain healthy. The whole life of healthy people would enrich the contents of environment. The healthy people would see the environment from their angle. It has been beautifully said in a poem.

In developing countries, we find people in the whole family suffering from virus fevers. Virus infection to one spreads to all in the family, then in the wider area. The only solution is to keep the environment clean through healthy people.

"As each beholds in cloud and Fire
The shape that answers his own desire."

All these prove that the Marginalised sections in the society are being greatly affected as they cannot insulate themselves from the health hazards on account of imperceptible damage to the environment. Market introduction in the healthcare industry, may protect those who have the affordability. On the other hand, it is the poor who are in large numbers take the adverse effect of deterioration in the environmental quality. It is obvious that when the nexus between environmental and health is analysed, theories of welfare of the poor does surface; both the environmentalists and healthcare planners have to interact for positive action in the above context.[1]

There are direct and indirect health effects of deteriorating environment and non-renewability of resources. Human activity is causing the extinction of animal, plant and microbiological organisms at rates which may eliminate one-forth of all species on Earth within the next 50 years. The incalculable human health consequences from the destruction include . . . the upsetting of the balance among ecosystems on which all life, including human life depends. Major efforts to protect natural habitats and to preserve biodiversity are required to prevent their medical catastrophes from occurring (Cherian, 1993). Many terminal disease threatening the survival of human race such as cancer, AIDS or arterioscteriotic heart diseases are the resultant effects of extinction of species and forests.[2]

HEALTHCARE ADMINISTRATION AS A COMPONENT OF SOCIO-ECONOMIC DEVELOPMENT

Environment hazards to health fall into two broad categories. On the one side is the lack of accessibility to basic environmental resources like sanitation, water, fresh air, shelter and like. On the other side is the exposure to hazardous environment. These hazards include biological agents viz., micro-organisms such as bacteria and viruses and parasites which contribute to the global burden of infectious disease; cause birth defects and damage the body immunity system and which render people susceptible to a variety of health risks.

The following table gives the principal health and productivity consequences of health mismanagement:

TABLE 3.1

Environmental problem	*Effect on health*	*Effect on productivity*
1	*2*	*3*
Water pollution and water scarcity	More than 2 million deaths and billions of illnesses a year attributable to pollution, poor household hygiene and added health risks caused by water scarcity.	Declining fisheries; rural household time and municipal costs of providing safe water; aquifer depletion leading to irreversible compaction; constraint on economic activity because of water shortage.

Air pollution	Many acute and chronic health impacts: excessive urban particulate matter levels are responsible for 300,000-700,000 premature deaths annually and for half of childhood chronic diseases; women and children in poor rural areas affected by smoky indoor air.	Restrictions on vehicle and industrial activity during critical episodes; effect of acid rain on forests and water bodies.
Solid and hazardous wastes	Diseases spread by rotting garbage and blocked drains. Risks from hazardous wastes typically local but often acute	Pollution of ground water resources.
Soil degradation	Reduced nutrition for poor farmers on depleted soils; greater susceptibility to drought.	Field productivity losses in range of 0.5-1.5 percent of gross national product (GNP) common on tropical soils; offsite siltation of reservoirs, river-transport channels, and other hydrologic investments.
Deforestation	Localized flooding, leading to death and disease.	Loss of sustainable logging potential and of erosion prevention, watershed stability, and carbon sequestration provided by forests.
Loss of bio-diversity	Potential loss of new drugs.	Reduction of ecosystem adaptability and loss of genetic resources.
Atmospheric changes	Possible shifts in vector-borne diseases; risks from climatic natural disasters; diseases attributable to ozone depletion (perhaps 300,000 additional cases of skin cancer a year worldwide; 1.7 million cases of cataracts).	Sea-rise damage to coastal investments; regional changes in agricultural productivity; disruption of marine food chain.

Source: World Development Report, 1992, p. 4.

The health component and other components of the socio-economic system necessarily interact. Health not only affects the remainder of the socio-economic complex, but is also affected by it, sometimes favourably, sometimes unfavourably. "The promotion and protection of the health of the people is essential to sustained economic and social development and

CHART 3.1

Socio-economic Development

Social Development
Social Services
Socio-economic Product (GNP)
Services
Goods
Social Welfare
Education
Health
Ensure activity of
Enhancement of
Improve Vitality of
Human Capital
Development of
Increase Production of
Exploitation of
Industry
Agri-culture
Natural Resources
Productive Services
Economic Development
Rehabilitation
Diagnostic Education
Curative
Preventive
Promotive

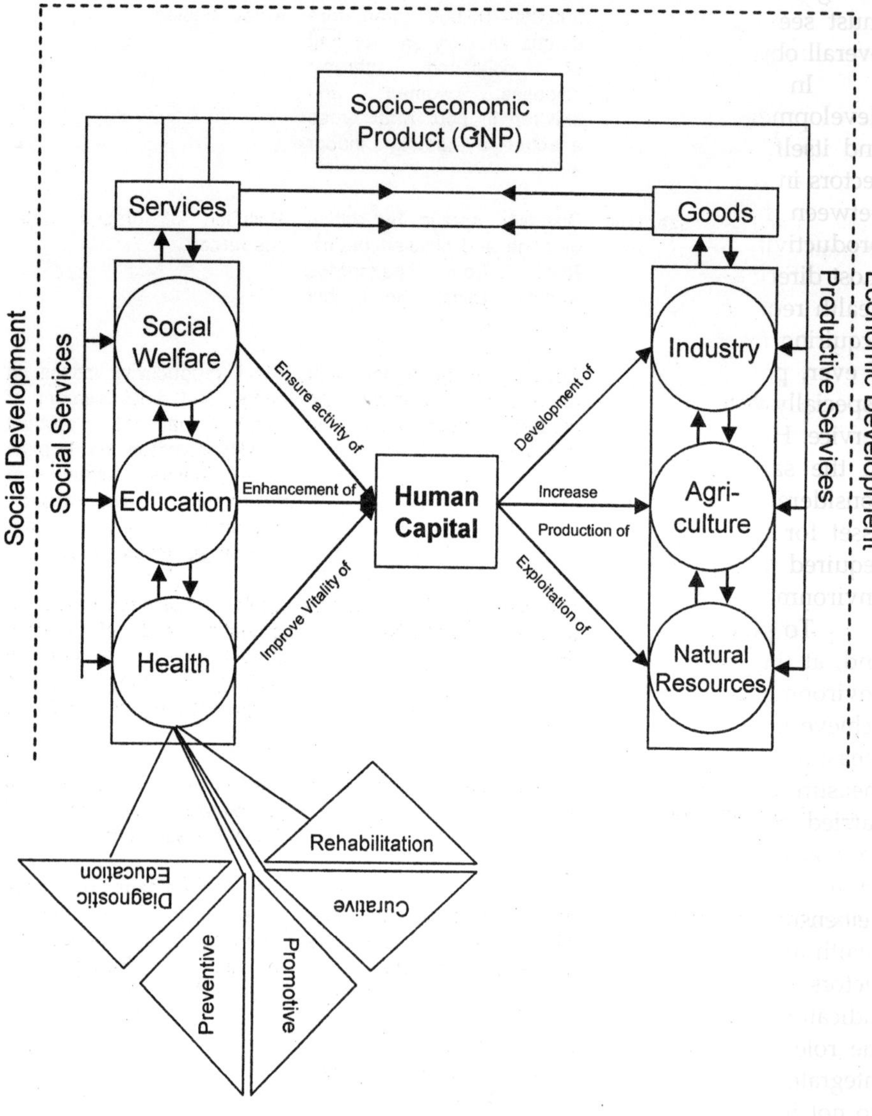

contribution to a better quality of life and to world peace and environment." The major areas in which health affects socio-economic development include problems arising out of the rate of population growth, rapid industrialisation and urbanisation, mental stress and social instability, environmental pollution and the growing disparity of living standards within and among nations, it needs to be reiterated here that social development not only continuously interacts with economic development but that the various aspects of social development keep on interacting with one another. 'A sound mind in a sound body' is an old proverb. Thus, changes in one sector of social activity produce changes in the other. We must see that these chain reactions are conducive to the attainment of overall objective of environment development.

In the overall and integrated concept of social and economic development of a country health cannot be considered exclusively as an end itself. One must take into account also its role as one of the social sectors in overall development and try to establish measurable relationships between health and the macroscopic variables, such as consumption, productivity and labour on which it depends or with which it is involved most directly. In other words, it is necessary to determine the investment in health required for development or the rate of development. The benefits acquiring from health programmes are less difficult to measure. It is rarely, if ever, possible to identify all the consequences of a health programme especially the long-term consequences. A healthcare is primarily a social service. Health programmes are mostly established because they contribute to the satisfaction of primary human needs, irrespective of economic considerations except in so far as they can be afforded and constitute an asset for the future. For this and other reasons the cost and other data required to evaluate the contribution made by health programmes to environmental development are essential.

To plan for health, that is, to meet the basic needs of the community and, at the same time, to satisfy the requirements of the overall pace for environmental development is a complex process. It will be possible to achieve it fully when the economic benefits obtained with a specific health measure can be expressed in quantitative terms and when it is possible to measure precisely the degree of benefit to health from activities which are carried on outside this direct operational sphere. While health planners have always assumed that there is a good correlation between health and environmental development. Research is still in its infancy in this area. H. Leibenstein has rightly said that data on general relationship indicated that health and education were the most evident among the large 'residual' of factors that proved statistically more important than the usual economic indicators in explaining environmental protection. Prof. D. Banerji stresses the role of health as a contributor to economic growth and the need to integrate health activities into general economic activities so that the former do not interfere with the latter or *vice-versa*. Dr. E.J. Thierry in his article, "Laying the foundations", succinctly remarked that,

"Health is man's most precious possession; it influences all his activities; it shapes the destinies of people. Without it, there can be no solid foundation for man's happiness. Nevertheless, all too often, social planners, forget this simple truth and leave health out of account. Integration of health schemes in overall development of environmental plans are of paramount importance.

Good health is a prerequisite to human productivity and the

"environmental development" process. It is essential to economic and technological development. A healthy community is the infrastructure upon which to build a sound and peaceful environment. The status of environment greatly depends on the quality of its people. Unhealthy people can hardly be expected to make any valid contribution towards environmental developmental programmes. Health is man's greatest possession, for it lays a solid foundation for his happiness. Charaka, the renowned Ayurvedic physician is known to have said: "Health was vital for ethical, artistic, material and spiritual development of man." (See Chart 3.2)

Buddha has said that of all the gains, the gains of health are the highest and the best. Health is not only basic to leading a happy life for an individual but it is also necessary for all productive activities in the society to make environment beautiful. Thus, no industry can expect the optimum output if it does not employ healthy workers or does not make and provide adequate facilities for proper maintenance of their health. Undoubtedly, good environment, professional efficiency, good health and productivity are inter-related. Yet, health cannot be bestowed upon people if they themselves do not make any effort to maintain a proper balance between their external and internal environments.

Whatever one may say, a disease-stricken society can hardly hope to extricate itself from the clutches of poverty and ignorance that keep it backward and underdeveloped in many areas of life. A nation can become truly healthy only when it succeeds in overcoming all these deficiencies stemming from cultural, social, economic and other causes in the environment. A nation that is ill-fed can hardly afford to exhibit efficiency in any field. In fact, an epidemic or endemic disease in any part of the world can pose a potential danger to all mankind and environment encompassing it and even a challenge to modern science. The Planning Commission has stressed the vital importance of public health in the enrichment of community life. It has been stated:

"Health is fundamental to the national progress in any sphere. In terms of resources for economic development, nothing can be considered of higher importance than the health of the people which is a measure of their energy and capacity as well as of the potential man-hours for productive work in relation to the total number of persons maintained by the nation. For the efficiency of industry and of agriculture, the health of the worker is an essential consideration."

In his address to 31st Session of WHO Regional Committee for South-East Asia held at Ulan Botor, Mongolia (22-28 Aug., 1978), Dr. Nyam-Osor, Minister of Public Health, Mongolia read a passage from a poem by Dashdorjiin Natragdorj, which glorifies "Health." It is being reproduced below.[3]

"Happiness, happiness, happiness
It may be of different origin on this earth

CHART 3.2

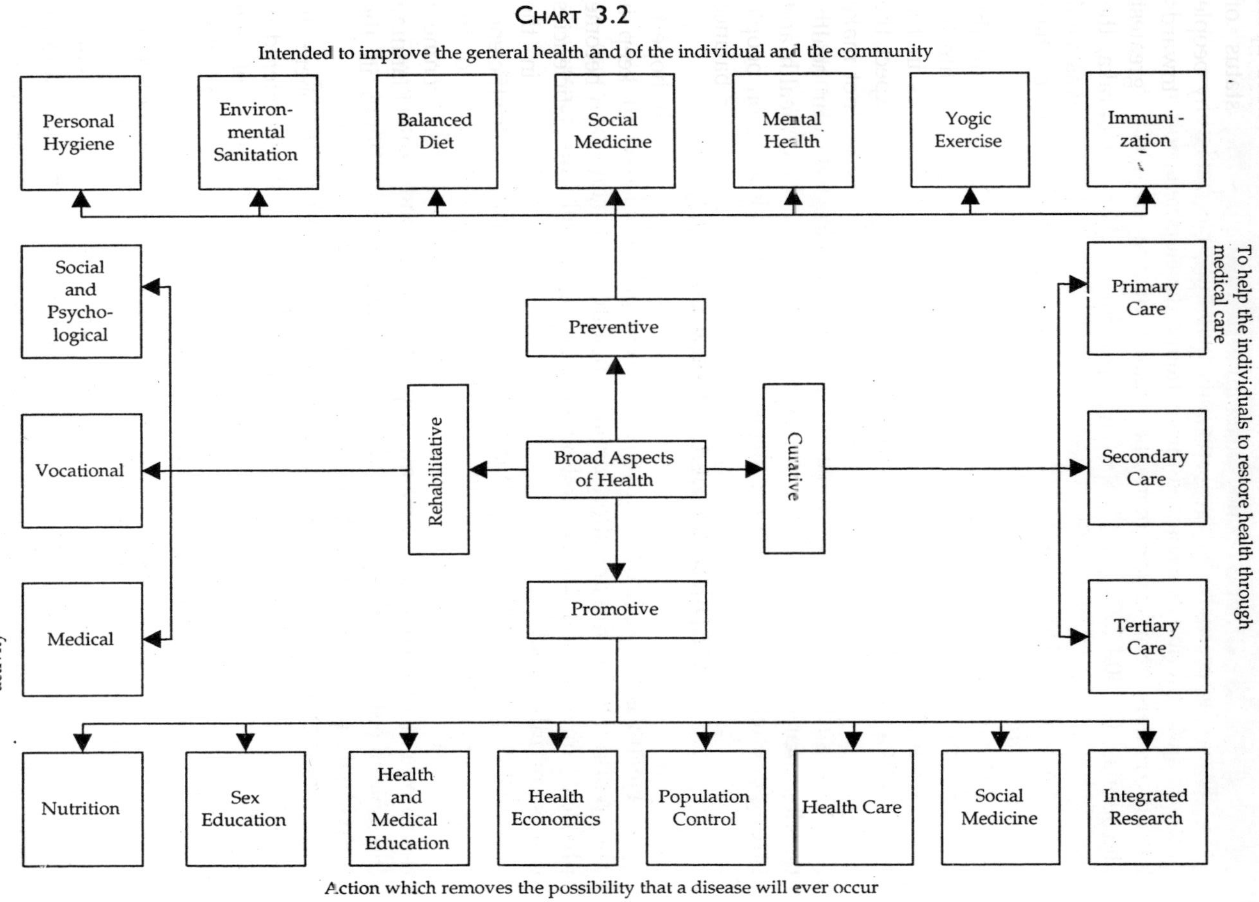
Intended to improve the general health and of the individual and the community
Personal Hygiene
Environ-mental Sanitation
Balanced Diet
Social Medicine
Mental Health
Yogic Exercise
Immuni-zation
Preventive
Broad Aspects of Health
Rehabilitative
Curative
Promotive
The combined and co- ordinated use of medical, social, educational measures for training and re-training the individual to the highest possible level of functional activity
Social and Psycho-logical
Vocational
Medical
To help the individuals to restore health through medical care
Primary Care
Secondary Care
Tertiary Care
Nutrition
Sex Education
Health and Medical Education
Health Economics
Population Control
Health Care
Social Medicine
Integrated Research
Action which removes the possibility that a disease will ever occur

But the happiness of being healthy
Is the real happiness."

Thus, there can be no two opinions that health is basic to national progress and in terms of resources for economic development nothing could be of greater significance than the health of the people. To quote Herophilas, C., 300 B.C.

"When health is absent
Wisdom cannot reveal itself
Art cannot manifest
Strength cannot fight,
Wealth becomes useless
And Intelligence cannot be applied."

As such, good health must be a primary objective of national development programmes. It is a precursor to improving the quality of life through better environment for a major portion of mankind.

MEANING OF HEALTH (See Chart 3.3)

Health is viewed differently by different people all over the world. The World Health Organisation defined health as "a state of complete physical, mental, and social well-being and not merely an absence of disease or infirmity.'

Thus, good health is a synthesis of physical, mental and social well-being of people and their adjustment with the environment.

"Health is a positive state of well-being in which harmonious development of mental and physical capacities of the individuals lead to the enjoyment of rich and full life . . . It implies adjustment of the individuals to his total environment—physical and social."

Some people even define it as a condition under which an individual is able to mobilise all his resources—intellectual, emotional, and environmental—for optimum living. Thus health is not static; on the contrary, it fluctuates on a scale which ranges between optimum health as defined by WHO to complete lack of health.

"We no longer ought to define health only in terms of sickness, but rather in relation to the harmonious development of every individual's personality and its impact on total environment. After all, it represents a balanced measure of a person's total potential—whether biological, psychological, environmental and social; and to the notion of individual health we should add the concepts of family and community health."

S.C. Seal, in his presidential address, defined health as:

"Flexible state of body and mind which may be described in terms of a range within which a person may sway from the condition wherein he is at the peak of enjoyment of physical, mental and emotional experiences,

CHART 3.3

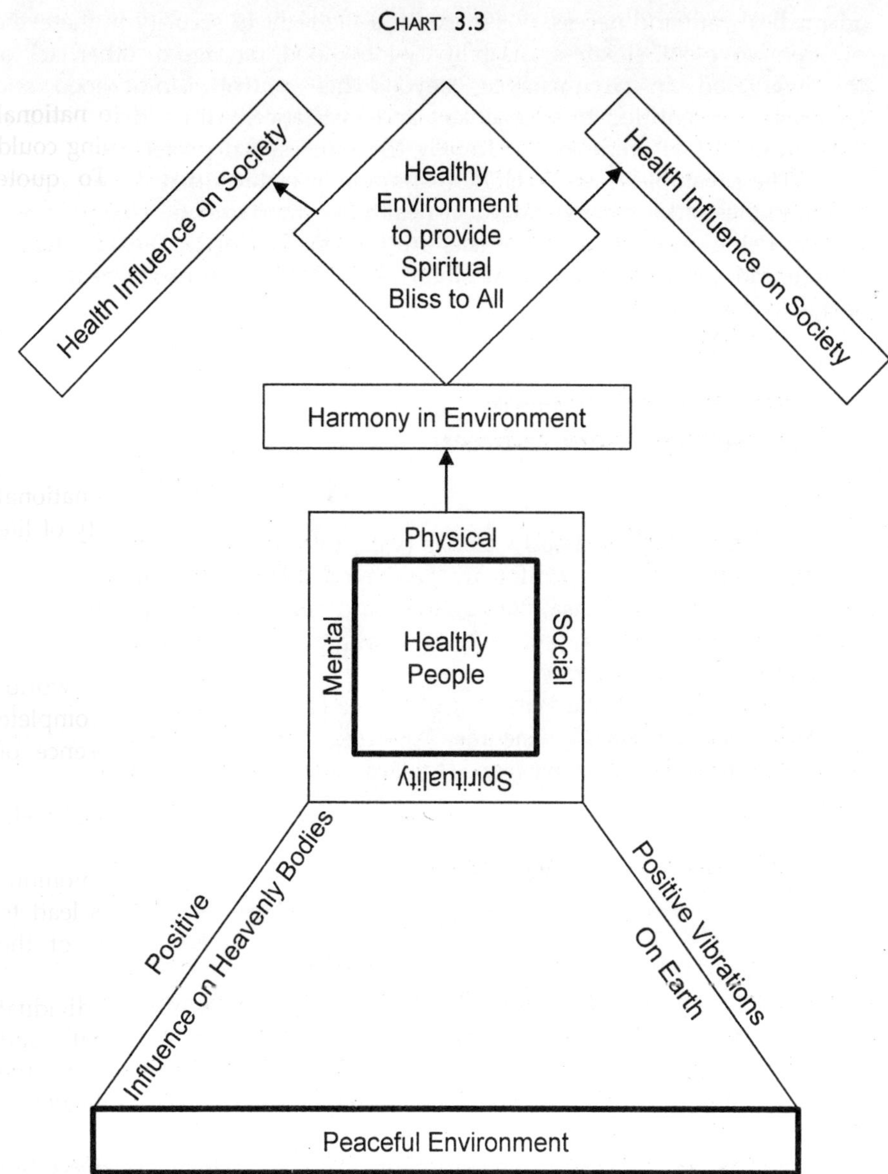

having regard to environment, age, sex and other biological characteristics due to the operation of internal or external stimuli and can regain that position without outside aid."[4]

"Health" has found an important place in the constitutions of all states and the UN agencies. Of the 30 Articles of the Universal Declaration of Human Rights, Art. 25 is particularly concerned with the right to health. Everyone has the right to a standard of living adequate for the health and well-being of himself and of his family, including food, clothing, housing ad medical care and necessary services and the right to security in the event of unemployment, sickness, disability, widowhood, old-age or other lack of the livelihood, in circumstances beyond his control. Motherhood and childhood are entitled to special care and assistance. All children whether born in or out of wedlock shall enjoy the same social protection.

The preamble to the WHO Constitution also states that the enjoyment of the highest attainable standard of health is a fundamental right of every human being and that governments are responsible for the health of their people and can fulfil that responsibility by taking appropriate health and social welfare measures.

According to Ayurveda:

समदोषः समाग्निश्य समधातुमलाक्रियः
प्रसन्नातमोन्द्रियमना स्वस्थ इल्यामिधीभते ।

—Ch. Su. Asthana: 15(41)

"A person whose bodily doshas (vata, pitta and kapha) are in a state of equilibrium with an uniformly healthy digestion, and in whom the functions of dhatus (Rasa, Rakta, etc.) and malas (waste products) are normal, accompanied by properly functioning senses, mind and body is said to be a healthy person."

Richard Hetzel, the President of Whole Health Institute, Australia, in his definition of health, includes positive, peaceful, caring attitudes expressed towards ourselves and towards the people and environment around us.

धर्मार्थ काममोक्षरनां आरोग्यम् लमत्तमम्

—Ch. Su. Asthana: 1(42)

Every body has three pursuits (esthana), i.e. pursuits of life (Pranaishana), pursuit of wealth (Dhanaishana) and pursuit of the after life (Parlokaishana). Out of all these pursuits, priority has been given to the desire for longevity and is the summum bonum for every body. It is so important and unavoidable that with the end of life, there is an end to everything in the world.

Ayurveda, through, encouraging simple habits protects the environment and also avoid exploitation of environment so that people in such an environment remain healthy.

Factors Influencing Health

A variety of factors influence human development both favourably and unfavourably. Some of these factors are; environmental—natural or man-made; physical, chemical, biological and social; economic, cultural factors; education, genetic factors; prenatal health development factors and nutritional factors. Thus the promotion of health cannot be achieved by measures that derive from any single health discipline, nor can health measures be considered independently of the broader educational, social, economic and administrative factors that are crucial to human development. Environment is the most important factor.

Obviously, he relationship between environment development and progress of health is of extreme importance. In fact, every aspect of economy has a health component which has an important bearing on the overall environmental development. Thus, as stated in a WHO paper on public health: "The health component and other components of the total system necessarily interact. Health not only affects the reminder of the socio-economic complex but is also affected by it, sometimes unfavourably."[5]

Because of this intimate relationship, it has been mentioned in the First Five-Year Plan, "If this subject is regarded in the proper light as one which is concerned with everything affecting the health of the community, it must be admitted to be the biggest and the most important problem of India."[6]

Socio-economic development consists of various components related to the productive shares of activities. Health programmes cannot be related unilaterally to either the economic or the social spheres as they influence both and are influenced by both in the context of environment.

There, obviously, is a need for a unified, integrated approach to public health, i.e., to combine services for nutrition improvement, communicable disease-control, better maternal and child-health and family welfare. Thus, conventional linear planning and the execution of separate programmes cannot meet the needs of human development. As stated by T. Adeoye Lambo in his article, "Total health" in *World Health,* "It is now apparent that a more balanced consideration of the biological, social and cultural aspects of health is needed. Life is a process and not a substance—a living system based upon the primacy of continuity and inter-relatedness throughout the universe. . . . If man and his family are to remain in empathy with the emerging necessities in the developing milieu, an adequate design of inter-disciplinary tools will have to be made to assist in this task of providing a total health package."[7]

In general, the factors influencing health could be classified into three broad categories: hereditary, environmental and personal. Similarly, the various conditions which play a vital role in determining one's health status can be put under three major areas, viz., mental health, spiritual health and physical health.

According to Advaita Saivism, every individual is a replica of Siva and Sakti Siva (pure consciousness) above the head of an individual. Here the term 'above' is used in a metaphorical sense to mean beyond empirical space and time. Sakti is present in an individual in the form of Kundalini (conscious pure energy). The kundalini is the source of creative upsurge in an individual. It is capable of transcending the barrier of myriadfold desires which permeates the body and the mind complex of an individual.[8]

The Upanisadic thinkers maintained that the health of an individual is sustained by prana (vital principle). Prana is the principle of life which enlivens the body of an individual. It steers an individual towards immortality.[9]

The Ayurveda, the age-old system of medicine is contained in great detail in ancient Sanskrit literature which believes that good health of the people make environment smooth.

Ayurveda the science of life, dealing with preventive, promotive, rehabilitative and curative, i.e. all aspects of mental and physical health of human being, considered in an upaveda of Atharvaveda or even fifth veda (ay. Equated with thumb and four vedas with four fingers of the palm), is divided in eight branches for its practical application; Kaumarabhrtya is one, having care of the child at its centre and physiopathologies of women from meno-ache to post-menopausal age around it, which was dealt by one specialist in its entirety. Technical advancements of twentieth century in health sector have made sky high longitudinal growth, squeezing horizontal field, Kaumarabhrtya was no exception, its dichotomy created two distinct specializations, i.e. obstetrics with gynoecology and neonatology with pediatrics. The neonate is snatched from the hands of obstetrician immediately after severing the cord, as that falls in the domain of neonatologist/pediatrician, who care the child generally upto twelve years of age, as after this age the drugs and doses become similar to the adult. Special attention to girl/women before marriage, fitness for marriage, care/advices before copulation for having progeny of better quality, and care of adolescent child was in wilderness, the mother was cared only after conception. Successive failures of various health scheme launched by the government for the care of women/mother and child, necessitated reconsideration of basic approach. The latest scheme is RCH (reproductive and child healthcare) launched with great fanfare, very much similar to Kaumarabhrtya.[10]

The concentration of Ayurveda is on holistic approach, i.e. complete equilibrium between individual and his environment.[11]

The scope of Ayurveda is not limited to physical health alone. It also seeks to promote a totality of physical, mental, and spiritual health in the context of man's interaction with his environment. Ayurveda is concerned with the origin of life and intelligence which are eternal. The wide scope of Ayurveda, in general, covers: (i) cosmological and ontological speculations about the intrinsic relationship between matter and life; (ii) biological theories concerning: (a) embryonic conception, (b) body, life, and soul, and (c) rules of genetics; (iii) physiological and pathological theories; (iv) food; (rules of health and longevity; (vi) diseases, their diagnosis and treatment; (vii) poisons and antidotes; and (viii) ethics.

Ayurveda makes a comprehensive holistic approach to the clinical examination of a patient and his diagnosis. The clinical Methodology in Ayurveda is two-fold designed to examine the "patient (Rogi)" and the "Disease (Roga)" separately. The examination of the "Patient" (Rogi Pariksa) comprises of a Ten-fold examination to ascertain the status of the genetic makeup of the individual and quantum of his 'remainder health'. The Ten-fold examination includes Prakrti, Vikrti, Sara, Samhanan, Sattva, Satmya, Pramana, Ahara Sakti, Vyayama Sakti and Vaya. The Examination of the disease (Roga Pariksa) aims to ascertain the nature of the disease and its aetiopathogenesis and Clinical manifestations. The Roga pariksa is ordinarily done through a general examination using Astavidha pariksa (Eight-fold examination) as well as a systematic examination through Sadanga Srotas Pariksa (Examination of different channels located over the Six parts of the body). The Astavidha pariksa includes: 1. Nadi (Pulse), 2. Mutra (Urine), 3. Mala (Stool), 4. Jihwa (Tongue) 5. Sabda (Speech), 6. Sparsa (Skin), 7. Drk (Eyes), and 8. Akriti (Facies). The examination of Pulse is an important component of the Clinical methodology in Ayurveda. The medieval texts on Ayurveda describe in detail the techniques of pulse reading and its diagnostic interpretations highlighting the characteristics of Vataja, Pittaja and Kaphaja Nadi as well as its diagnostic and prognostic implications. Ayurveda considers Health of Arogya as the state of Dhatu Samya, i.c. Biobalancc of cquilibrium of milicu intcrior whilc it considcrs the disease as the state of Vaisamya or imbalance. Accordingly the goal of treatment of a sick person is to restore the balance. Ayurveda conceives that the human body-mind has inherent natural power to fight with the cause of disease and to heal the loss as per the Doctrine of Swabhaoparam Vada with the help of Oja Bala and Vyadhiksamatva, i.e. Immunity.[12]

The vast ocean of Ancient Sanskrit learning deals with the well-being of mankind which is universally considered as the essence of positive health. So the present Medical Science defines the term health as follows— "Health is a state of complete physical, mental and social well-being and not merely absence of disease or infirmity. So far as healthcare is concerned modern medical Technology helps a lot to reduce physical pain through surgical operation, preventive and curative medicines and some other medical devices. But when the problem of mental and social disorder arises modern medical science becomes silent. It fails to extend all-round service in the field of healthcare. In fact, it becomes a challenge to medical science. So in order to solve such problem modern man comes to the door of Yoga Darshana and other branches of Sanskrit learning which can help in a scientific way to face this challenge and to promote social well-being and positive health of mind as well as body. In fact Yoga therapy, as a contribution of Sanskrit has been well accepted in the world as a complement to modern medical Technology.[13]

Ayurveda is a daily balance between individual and environment through daily chores of life.

Mira Roy in an Article, "Ayurveda" in *Cultural Heritage of India*, Vol. VI, 2001, states:

Physical and metaphysical speculations about matter and life form the philosophical basis of Ayurveda. It accepts that man, the subject of its treatment, is a part of the cosmic existence and represents the cosmos in miniature. In this respect, the Samkhya-Vedanta view of cosmogony and the allied Vaisesika view of inherent nature of substances have been incorporated in Ayurvedic treatises. All material bodies, according to Samkhya and Vedanta, are evolved from the interaction of Prakrti and Purusa, the dynamic (also material) and static (also conscious) principles of the universe respectively. Prakrti is the substratum of three elementary components (gunas) of creation: sattva (intelligence stuff), rajas (energy stuff), and tamas (matter stuff). The process of creation is said to be initiated in Prakrti by the transcendental Purusa through a disturbance in the equilibrium of the three gunas. The gunas thus form the inherent components, though in varying degrees, of every living object.

Every living being may be represented as karmapurusa (individuated soul) in union with mind, sense-organs, and material body. This material body is composed of gross elements in the form of kala (protective layer), dhatu (component matter), mala (eliminations), three dosas (humours), agni (digestive fire), and kriya. Each of the fundamental components and primary elements constitutes the living organism, imparting its specific nature and properties to the individual in the proportion in which it is present. The materials (dravya) which form food and drugs, being compounds of the five mahabhutas, are also mutations of Prakrti.

The literary treasurers of Sanskrit are not mere eulogies of Gods or philosophical explanations and codes of conduct. They possess answers to all our queries—be it vague or scientific. The twenty-first century world is a technological and space research-oriented world. The vast advances in the scientific sphere have emancipated man from his subjection to nature. Unfortunately due to various reasons, at present peace of mind and good health have become a rare feature of man to protect pollution of environment. At this juncture he seeks guidance to restore good health and through that mental peace. The growing popularity of Yoga and awareness in the concepts of Hindu medicinal treatments show that the entire world looks to India for enduring solutions to maintain good healthy environment. Ayurveda gives the solution. Ayurveda is not merely a method of medical treatment but a way of life. Simple methods of maintaining good health as shown in Ayurveda, like proper diet, proper maintenance of parts of the body such as teeth, eye, hair, etc. as well as to be in harmony with environment.[14]

If we look into this with deep insight, the major factors responsible for all these are disturbances in environment and its degradation, untoward interference with natural laws of Nature, non-practice of daily and seasonal regimen, not following sadavritta, unawareness of preventive, promotive, prophylactic home care, changed style of life, uncontrolled food habits and suppression of morality. If the world community do not change its style of life and ignore the rules laid down in Ayurveda—thousand years ago, the situation of healthcare will be threatened and worsen in the new millennium, resulting into polluted environment.[15]

Ayurveda is time tested treasury house of knowledge and is not just a medical science. Charaka said:

विषम स्वस्थवशतानां ऐते रोगस्तथोपरे ।
जयन्ते अनातुरस्तस्मात् स्वस्थवशतपरो भवेत् ।।

—Ch. Su. Ashtana: 7 (44)

Ayurveda has laid down some specific measures/methods of Swastha-vritta to provide a preventive, promotive, curative and rehabilitative healthcare as well as pure environment. These are the only answers to all the diseases in the 21st century.

(A) PREVENTIVE MEASURES

Ayurveda's prime objective is:

स्वस्थस्य स्वास्थ्य रक्षणं ।
आतुरस्य विकार प्रशमनं च ।।

—Ch. Su. Asthana: 29 (24)

which means, the preservation of health and cure of diseases.[16]

The Ayurveda physicians of ancient India had a well-defined medical ethics. According to Ayurveda system of medicine, longivity is necessary for an individual so that he may realize the supreme ideals of righteousness, love, affluence and liberation from ignorance and suffering. He must be, therefore, free from disease so that he may realize his supreme ideals in his life. He must be healthy and happy in order to fulfil his mission in his life.

Charaka maintains that well-educated and well-trained physicians cure patients from diseases.[17]

According to Charaka, excellence in knowledge, extensive practical experience, dexterity and purity of the mind are the four essential characteristics of an Ayurvedic physicians. A physician's purity of mind helps a patient in combating against the latter's disease.

All of us in life experience moments of disharmony. We find we are often at cross-purposes with life, with events, with daily happening, with others. Out of all this disorder and disharmony, if we can build lives of harmony and orderliness, we will succeed if not at all times at least in the most crucial moments in stilling the chattering of our minds. (See Chart 3.4).

For harmony in Environment and Health of the people we suggest the following technique:

1. Yoga Therapy

Swami Satyananda Sanswati in his book, "Asana Pranayama Mudra Bandha, (Bihar School of Yoga, Munger, Bihar, India, 1999) suggests the Yoga as has been put in our ancient Sanskrit Literature.

"Yoga is not an ancient myth buried in oblivion. It is the most valuable inheritance of the present. It is the essential need of today and the culture of tomorrow."

CHART 3.4

Healthy People
Absence of Diseases and Positive Attitudes leading to Socio-economic Development
Avoid Exploitation of Environment
Emit Good Vibrations and Pure Air good for Life Support System
Purifies and Strengthens Good Environment
Life of Harmony and Environmental Peace—Physical, Mental and Spiritual
Stimulating and Enjoyable Environment
Positive Attitude to Work

For most people, however, yoga is simply a means of maintaining health and well-being in an increasingly stressful society. Asanas remove the physical discomfort accumulated during a day at the office sitting in a chair, hunched over a desk. Relaxation techniques help maximize the effectiveness of ever-diminishing time off. In an age of mobile phones, beepers and twenty-four hour shopping, yogic practices make great personal and even business sense.

Yoga is a part of Ayurveda. The word yoga is derived from the Sanskrit root 'yuj' meaning 'to unite', 'to combine', and 'to integrate', which means total integration of the physical, mental, intellectual and spiritual aspects of the human personality.[22] Yoga is a way of life, propounded by Patanjali in a systematic form. It consists of 8 steps, namely, restraint, observance of austerity, physical postures, breathing exercise, restraining sense organs, contemplation, meditation and samadhi.

यम - नियामासन - प्राणायाम - प्रत्याहार; धारणा - ध्यान - समाधयोडष्टावङ्गानि

—Pantajali-Yogasutra 2.2.9

They are controlled by means of practice and non-attachment. Patanjli. Yogasutras.[12]

Practice is the repeated effort to follow the disciplines which give permanent control of the thought-waves of the mind. *Ibid.*[13]

Practice becomes firmly grounded when it has been cultivated for a long time, uninterruptedly, with earnest devotion. *Ibid.*[14]

The practice of yoga prevents psychosomatic disorders/diseases and improve individual's resistance and ability to endure stressful situations. As a primary prevention, yogic exercises should be advised to drive the benefits of prevention of diseases, promotion of health and for therapeutic purposes.

Swami Harshananda in his Article, "attainment of yoga" mentions that knowingly or unknowingly, all of us are struggling to get peace. As long as our mind is in pieces and the pieces are in ceaseless mutual conflict, peace eludes us. It is only when we learn to put these pieces together so as to make the mind whole and integrated that we gain the peace of Kaivalya.

This is easier said than done. However, with competent guides like Patanjali who are ever eager to help out of infinite compassion, this task should not be that difficult.

Patanjali, the great master of the Yoga system, calls these pieces of the mind as vrttis, modifications, which are ever arising and never subsiding. Yoga or union (uyj = to yoke) of the individual self with the Supreme Self will result through Yoga or Samadhi, (yuj = to get samadhi or perfect concentration) when these Vrttis are controlled, suppressed and eliminated, by the right kind of discipline and training. This discipline and training is also Yoga.[18]

Dr. S.C. Manchanda, Professor and Head; Department of Cardiology, All India Institute of Medical Sciences, New Delhi has depicted the role of Yoga lifestyle in Coronary Artery diseases in his "Research Study of Reversal of Coronary Heart Disease through Preksha Meditation with Reference to: Coronary Atherosclerotic Reversal Potential of Yoga Lifestyle Intervention." According to the study, forty-two male patients (mean age 51.0 + 9.5 range 32-72 years) with angiographically proven CAD were included. Patients in the control group (n=21) were managed on conventional medical therapy (with control of risk factors, AHA step 1 diet, moderate aerobic exertion), while those in the yoga group (n=21) were advised strict lifestyle modifications and yogic exercises as detailed below. The yogic lifestyle intervention programme consisted of:

(a) Yogic lifestyle methods:
   - (i) Health rejuvenating exercises: a set of movements for improving the general tone of the body and to improve coordination.
   - (ii) Relaxation exercise (Kayotsarg): a method of complete relaxation to prepare the body and mind for mediation.
   - (iii) Breathing exercises (Pranayama).
   - (iv) Yogic postures for stretch relaxation (Asanas).

(v) Preksha meditation (preksha means seeing deeply within).
(vi) Reflection on moral values (Anuvrat and Anupreksha.)

(b) Stress Management (relaxation, breathing exercises and Preksha meditation).

(c) Dietary control.

(d) Moderate aerobic exercises.

The change in the lesion severity was classified into regression (10% absolute reduction in diameter stenosis), no significant change (<10% change in diameter stenosis) or progression (>10% absolute increase in diameter stenosis). In the Yoga group, 3 (5%) lesion showed progression, 46 (75%) lesion showed no change while 12 (20%) lesion showed regression. In the control group 22 (37%) lesions showed progression, 36 (61%) showed no change while 1 (2%) showed regression.

Yoga lifestyle intervention is beneficial in improving the symptoms and exercise capacity, lowering weight and serum lipid levels. It also retards the progression of coronary atherosclerosis in patients with severe coronary artery diseases and reduces revasularisation procedures.

Yoga is a system of physical, mental and spiritual training. It originated in India thousands of years ago. It is not a cult nor a creed. But it is a method of self-realisation which starts with the purification of the body and ends with the unfoldment of the spirit.

In ancient India the early Yogis were a group of mystics and scientists to whom the relationship between the mortal man and an immortal spirit was of great interest. They set about to find ways and means of uniting these two during the earthly life of man. They spent not decades but centuries in making their experiments with different methods of concentration, meditation and relaxation; with various breathing processes, postures and foods. When they finally succeeded in their experiments, they systematized the result of their findings and called it the science of Yoga. The aim of Yoga is to achieve reintegration of the individual consciousness with the cosmic consciousness.[19]

Yoga pays particular care and attention to the purification of the body. It is often asked, why Yoga bestows so much attention on the body, when its aim is a spiritual union with the Divine. Yoga regards the body as a vehicle through which the spirit manifests itself. Just as a violinist takes care of his violin without which he would not be able to express his art, so the Yogi takes care of his body as the only instrument through which he can express the spiritual powers.

In our daily life tensions accumulate, increasing our mental burden. This makes us prone to depression, anger toward others, aggressive behaviour, guilt consciousness and self-pity. Our personality contracts under these inner pressures and as a result we are miserable and insecure. Loneliness and lack of support often plague us. We feel we are drifting, lost at sea.

We have to steer our ship though all these tempestuous waters of life in order to reach the safety and security of the shore. Gradually it becomes evident that our search is for something infinite, permanent, but nevertheless inextricably interwoven with our every day life. It is essential to learn to utilize every experience, pleasant or unpleasant, big or small to mould our character and expand our consciousness. Every one of these situations should draw us closer to the goal, which according to Vedantic thought is coming face to face with one's own Divine nature, or "to discover the eternal relationship between the eternal Soul and the eternal God. Becoming perfect or going toward God simply means realizing what is already within ourselves. This journey is termed variously as going back home, meeting a long-lost beloved friend, or attaining our own empire. It should be a lively, natural and joyful undertaking."

With resolute hearts we adopt some time-tested techniques in our daily life, and though assiduous practice we ultimately realize the Truth. This realization transforms our life, changes our perspective, and reveals the profound significance of everything we experience. We will then see one indivisible light shining inside and outside ourselves. We become the embodiment of love, peace, fearlessness and strength. How to accomplish this journey smoothly with conservation of time and energy, and with the maximum benefit to oneself and others is the theme of Yoga?

Thus the aim of Yoga is to completely alter one's personality and outlook so that he is able to face all problems of life with equanimity, while pursuing to achieve the ideals which he cherishes. It is a complete break with normal waking consciousness. It is neither a condition of vain pursuits and frustrations of waking life, nor a condition of mere dreaming, nor even condition of absence of quality as in deep sleep, but a condition of calmness and tranquility of mind in daily pursuits. As the Gita describes with an analogy, he is one in to whom all desires enter as waters into these and is ever motionless though constantly being filled (II.70). He enjoys and suffers like all human beings; he has passions, fears and rages like all human beings; but unlike the ordinary human beings, he is able to maintain tranquility through them all.[20]

2. Mantras

Mantra is a mystic syllable with esoteric meaning. It is extremely efficatious when it is pronounced properly with clear awareness of its esoteric meaning. It produces certain vibrations which alter the organic and mental states of an individual. It is also capable of altering the organic and mental states of other person. It is even capable of producing changes in the environment. Patanjali in Yogasutra 1.29 speaks that mantras leads to the awareness of the indwelling spirit.[21]

Swami Vishnu Devananda states that Mantras are Sanskrit-invocations of the Supereme Being. Reinforced and propelled by japa, meditation, they pass from the verbal level though the mental and telepathic states, and on to pure thought energy. Of all languages Sanskrit most closely approaches telepathic language because of its affinity to the fifty primeval sounds. It is the most direct way to approach the transcendental state.[22]

Swami Rama in his book, living with Himalayan masters states that Mantra is a syllable, a sound, a word, or set of words found in the deep state of meditation by the great sages. It is not the language in which human beings speak. Those sounds which are received from the super conscious state lead the seeker higher and higher until he reaches the perfect silence. The more awareness is increased, the more mantra reveals new meaning. It makes one aware of a higher dimensions of consciousness. Exploiting the noble tradition by selling mantras in the marketplace is absurd.[23]

OM is the primordial spanda (vibration). All mantras have emerged out of it. OM is of the nature of pure light. All other mantras are also of the nature of light waves. A Yogi who frequently pronounces mantras and is conscious of their esoteric meanings comes to possess a radient and luminous body full of glowing health.[24]

Mahesh Chandra Pal observes that Gayatri Mantra may be called 'supreme medicine' (manausadhi) because it heals all diseases. In his view, any sick person may be cured of his disease by just regularly reciting Gayatri mantra. The ancient Vedic seers never fell ill because they used to regularly recite Gayatri mantra by becoming fully aware of its esoteric meaning. There are several other mantras which have healing power. These mantras spread vibrations in the environment which make it fit as these vibrations enter other individuals.

OM is the first syllable of the Gayatri mantra which the ancient Vedic seers used to recite. It symbolizes the first rhythm through the medium of which the universe was created. The next few syllables which follow the syllable OM are Bhurbhuva svah. Here the syllable 'svah' means 'heaven'. This heaven has two regions, viz., the lower and the upper, the lower region of the heaven is known as 'Indraloka' where deities reside and enjoy happiness. The heaven of the upper region is permeated by truth. Wise persons prefer to enter into the upper region of heaven which is permeated by truth.

Pure consciousness (Siva) is the source of Gayatri mantra. Gayatri mantra symbolizes the sun. Anybody who habitually recites the Gayatri mantra gets purified in his body and mind because the radient energy of this mantra burns all the blemishes in his personality.

Swami Sivananda in his "Practice of Yoga" rightly suggests:

OM and the Gayatri-Mantra have acquired such great importance that they are often referred to as the Pranaya and the Gayatri just as the Bhagavad Gita is referred to as the Gita. In the Vedas, Upanisads, the Gita, and the later literature, there are numerous references to the holiness, importance, and significance of the Pranaya and the Gayatri. The whole of the Mandukya Upanisad is devoted to the delineation of the spirituo-philosophical significance of OM. Though the Upanisad contains only twelve verses, it is considered so important that numerous commentaries are written on it. Sri Gaudapada-acarya, the grand Guru of Sri Sankaracarya, has written an extremely subtle and revolutionary philosophical work called the Mandukya-karika to elucidate the high philosophy of this Upanisad which establishes the supremacy and ultimacy of the Non-dual Reality (Advaita) Sri Sankaracharya has commented on both the Upanisad and the Karika.[25]

The efficiency of the Japa is accentuated according to the degree of concentration. The mind should be fixed on the Source. Then only you will realize the maximum benefits of a Mantra. Every Mantra has got tremendous force. A Mantra is a mass of Tejas or radiant energy. It transforms the mental substance by producing a particular thought movement. The rhythmical vibrations produced by repeating the Mantra, regulate the unsteady vibrations of the five sheaths. It checks the natural tendencies of objective thoughts of the mind. It helps the spiritual power and reinforces it.[26]

3. Role of Pranayama

The term pranayama is derived from the Sanskrit term 'prana' which means the 'vital principle.' The vital principle permeates the brain and the nervous system of an individual. It is the source of volition, enthusiasm, spontaneity and happiness in an individual. He spreads the same in the environment which also becomes pure.

Pranayama is the method of rhythmic regulation of breath. It produces stability in the body, and equanimity in the mind of an individual. The subtle physiology of an individual gets purified through regular practice of pranayama. The body of an individual becomes free from leanness, obesity, crookedness, etc. through regular practise of pranayama. It becomes exceedingly beautiful and fragrant through regular practise of pranayama. It becomes very light. It can even violate the law of gravitation. Swami Vishnu Devananda states:

Pracchardana-vidharanabhayam va pranasya

It is also achieved by the expulsion and retention of the breath.

This is a reference to the practice of pranayama as a method of purification. Regulation of the breath gives control over the thought waves, for control of breath is directly related to control of mind. There are many pranayama exercises, each of which has a special effect on the autonomic nervous system and the psyche.[27]

We do not pay any serious attention to breathing, the most important of all our bodily functions. It has never occurred to many of us that a great deal of our physical and mental troubles are due to the fact that we do not breathe correctly. Life and breath are synonymous. We live as long as we breathe. We start our life with the first breath and end it with the last breath. We never stop breathing whether we are awake or asleep. We can exist without food for weeks and without water for a few days but without air we cannot exist even for a few minutes. Air is the most important nourishment for our blood. All the activities of body from digestion to creative thinking depend upon the oxygen supply through breathing; yet we treat breathing with utter indifference. If there is a deficiency in the supply of oxygen, the process of ionization will be incomplete and the food is partially assimilated. Nearly 50 percent of delinquency in minors is due to oxygen starvation which is the result of shallow breathing and lack of fresh air.

The habit of shallow breathing is one of many unnatural habits that modern civilization has forced upon us. It has been proved that in the civilized world only babies can breathe in a natural way. In order to enjoy good breaths in a day. Shallow breathing is directly or indirectly responsible for a number of physical and mental diseases ranging from nervous disorders to common colds. To function properly the brain requires three times more oxygen than the rest of the body. If it does not get its due allotment, it exacts it from the body supply. That is why brain workers often possess a poor physic and a bad health. Deep breathing not only nourishes the whole system but also cleanses it. Kiran Bedi in her Article in *The Tribune* (Sept. 7, 2000). "The Miracles of Dhamma", i.e. Vipasana advocated by Lord Buddha has been deeply impressed by the impact of Vipasana (a type of Pranayama) on Police Officers.[28]

After taking the feedback of our silver jubilee Vipassana course on police officers the teacher Sri Bhanwar Singh Sahwal who conducted the course shared his experiences about Vipasana.

Narration of this personal account of the teacher was an eye-opener for 55 police officers sitting in the meditation hall. It was experienced that we do not have to wait for depressions and fears to overpower us. Solutions are amongst us here and now. We only have to seek them, learn them and practice them.

Dhamma is one of our richest heritages. It is for us to convert it from a distant archaeological monument into a holistic dwelling.

Prana is not mere breath but it is cosmic energy. It is a life giving principle which pervades the whole atmosphere. It is manifested in every form of existence—organic and inorganic. By breathing exercises it is possible to raise the degree of circulation of Prana in the body. The surplus of Prana is stored in the solar plexus which is the battery of human body.

4. Nutrition and Health

Swami Vishnu Devananda in his book Meditation and Mantras has rightly said that, What is consumed by the human body correlates directly to the efficiency with which the brain functions. Recent studies show that certain red food colouring creates hyperactivity in children, and that refined sugar can cause emotional instability. These are just two examples of substances that are often heedlessly consumed without understanding their effect on the body and mind.

Several years ago vegetarianism was, in a sense, an underground practice. A person who refrained from eating meat was viewed with a certain amount of curiosity, if not suspicion. Today it is quite a different story. Health food stores and vegetarian restaurants are prevalent. There is a growing awareness that our health is directly affected by what we eat. Many diseases can be cured by a change in diet or a short period of fasting, with no medications at all. This is true not only of physical disorders, but of many mental difficulties as well. It is particularly important that pregnant mothers have this awareness; too often they do not realize the effect of their diet on the developing fetus.

There is no doubt that, "You are what you eat", a subtle part of what is consumed becomes the consciousness. Those who have changed from a meat to vegetarian diet notice a corresponding change in consciousness. There is a certain grossness that disappears, and the awareness becomes finely tuned.[29]

In the Bhagavad Gita three types of food have been mentioned which produce three different types of dispositions in individuals.

A person becomes healthy, moral, religious, intelligent and creative by regularly taking, satvika food.

Satvika spreads satvika and the Cumulative effect is purity of environment:

आयु: सत्त्वबलारोग्यसुखप्रीतिविवर्धना: ।
रस्या: स्निग्धा: स्थिरा हृद्या आहारा: सात्त्विकप्रिया: ।। (XVII/8)

Foods which promote longevity, intelligence, vigour, health, happiness and cheerfulness, and which are sweet, bland, substantial and naturally agreeable, are dear to the Sattvika type of men."[30]

कट्वम्ललवणात्युष्णतीक्ष्णरुक्षविदाहिन: ।
आहारा राजसस्येष्टा दु:खशोकामयप्रदा: ।। (XVII/9)[31]

Foods which are bitter, acid, salty, overhot, pungent, dry and burning, and which cause suffering, grief and sickness, are dear to the Rajasika type of men.

यातयामं गतरसं पूति पर्युषितं च यत्
उच्छिष्टमपि चामेध्यं भोजनं तामसप्रियम् ।। (XVII/10)[32]

Food which is half-cooked or half-ripe, insipid, putrid, stale and polluted, and which is impure too, is dear to men of a Tamasika disposition.

5. Power of Music

The atmosphere has two aspects; physical and spiritual. The physical ecosystem depends on the spiritual ecosystem. If the spiritual ecosystem of a place gets spoilt then the physical ecosystem cannot improve either. If the people here become too headstrong then nothing will work. However, when there is chanting of the Lord's name by hundreds of thousands of people every day, then there will be peace in all four directions.

Pravrajika Varadaprana in his Article, "The power of music" states quoted in values, "the key to a meaningful life" states that: When one is feeling low or depressed, listening to music can help change the mood when nothing else helps. We can consider the effect of music on the mind from the standpoint of the gunas, the three qualities that affect the moods of our minds. When we are feeling dull and lethargic (tamasic), music of a lively, vibrant nature (rajasic) can pull us out of that mood. When we are feeling restless and agitated (rajasic) we can be calmed down by music that is serene and peaceful (satvic).

Music can draw the mind out of the world of maya, or it can concentrate the mind and elevate it to a higher level of consciousness. The test of good music for the spiritual aspirant is whether or not it is compatible with the thought of god.[33]

Those who can follow the words of the song can sing in the chorus and those who cannot follow the words can lose themselves in the bhava, the mood of devout surrender, which it expresses. The words of the song are:

Lord, let me see your face in every face I see,
Lord, let me feel your grace, feel your grace in me,
Lord, let me find the place where you want me to be,
And Lord, let me find the space that brings me
Nearer to Thee.

This song means that wherever I look, You and only You are there. Wherever I turn my eyes, I find You and You alone. Every flower has Your fragrance. It is not necessary to tell a bee to go to jaggery; wherever there is jaggery a bee will be attracted to it. Wherever a bhajan is sung, the mind will be attracted to it. Wherever a bhajan is sung, the mind will be attracted and engrossed by it. Even a cow becomes engrossed in a bhajan.

6. Non-Violence

Violence has become a greatest pollutant of this life. People do violences in the name of religion, fundamentalism and personal gains creating permanent scars on this globe. Gujarat violence is a recent example. Such incidences spoil the environment and disturb its peace causing enmity, hatred and jealousy among people causing a great danger to environment. Swami Rama has laid down some principles, based on Gandhiji ideology which if followed can bring communal harmony, national integration and international brotherhood. All these principles are based upon the philosophy of Shrimad Bhagavad Gita, Vedas, etc. To quote:

1. Non-violence and cowardice cannot go together, because non-violence is a perfect expression of love that casts our fear. To be

brave because one is armed implies an element of fear. The power of ahimsa is an extremely vital and active force which does not come from physical strength.

2. A true follower of ahimsa does not believe in disappointment. He dwells above in perennial happiness and peace. That peace and joy do not come to him who is proud of his intellect or learning; they come to him who is full of faith and has an undivided and single-pointed mind.
3. The intellect can produce many wonders, but non-violence is a matter of the heart. It does not come through intellectual exercises.
4. Hatred is not overcome by hatred, but rather by love. This is an unalterable law.
5. Devotion is not mere worship with the lips. It is self-surrender with mind, action, and speech.
6. Gandhi did not believe in the barriers created by religions, cultures, superstitions, and mistrust. He taught and lived the brotherhood of all religions.
7. Gandhi believed in the art of living without concern for the fruits of ones actions. He practiced not worrying about success or failure, but paid attention to the work at hand without feeling the slightest anxiety or fatigue.
8. In order to enjoy life one should not be selfishly attached to anything. Non-attachment means to have a pure motive and a correct means without any worry or desired result. He who gives up action falls, but he who gives up the reward rises and is liberated.
9. Yoga is the complete re-integration of all the states of mind, the intellect, senses, emotions, instincts, and every level of personality. It is a process of becoming whole.
10. One's mantra becomes one's staff of life and carries one through every ordeal. Each repetition has a new meaning and carries one nearer and nearer to God. It is capable of transforming that which is negative in the personality into that which is positive, and it can gradually integrate divided and opposing thoughts at deeper and deeper levels of consciousness (Based on Gandhiji Ideals).[34]

If you practice non-violence out of cowardice, it is no merit at all. Real non violence means the greatest strength and power of endurance that a man can attain to. It means the greatest courage coupled with the greatest love. It means total absence of hatred. That is what Sri Krsna tried to teach Arjuna in the Gita. He exhorted him to do his duty, which in his case happened to be fighting, without hating others.[35]

The ahimsa is a high ideal. We must proceed step by step towards that ideal. The mind must be cleansed of all unclean, we get some real spiritual experience. Ahimsa as a theory and ahimsa as practised in one's own life are wide apart. In the Isavasya Upanisad you read, 'When a person sees the Self in all people and all people in the Self, then he hates no one. This is a recurring idea in the Upanisads—that self-realization is the basis of true ahimsa. When one realizes the Self, one hates none.

7. Company of Good People

Swami Ashokananda says, "Another remedy for a restless mind is the companionship of those who have already reached a high state. In their company you will find that your mind will gradually be withdrawn from the gross things of the world. Seek out such holy people. I will admit they are not easily obtainable, but that which you are seeking is not a small things, the company of the spiritually enlightened will make of a mortal man an immortal god. Search for such people. In the company of god there is a possibility that you will come across them if you are earnest. Keep company with them, and you will find your mind has withdrawn from the sense world and a deep and calm state has come."

8. Meditation

Meditation is the process where the mind of a person is attracted towards God without interruption and is always keen to sit in prayer from the core of heart. Prayer and Japa always help in supplementing and complementing meditation.

It is important to know the difference between ordinary concentration and meditation. By the word 'meditation' we mean dhyana or contemplation. It is not just ordinary concentration. It is a special type of concentration. In the first place, meditation is a fully conscious process, an exercise of the will. Secondly, meditation means concentration on a spiritual ideal which presupposes that the aspirant is capable of rising above worldly ideas. And finally, meditation is done usually at a particular centre of consciousness. It is clear that true meditation is a fairly advanced state, attained after long practice. It is the result of long years of discipline.[36]

Meditation is the practice by which there is constant observation of the mind. It involves setting aside a regular time and place for the specific purpose of discovering that infinite well of wisdom which lies within.[37]

Without the help of meditation, you cannot attain knowledge of the self. Without its aid, you cannot grow into the divine state. Without it, you cannot liberate yourself from the trammels of the mind and attain immortality.

Meditation is the only royal road to the attainment of freedom. It is a mysterious ladder which reaches from earth to heaven, from error to truth, from darkness to light, from pain to bliss, from restlessness to abiding peace, from ignorance to knowledge. From mortality to immortality.[38] To quote Swami Vishnu Nanda,

> Dukha-daurmanasyangamejayatva-svasa-prasvasa
> viksepa-sahabhuvah

Mental pain, depression, physical nervousness, and irregular breathing are the symptoms of a distracted state of mind.

These are outward manifestations of an internal state of being. They are the result of the above-mentioned obstacles to meditation. They are also a way of life for many thousands who never undertake spiritual disciplines such as meditation and Yoga. But they can be thoroughly remedied by repetition of OM, surrender to the Lord, and regularity in practice. Even during periods when ones original enthusiasm wanes, continuing in the daily schedule of spiritual practice strengthens the will and builds positive spiritual habits, or samskaras. In due time, each test is passed and meditation is approached with renewed vigour.[39]

Tat-pratisedhartham eka-tattvabhayasah

In order to remove these obstacles, one should meditate on one aspect of Truth.[40]

Practise japa and meditation regularly. Do not miss even one day. The mind is like a spoiled child—always restless. Try repeatedly to steady it, by fixing it on the Chosen Ideal and at practice for two or three years, you will begin to feel an unspeakable joy and the mind will become steady. In the beginning the practice of japa and meditation seems dry. It is like taking bitter medicine. You must forcibly pour the thought of God into your mind, then as you persist, you will be flooded with joy. What a terrible ordeal a student undergoes to pass his examination. To realize God is a far easier task. Call on Him sincerely with a tranquil heart.[41]

Once we have overcome tension we reach a dimension of inner bliss as is expressed in the immortal verse of the poet Rabindranath Tagore:

Remain in bliss in this world/Fearless, pure in heart
wake up in bliss every morning,
Carry out all your duties in bliss
Remain in bliss in weal and woe
In criticism and insult,
Remain in bliss unaffected,
Remain in bliss pardoning everybody.[42]

Swami Sivananda in his article, "Religious Education and Practice of Yoga" mentions the causes of stresses and strains and suggest meditation as has been laid down in all our ancient Sanskrit scriptures.

"Watch your mind very carefully. Be vigilant. Be on the alert. Do not allow the waves of irritability, jealousy, hatred and lust to disturb you. These dark waves are enemies of peaceful living, meditation and wisdom. To some it is very difficult to keep the mind unruffled and pure, the causes being deep-rooted worldly Samskaras, unfavourable surroundings, and the predominance of extrovert tendencies. To some, of course, evil thoughts are not a problem at all. They appear occasionally as a passing phase without doing much havoc. The very fact that evil thoughts give you mental suffering is a sign of spiritual progress; for many do not have that much of sensitiveness."

Put a piece of iron-rod in the blazing furnace. It becomes red as fire. Remove it. It loses its red colour. If you want to keep it always red, you must always keep it in the fire. So also, if you want to keep the mind charged with the fire of Brahmic wisdom, you must keep it always in contact with the Brahmic fire of knowledge through constant and intense meditation. You must keep an unceasing flow of the Brahmic consciousness. If you can meditate for half an hour, you will be able to engage yourself with peace and spiritual strength. Such is the beneficial result of meditation. As you have to move with different minds of peculiar nature in your daily life, get the strength and peace from meditation. Then you will have no trouble or worry.[43]

The same fate may overtake India if it neglects its spirituality. Through perfect moral life and intense spiritual practice the great spiritual reserves of the nation must be constantly replenished. The heritage of countless rsis, sages and saints should not be frittered away. Everyman must contribute something to the common spiritual atmosphere. This is the duty of all thoughtful Indians.[44]

In nutshell Meditation is the process where the mind of a person attracted towards God without interruption and is always keen to set in prayer from the core of heart. Prayer and Japa always help in supplementing and complementing meditation

8. Naturopathy

Naturopathy is not only a system of treatment but also a way of life. It is often referred to as a drugless treatment of diseases. It is based mainly on the ancient practice of the application of the simple laws of nature. The system is closely allied to Ayurveda. There are two schools of thought regarding the approach to naturopathy. One group believes in the ancient Indian methods while the other mainly adopts western methods which are more akin to modern physiotherapy.

The advocates of Naturopathy pay particular attention to eating and living habits, adoption of pacificator measures, use of hydrotherapy, cold packs, mud packs, baths, massage and a variety of method/measures based on various innovations.

A carefully supervised fast or partial fast is advocated to clear the system of its toxic build up. Water and/or diluted fruit juices are permitted during the period of fast. A strict supervision during the period is kept lest the patient develop untoward physical and emotional effects. The system believes that the way of life, if properly organised and if one does not retaliate, one can get the bounties of energy, health and happiness from the benevolent nature. For prevention of diseases, promotion of health and to get therapeutic advantages, it is required to adopt natural means.

Swami Abhedananda in his book, Science of Psychic Phenomena rightly states:

Mind has the power to cure disease, and in fact, the healing power can be strengthened and increased by correct breathing and right-thinking. Ordinarily, people do not breathe properly and pay no attention to their mental conditions, but encourage hatred, jealousy, malice, greed, lust, fear and other destructive forces; and they do not realize that all these produce abnormal activities of the subtle body first, and then of the organic functions, and consequently, they suffer. Therefore, instead of encouraging those causes of abnormal conditions of mind and body, we should encourage good thoughts, and develop friendliness, purity and chastity.

All the abnormal mental states like anger, hatred, jealousy, malice, fear, passion, greed, vanity, pride, self-conceit and egotism are the diseases of the mind. Therefore, these should never be cultivated. They poison the system and create wrong vibration in the atmosphere of the place, and influence other minds. A great disturbance in a family or in a community is caused by such destructive thought currents. Therefore, cultivate the opposite constructive thoughts, which will bring health, prosperity and happiness.[45]

G.C. Pande in his paper, "Neurosciences and Philosophy—Some Problems in the Light of Indian and Buddhist Philosophy" presented at the National Seminar Science, Society values and consciousness, held on 27th and 28th May, 2002 at Panjab University, Chandigarh stated . . .[46]

Philosophical enquiry was accompanied by meditational praxis and so the science of Yoga developed as the science of consciousness. The states of consciousness are as objective, transient and causally determined as the states of the body but being inherently imperceptible by sensory means they can be correlated with but not identified with the states of the brain and nervous system. Freedom, truth, goodness and other such ideal values are manifested only in consciousness for the self. The self revealed in the subjectivity of self-consciousness can neither be a fleeting object nor a deniable illusion. Such a philosophical interpretation of the nature of man is perfectly consistent with the findings of neuroscience though not with naturalistic humanism. This theory of man or a self or spirit revealed in consciousness but different from changing states of consciousness is confirmable by Yogic science which relies on introspection, intuition, inter-subjective agreement and predictable practical consequences.

The science of yoga grapples with this problem of self-realization. It distinguishes two elements in experience namely, its objective and changing content which represents the external reality and the pure subject or consciousness that witnesses this content. Just as a complex of pure consciousness and changing mental states. Consciousness, mind and body, however normally function as if they were one.

The methods of yoga are specialized techniques of introspection which are tested by inter-subjective agreement and predicable behavioural changes. The yogic science constitutes a coherent and growing tradition which is still hiring and flourishing.

Her holiness Rajyogini Prakashmani, in her learned writing on

"Global Peace and Harmony through Spiritual Education" rightly advises as:[47]

Many people today think that spiritual knowledge and moral principles are only for personal progress and that it does not apply to resolving the problems facing society as a whole. Spiritual knowledge brings about self-change, therefore, it is an effective tool for social transformation at all levels and establishing sustainable peace and prosperity for everyone.

At this time we are seeing the beginnings of a synthesis of science and spirituality. The aim of science and technology has always been to improve the quality of life and make the world a better place physically. In the hands of individuals under these ways of negativity, insecurity and greed and lust for power it has become a tool of destruction. However in the hands of an enlightened, spiritually aware leadership, motivated by feelings of benefit and love, science and technology can create the physical expression of a new civilization, clean renewable energy, pollution-free, fast and silent transportation, environmentally friendly infrastructure, architecture and communication systems, etc.[48]

CONCLUSION

A large section of civil service are not interested in discharging their duties at all levels except drawing their salaries. It is high time that we should through training and circulating written material about our Sanskrit literature, which is our heritage, teach them the benefits of working whole heartedly and with devotion. Besides, we may teach them how to keep fit through various physical, mental and spiritual techniques to achieve happiness in this life and beyond. This will also make our country the best in the world as we want to develop on moral and spiritual principles. The world is looking towards India for its philosophical values. We should first practice them in our country and then show to the world our rich cultural heritage

Notes and References

1. B. Dharmambal, Environmental Health Indicators, some issues in Environmental Challenges of the 21st century, editors, S. Radha-Amar Singh Sankhyan, New Delhi, Deep & Deep, 2002, p. 175.
2. S. Radha, Environment Impact on Health in the 21st century, *Ibid.*, pp. 187-88 and 200.
3. WHO, SEARO, S.E./ RC/31, p. 59.
4. Seal, S.C. (1963), Presidential Address, 50th Science Congress, Delhi.
5. WHO, Public Health Papers, No. 49, 1973, p. 9.
6. Govt. of India, First Five Year Plan, p. 511.
7. WHO, *World Health*, December, 1975, p. 3.
8. A.K. Sinha, Philosophy of Health and Medical Sciences, Ambala Cantt. Associated, 1983, p. 10.

9. Prashna Upanisad, III, 12.
10. P.V. Asha Kumari Tewari, Universal Relevance of Kaumarabhartya, in Vachaspati Upadhyaya, *op. cit.*, p. 129.
11. R.H. Singh "The Unique Holistic Approach of Ayurvedic" Diagnostic and Cure in Vachaspati Upadhyaya, *op. cit.*, pp. 123-24.
12. R.H. Singh, *op. cit.*, pp. 123-24.
13. Khagendra Patra, Sanskrit and Contemporary Challenge to Medical Science—A study, in Vachaspati Upadhyaya, *op. cit.*, p. 104.
14. Jayalakhasmi Balasubramanium, Ayurveda: A way of Life, in Vachaspati Upadhyaya, *op. cit.*, p. 58.
15. Charaka Samahita, Charaka Sutra Asthana: 7(44).
16. *Ibid.*, 29 (24), it gives more importance to the prevention of disease.
17. Agnivesa's Caraka Samhita, Varansai, Chowkhamba Sanskrit Series, 1976, Vol. I, XXIX, 7.
18. Swami Harshananda, 'Attainment of Yoga Malodies and Remedies' in *Yoga: Its Various Aspects*, Sri Ramakrishna Math, Madras, pp. 203-04.
19. Manchanda, S.C. *et. al.*, "Research Study of Reversal of Coronary Heart Disease through Preksha Meditation with reference to coronary atherosclerotic reversal potential of yoga lifestyle intervention", A Research Study conducted by AIIMS, Deptt. of Cardiology, New Delhi, pp. 1-8.
20. Swami Prabuddhananda, Yoga in Daily Life, In *Yoga: Its Various Aspects*, Shri Ramakrishna Math, Madras, pp. 121-22 and 70-71
21. Swami Rama, *Ibid.*, 79.
22. Swami Vishnu Devananda, *op. cit.*, p. 60.
23. A.K. Sinha; *op. cit.*, pp. 36-37.
24. Swami Mukhyananda, Om Gayatri and Sandhya, Ramkrishna Math, Madras, p. 20.
25. Swami Sivananda, Practice of Yoga Quoted in Swami Vishnu Devananda, *op. cit.*, p. 60.
26. Swami Vishnu Devananda, *op. cit.*, p. 161.
27. Swami Vishnu Devananda, *op. cit.*, pp. 15-17.
28. The Daily Tribune, Sept. 7, 2002
29. Bhagavad Gita XVII/8, Jayadayal Goyandka, Gita Press Gorakhpur.
30. *Ibid.*, XVII/9.
31. *Ibid.*, XVII/9.
32. *Ibid.*, XVII/10.
33. Pravrajika Varadaprana, The Power of Music, pp. 127-28. Quoted in "Values: The Key to a Meaningful Life", Ramakrishna Math, Madras.
34. Swami Rama, *op. cit.*, pp. 219-20.
35. Swami Yatiswarananda, *op. cit.*, p. 324.
36. *Ibid.*, p. 324.
37. Swami Vishnu Nanda, *op. cit.*, p. 1.
38. Swami Sivananda, Bliss Divine, Quoted in Swami Vishnu Nanda, *op. cit.*, p. 1.
39. Swami Vishnu Nanda, *op. cit.*, p. 160.
40. Swami Prabhavananda, The Eternal Companion, Madras, Sri Ramkrishna Mission, 1971, pp. 335-36.
41. Swami Gokulnanda, preface, IX.
42. Swami Swami Sivananda, Practice of Yoga, Quoted in Swami Devananda, *op. cit.*, p. 34.
43. Swami Yateshwarananda, *op. cit.*, p. 671.
44. Swami Abhedananda, Science of Psychic Phenomena, Ramakrishna Vedanta Math, Calcutta, 1993, pp. 96-97.

45. G.C. Pande, "Neurosciences and Philosophy—Some Problems in the light of Indian and Buddhist Philosophy, National Seminar, "Science Society, Values and Consciousness" 27th and 28th May, 2002, P.U., Chandigarh.
46. Aliyar, 2002, p. 50.
47. *Ibid.*, p. 80.
48. *Ibid.*, pp. 15-16.

CHAPTER 4

ENVIRONMENT POLLUTION AND HEALTH EDUCATION

The objective of water management is to maintain adequate supplies of water of a good quality for the entire population, while preserving the hydrological, biological and chemical functions of ecosystems, adapting human activities within the capacity limits of nature and combating vectors of water-related diseaes.
Agenda 21—An Assessment, Ministry of Environment and Forests, Government of India.

"O Mother Earth! You are the world for us and we are your children; let us speak in one accord; let us come together so that we live in peace and harmony".

—*Atharva Veda* (c 1200 B.C.)

Environment Pollution and Health Education

INTRODUCTION

No country on the globe except India has given a constitutional status to the law relating to environmental control, protection and preservation. Specific provisions were already there. But recently more provision through 42nd amendment have been added in the body of the constitution thereby making it obligatory on the State and every citizen to protect and improve the environment.

Right to breath in free and fresh air, consume contamination free potable drinking water, reside, walk and travel in noise-free environment is guaranteed by Article 21 to all the residents of India. In fact the right to life takes within its sweep the right to food, the right to clothing, the right to decent environment and reasonable accommodation to live in. Thus constitution provides decency to life.

STATUS OF INDIA'S ENVIRONMENT

The urban areas represent complex environmental problems. The living conditions of millions of urban poor are such that they pose a threat to their health and have potentially catastrophic social consequences. For the urban poor, the living conditions are the worst. If these problems are not addressed to in an adequate and timely manner, serious environmental and associated health consequences will 'follow'. Burgeoning urban population beyond the carrying capacity of the different components of urban eco-systems, coupled with indifferent urban governance, are the root causes for urban environmental problems. Air pollution can cause chronic and acute respiratory diseases, ventilatory malfunction, heart diseases, cancer of the lungs and even death. The blood lead levels of persons in

Ahmedabad, Bombay and Calcutta have been reported to be higher than the corresponding levels of persons in lead-free gasoline areas. The details of ambient air quality status in ten large cities/towns are at Table 4.1. In most of the cities, while the SPM levels are significantly higher than the CPCB standards, the levels of SO_2 and NOx are within the CPCB standards.

TABLE 4.1

Ambinet Air Quality Status in some Cities/Towns During 1998

City	SPM			SO_2			Nox		
	R	C	I	R	C	I	R	C	I
CPCB Standards	140	140	360	60.0	60.0	80.0	60.0	60.0	80.0
Delhi	284	272	305	15.2	17.4	18.6	22.4	37.3	37.5
Mumbai	340	Na	308	40.7	Nil	39.1	24.9	Na	30.4
Howarah	469	570	835	12.1	53.4	46.7	37.6	64.7	67.7
Chennai	60	156	85	9.2	10.0	11.0	8.1	16.9	6.8
Hyderabad	129	187	100	6.5	7.1	6.0	23.3	48.0	15.7
Ahmedabad	239	550	305	9.0	19.3	27.6	17.7	30.9	29.4
Cochin	133	131	116	8.8	9.8	10.5	13.8	19.9	9.9
Nagpur	236	157	162	4.7	5.7	4.0	20.0	15.5	9.2
Jaipur	207	226	302	6.8	6.4	7.5	10.6	9.9	11.5
Kanpur	433	495	451	1.59	18.6	17.1	15.6	18.3	17.1

R = Residential
C = Commercial/Residential
I = Industrial

SPM = Suspended Particular Matter
SO_2 = Sulphur Dioxide
Nox = Nitrogen Oxides (as NO_2)
Unit = Mg/m^3

Source: Central Pollution Board and National Environmental Engineering Research Institute.

The rural population uses substantial quantities of non-commercial fuel, i.e. crop residues, animal dung or wood. Although their share in total fuel consumption is decreasing, these still provide 80 per cent of rural energy for cooking. Several adverse health effects are suspected to arise due to indoor pollution especially where conventional 'sigri' has not been replaced with smokeless chulha. Respiratory infection in children, chronic lung disease, lung cancer in adults and adverse pregnancy outcomes, such as low birth weight and still birth of the child, for women exposed during pregnancy, are some of the diseases associated with indoor pollution.[1]

Current Situation

Global environmental issues, such as ozone depletion, climate change due to accumulation of Greenhouse Gases (GHGs), bio-diversity loss, etc. are largely due to the rapid industrialisation of the developed nations. India is an insignificant contributor to the GHG emissions as can be seen from the Table 4.2.

The main environmental problems in India relate to air and water pollution, degradation of common property resources, threat to biological

CHART 4.1

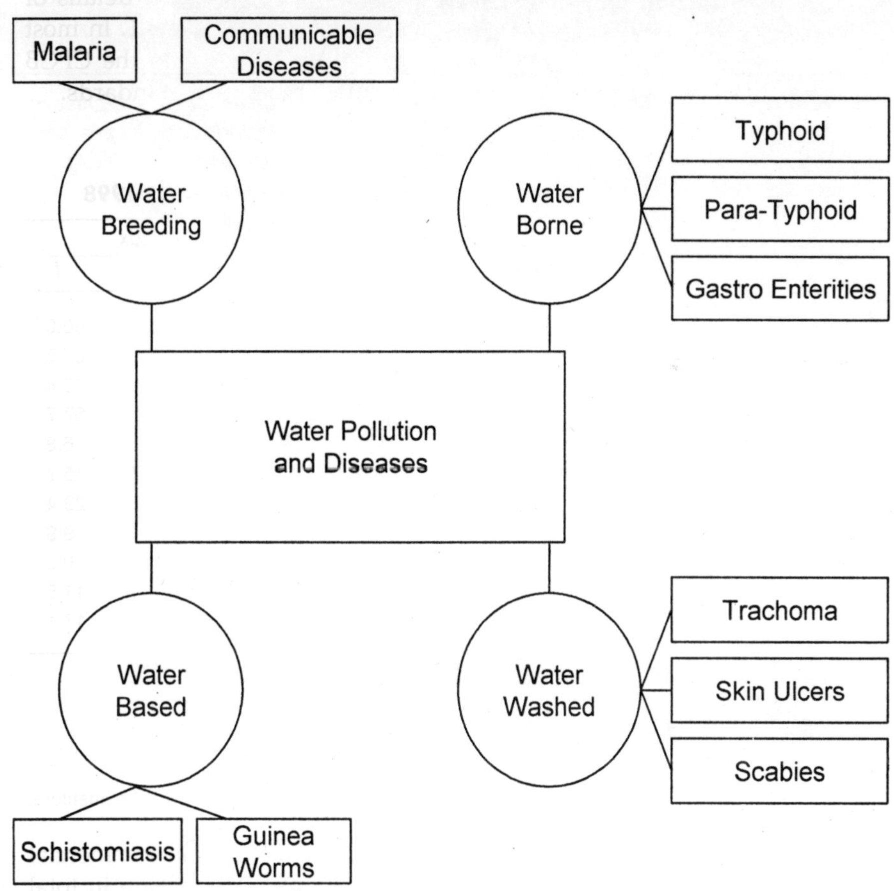

diversity, solid waste disposal and sanitation. Increasing deforestation, industrialisation, urbanisation, transportation and input-intensive agriculture are some of the other major causes of environmental problems being faced by the country. Poverty presents special problems for a heavily populated country with limited resources.

The daily chore of life of the people was based on the inscriptions in ancient literature. People would get up early in the morning and go out for a walk to breathe in fresh air after freeing one self from bowel's movements (शोचय). After walking and exercise, bathing was essential to cleanse the body followed by daily chores of life.

People were taught to keep their house, Mohalla and village/city clean so that they can lead pollution free life. There were codes of conduct and if these were not followed, punishment was imposed.

Hence in the ancient India there were well laid out practices for environmental sanitation, i.e. pure air, potable drinking water and

TABLE 4.2

Carbon Emissions Levels in Selected Countries

(million tonnes)

Country	*Share of World Population 1996*	*Share of Gross World Product 1994*	*Share of World Carbon Emissions 1995*	*Emissions per capita*
United States	5	26	23	5.3
Russia	3	2	7	2.9
Japan	2	17	5	2.4
Germany	1	8	4	2.9
China	21	2	13	0.7
India	17	1	4	0.3
Indonesia	4	1	1	0.3
Brazil	3	2	1	0.4
Total	56	59	58	0.9

Source: Compilation from several international published sources.

sanitation. In the schools of learning called 'Gurukuls' emphasis was laid on cleanliness in daily life.

Mahatama Gandhi, the embodiment of Ancient India, preached simplicity, cleanliness, sanitation, in the house and street. He did not only believe in these principles but practiced them with his own hands and through his associates. He believed in simplicity.

Air Pollution

The ambient air quality has deteriorated all over the country, especially in the semi-urban and urban areas. Anthropogenic activities result in the air pollution on account of 3 major sources: stationary sources (use of fossil fuels in industries and thermal power plants), mobile sources (vehicles) and in-door sources (burning of bio-mass). The relative contribution of the 3 sources varies across the country depending upon various factors. It is estimated that indoor air pollution in India's rural areas is primarily responsible for 500,000 deaths annually, mostly of women and children under 5.

Impure environment produce output which leads to many problems. (Refer Table 4.3)

The Tribune Editorial dated Oct. 16, 2001, has warned the people to be careful of the impurities of air created through burning paddy. To quote: The burning of paddy and wheat stalks after harvesting was always a nuisance, causing numerous eye and breathing difficulties to the people living nearby. But the practice has now become so widespread that it is threatening the very weather pattern of the continent. Last week's darkness at noon rain has been directly attributed to it and it also seems to have a lot to do with the brown cloud hovering over the entire Asian continent. Debilitating influence that it has on the environment is only now being fully understood. Worse, these effects are going to last decades, if not centuries. Provided we stop forth with, that is! The chilling fact is that the whole approach still continues to be causal, despite the fact that the Press with *The Tribune* in the lead—has been shouting from the housetops about the critical dangers involved. The carbon dioxide that we are mindlessly sending into the atmosphere might stay there for more than a century, endangering the life and health of even future generations.

Pollution can be mitigated by planting good biomass-producing trees like Arjun, jamun, karanj, neem, guava, siris, aonla, babool, sheesham, ironwood, bamboo, khamer, etc.

There are certain medicinal herbs like milk thistle, dandelion turmeric, picrorhiza, phyllanthus and green tea, which can help you rise above a toxic environment. Fortunately, we have the tools for heading off this disaster. It only remains for us to use them.

Recently the Punjab and Haryana High Court has directed the Punjab Government to get in touch with the Punjab School Education Board authorities for incorporating environment studies in the syllabi for classes VI to X.

Issuing the direction, a Division Bench of the Punjab and Haryana High Court, comprising Mr. Justice G.S. Singhvi and Ms. Justice Kiran Anand Lall, added: It would be appreciated if environment experts are associated for the purpose of formulating a model syllabus for the academic session 2003-04.

Air Pollution and Its Management

In Samaveda Air is addressed as father brother and friend (Sam. 1841). Air has medicinal qualities and bring welfare and happiness (Sam. 1840). Gita in chapter 9 sloka 6 states that air above the earth surface has spread everywhere in the sky. There was a provision for yajna which was performed in every house. This killed the harmful germs in the air. Agni was considered to be the best purifier of Air.

The basic input of human life is fresh air. No life on earth can exist without oxygen. Food, water, and sunlight, are also very essential, but the breathing exercise in the human and animal life is going on every time. It ceases only when the individual is pronounced as dead.

We can live without food and water for days together but for only five minutes without air. On an average a man needs 30 lbs of air every day.

The rapid increase in private motorized transport, coupled with poor and infrastructure has led to a congestion and severe air pollution. The concentration of air pollutants exceeded the World Health Organization (WHO) guidelines in many urban centers in India. Long-term exposure to soot, dust, sulphur and dioxide and small particles in the air causes a wide range of chronic respiratory diseases and exacerbates hearts disease and other conditions. Heavy reliance on oil, particularly for transport, contributes to pollution-related health problems in large cities. In India, the death rate due to cancer increased by 3 percent and that of lung cancer by 9 percent since 1990. Even in smaller cities in India the environmental impact of rapid urbanization is increasing significantly.[2]

Air pollution may be defined as the presence of one or more pollutants or combinations of these pollutants in such quality and for such duration which may prove to be injurious to human, plant or animal life or to property. Air pollution occurs when the capacity of the atmosphere to dilute the pollutants is not within its capacity.

Let us discuss the important pollutants in air:

1. Inhalation of Carbon Monoxide—When carbon monoxide is inhaled, it absorbs oxygen from blood and comes out as carbon dioxide causing many disorders like mental stress, laziness. It affects lungs and cardio-vascular system.

2. Sulphur dioxide can cause problems in respiratory system, lung tissues, eye irritations, etc.

3. Flyash, an emission of thermal plants causes serious air and water pollution. This need be controlled by pollution control instruments. Those who live near the thermal plants are seriously affect.

4. Burning of Agricultural wastes like straw, husk, and animal wastes like cow/buffalo dung inside the house—These cause suffocation leading to breathing problems and irritation to eyes, etc.

5. Automobile Exhaust—Pollution from automobiles is very serious as it releases poisonous gases partly because of poor quality of fuel, partly old vehicles and road conditions. The emission gets converted into unbearable gases causing stress and strain. Things are being improved through the intervention of the Supreme Court. In Delhi, Supreme Court has banned the use of vehicles older than 15 years and many other measures have been imposed to improve environment.

The Air Act defines air pollution as the presence in the atmosphere of any air pollutant, which means any solid, liquid or gaseous substance present in the atmosphere in such concentration as may be or tend to be injurious to human being or other living creatures or plants or property or environment.[3]

Rgveda says that pure air is a boon to good health and happiness:

वात आ वातु भेषजं शंभु मयोभु नो हृदे । प्रण आयूंषि तारिषत् ।
उत वात पितासि नः उत भ्रातोत नः सखा । स नो जीवात वेकृधि ।
यददो वात ते गश्हेऽमृतस्य निधिर्हितः । ततो नो देहि जीवसे ।।
ऋक् 10-86, 1-3

In Rgveda, Air is considered as the agent for the welfare of the people, Air is addressed differently as father, brother, and friend. Vayu is prayed to impart good health and eternal happiness and blessings.

"Vayu is that sutra, for his power are held up all these beings and their birth. That is why, O, Gautama, when a man dies, that is when the Vayu leaves him, all his limbs become powerless."[4]

AV IV 5.25.1 states that air is the support of all beings. We sing the praises at Vayu and Savitri, who protect us and who surround (i.e. parvade) the whole world. May they free us from sin.)

वायोः सवितुविदथानि मन्महे चावात्मवद् विशायौ यो च रक्षयः ।
यौ विद्यस्य परिभु बभुवयुस्तौ नौ मुच्चतमहंसः ।।

The Vedic Rsis recognized Air as a vital cosmic constituent and included it in the five elements. Vayu is termed to as a deity presiding over the mid-region. (इमानि पञ्च महाभूतानि पृथिवी वायुः आकाश आप ज्योतीर्णि । Ait Up. 3.3)

(वायुर्वा अन्तरिक्षस्याध्यक्षः । MS 4.1.1; KS-30-10, etc. अथातो मध्य-स्थानाः देवताः-तासां वायुः प्रथमगामी ।)

That the pure, and clean air is a source of health, happiness and consequently of long life, was also mentioned by the Vedic Rsis. Two small Rgvedic Suktas viz. X.186 and X.137 may be regarded of great significance from this point of view of the importance of Air.

In Rg. X.186, Vata is referred to as causing welfare and happiness. The Rsi is so emotional of this element that he addresses Vata as his father, brother and friend. Vata is a store-house of ambroisa for him and requests it, to bestow its medicinal qualities. (11. वात आ वातु भेषजं शंभु मयोभु नो हृदे। प्रण आयूषि तारिषत् । उत वात पितासि नः उत भ्रातोत नः सखा । स नो जीवात वे कृधि । यददो वात ते गृहेऽमृतस्य निधिर्हितः । ततो नो देहि जीवसे ।। Rg. X.186.1-3)

Rg. X.137 divides the wind into two categories , the one bringing vigour and other blowing away the evil. Since Vata is the Universal medicine, he prays the wind to blow with its medicinal qualities.

Further TS and MS positively state that, whatever smells ill, spreads out in a windy place, for Vayu is its purifier.

द्वाविमौ वातौ वातः आ सिन्धोरा परावतः । दक्षं ते अन्य आ वातु परान्यो वातु यद् रपः । आ वात वाहि भेषजं नि वात यद् रपः । त्वं हि विश्वभेषजो देवानां दूत ईयते ॥ Rg. X.137.2-3.

Thus the Vedic Rsis were so fully aware of the medicinal qualities and the intrinsic worth of this environmental element, that they eulogized it to the extent that it forms an integral part of Prajapati. अर्धं ह प्रजापतेर्वायुः अर्धं प्रजापतिः (SBr 6.2 2.11) (They further wished that the Air should provide sweet essence.

(मधु वाता ऋतायते (Rg. 1.90-6)

In the older times, many types of Yagnas were performed which used to purify air. However, there was not much problem regarding Air pollution in ancient times.

Many times Kariri Yajnas (इष्टि) were performed to bring rain which purified the air. अपां धारां भिन्धि - पुरो वातो वर्णन् जिन्वरावण्तं स्वाहा । तै.स. 2-4-7

वायुर्वै वृष्ट्या ईशे स एवास्मै पर्जन्यं वर्षयति । (तै.सं 2-4-9)

Rigveda says that pure air is a boon to good health and happiness.

Bhagavad Gita in Chapter 9 sloka 6 has observed that air has its origin in ether and also disappears in ether, spring from ether, remaining in and finally disappearing into ether and under no circumstances remain apart from ether but never remains in it and yet ether has no connection what so ever with the air of its movement and other changes in it, and is always beyond it.

There are seven layers of Air in the sky.

The Taittiriya Upanisad indicates about various types of wind in the human body (Shikshawali—18)

अथध्या' त्मन् । प्राणो व्यानेऽपान उदानःसमानः ।

Let us discuss some of the methods mentioned in Ancient Sanskrit Literature to get the supply of pure Air (Oxygen):

1. Ancient Sanskrit Literature suggests to people to get early in the morning and go out for the morning walk. Since, the morning, there is less pollution and plenty of oxygen can be inhaled by us during the morning as well as good blood circulation can be ensured.
2. Ancient Sanskrit literature suggests pranayama which is a method of getting good supply of oxygen and cultivating equanimity through balanced breathing.

Intake of Food	Prana Vayu	Heart/Stomach
Digestion of Food	Samana Vayu	The Naval
Speech	Udana Vayu	Throat
Excretion	Apana Vayu	Anus
Oxygen Supply	Vyana Vayu	Throughout the Body

3. Japa and meditation also help in getting pure air.
4. Yoga exercises in the morning increase oxygen intake
5. Houses were not stuffed with materials which emits foul smell as air mixes with organic material in the house and causes pollution.

In our ancient Indian culture, we find many verses in our Vedas indicating the importance of rainfall water in our life as rain water was the main source of water.

Problem of water can be solved through the yajnas to bring water available at great length on the earth and in the sky (Yajurveda 18/36).

Life prospers only because of food and water. (Atharvaveda, 11/4-5)

Mother earth gets satisfied through rain and the sky satisfies through fire. (Rigveda, 1/164-51)

> Bearer of all things, hoard of treasures rare, sustaining, Mother Earth. What of thee I dig out, let that quickly grow over. Let me not hurt thy vitals, or the heart.
>
> —Atharva Veda (c 1200 BC)

WATER POLLUTION AND MANAGEMENT

In earlier times the state took care of the water supply to a large extent by the development and maintenance of several ingenious and indigenous ways of storing rain and floodwaters. The concentration of rainfall in the monsoon season and the variation in extent of precipitation over space compelled the storage of rain water in order to spread the resource availability into the lean season. It was the dharma of the ruler to support and execute water storage structures. Urban planning took into consideration natural catchments and focused on enhancing the water harvesting systems. The tank system was so well developed in many watersheds of Karnataka that it was estimated that hardly any runoff waters escaped from the catchment. Settlements like Jodhpur, Coimbatore were based around their water tanks and their associated catchments. The city of Jodhpur was built around the catchments of 35 tanks and Coimbatore around 24 tanks. Such examples abound in the historical annals of our country.

Air and water were held in high esteem in Ancient India. They were worshipped like god. (वातो देवता) Rivers are named with respect like Ganga Maya (mother Ganga). For all rivers Artis (songs) are sung in the morning and evening so that people treat them like god and not make them dirty.

Swamy Ram Tirtha has a great reverence for the Ganga—To quote him:

> O river Ganga let me sacrifice myself for you
> this body of the flash and bones
> Let me surrender it to you
> (आपः मानुषी) Oh Water, you are for the welfare of mankind

In Ancient India, water was considered as an inexhaustible gift of God and water was pure because the affluent at that time were limited. Beside people used water only when needed, i.e. no wastage. But today, the position is altogether different as the total amount of water available to the human race is not only limited but is fixed and cannot cater to the requirement for all times to come. In addition, pure water is very difficult to attain.

Quantities of pure water: Acharya Sushruta has written that water which is devoid of all smell and taste and is pure, cool, transparent and pleasant should be considered ambrosia for life. Saying that water is best among all food articles, he adds that pure water is life-giving and always helpful to human body.

Importance of Water

Water is life. It is therefore found that crisis of water brings crisis in life. In our ancient Indian culture, we find many verses in our Vedas indicating the importance of rainfall water in our life as rain water was the main source of water.

Problem of water can be solved through the yajnas to bring water available at great length on the earth and in the sky (Yajurveda 18/36). Life prospers only because of food and water (Atharvaveda, 11/4-5)

Mother earth gets satisfied through rain and the sky satisfies through fire. (Rigveda, 1/164-51)[5]

(A) (a) General

Water is the main source of the needs of life like vegetation, insects, animals, birds and hence the rain is welcome. To quote from Chandogya Upanisad:

> आपो वाव अन्नाद भूयस्यः तस्माद्यदा सुवृष्टिर्न भवति व्याधीयन्ते प्राणाः अन्नो कनीयो भविष्यतीति । अथ यदा सुवृष्टिः भवति आनन्दिनः प्राणा ह भवत्यन्नं बहु भविष्यतीति।

आप एवेमा मूर्ता येयं पृथिवी यदन्तरिक्षं यद् द्यौर्यत्पर्वता यद्देवमनुष्या यत्पशव वयांसि च तृण वनस्पतय: श्वापदान्या कीटपतङ्गपिपीलक्म । आप एवेमा मूर्ता: ।

Water, verily, is greater than food. Therefore, when there is no good (sufficient) rain, living creatures sicken with the thought that food will become scarce. But when there is good rain, living creatures rejoice in the thought that food will become abundant. It is just water that assumes different forms of this earth, this atmosphere, this sky, the mountains, gods and men, beasts and birds, grass and trees, animals together with worms, flies and ants, water indeed is all these forms.

—Chandogya—VII.10.1

Water is for the welfare of mankind (आप: मानुषि)

Let mother water purify us (आपो अस्मान्मातर: शुन्धयन्तु (यजुर्वेद 11-50)

With pure water

Oh Goddess water give us blessings to make our life sublime.

आपो देवी: बृहती: विश्वशंभुव: (यजु: 4.7)

आपो हि ष्ठा मयो भुव: (यजु: 11-50)

As already explained in the previous chapter.

According to our ancient Sanskrit Literature the universe is made of five basic elements viz. (1) ksiti (earth), (2) apah (water), (3) tejah (light), (4) marut (air), and (5) vyoma (ether). Thus apah or water plays a cosmic role in our living organism and brings bliss and purity in life..

In Taittiriya Samhita (1.2.1.1), it is mentioned that water is a source of life, lustre, beauty and radiance.

Water has been mentioned as a cleaning object in the Vajasaneyi samhita (4.2). Water is also a dirt cleaner has been mentioned in the same text (6.17). It reads: "idam apah pravahatavadyam ca malam ca yat." Taittiriya Sam. also stresses the same in its mantra—"yadevasya amedhyam tad apa hanty apo avoksati santyai."

(b) Promotion and Preservation of Natural Environment

Water is the most essential for keeping a balance in environment. The natural environment of any place is dependable by the land-water relation of that area. The land consisting mostly of earth and trees, is dependent on water and *vice-versa*. So Rta was also identified with water, the most important ingredient of nature. The rivers flow following Rta (II 28. 4; X 139. 4). Thus water is an important principle, which determines the regularity of rains, crops, etc. and maintains the balance in the universe.

(c) Medicinal Value—(Yajurveda 9-6) RK (23-19)

In vedic texts, water has the quality of forceful medicinal curing substance, a great healer and remedy. Rgveda (1.23.20) mention water to be the abode of all medicines. It says:

"apsu me somo abravid antar visvani bhesaja /
agnim ca visvasambhuvam apas ca visvabhesajih // (1.23.20)

In Hungary, there are large number of places where bathing can cure many diseases. Blatona lake is famous for that. Our revered, Rabinder Nath Tagore got treatment at this lake. Even our hill stations have places where water has many medicinal qualities.

All medicines are also present in it (apsu antar amrtam apsu bhesajam apam uta prasastaye). The Vajasaneyi Smhita (4.12) establishes the medicinal utility of water in all clear cut terms. It says: "Svatrah pita bhavata yuyam apo asmakam antar udare susevah/ta asmabhyam ayaksma anamiva anagasah svadantu devir amrta rtavrdhah.[6]

Let us give some examples from Ayurveda. Ayurveda has clearly advised against using contaminated water for all purposes. It says that a man who drinks or bathes in contaminated water, incurs the risk of being affected with edema, jaundice, abdominal worms, skin infections, indigestion, colic, ascetic and many other dreadful diseases. Ancient author Pandit Bhavaprakash has advised that water which is pure and is kept overnight in a copper vessel should be the first drink of the day. Perhaps, he was also hinting that copper as a trace element is essential for the body.

(d) Bestow Peace and Tranquility

Mind of a person gets peace by using pure water. Satapatha Brahmana (1.2.2.11) mentions apah as a source of great peace. It says: "santir apas tad adbhih sanatya samayati"

(a) *Promotes good health.* Inadequacy in the availability of safe drinking water, unfavourable environmental conditions and lack of personal hygiene have been the major causes of disease and disability among people. As per WHO statistics, 80 per cent of diseases in the developing countries are related to unsafe water supply and inadequate sanitation causing high child mortality, low life expectancy and poor quality of life. In India, more than one million children below 5 years died from dehydration caused by diarrhoea annually, while another 250 thousand are victims of tetanus. Poliomyelitis has been a cause of lameness among 170 thousand children per year. There is also a very high rate of occurrence of intestinal worms, particularly in West Bengal, Bihar, Orissa, Andhra Pradesh, Tamil Nadu, Kerala and Maharashtra. The national goal to reduce child mortality from 146 per thousand to 125 by 1995 and 70 per thousand by 2000 cannot possibly be achieved without a significant change in the existing mortality/morbidity related to water and sanitation. Also important is to change the peoples' perception about the link between sanitation and health. According to a recent KAP survey in the country, 37 per cent people do not know/do not believe that exposed excreta can harm health. Outdoor defecation is not generally seen as a problem except in terms of inconvenience during rain, night or winter to women.

Dr. H. Mahler, former WHO Director-General, has rightly said that,

I am utterly convinced that the number of water taps per 1,000 population will be an infinitely more meaningful health indicator than the number of hospital beds per 1,000 population. Mr. Kurt Waldhelm, former UN Secretary-General also stressed that, the provision of safe water and sanitation does not merely mean happier, healthier citizens; it also means increased economic productivity.

Nikolas P. Napulbow in his editorial "Water For All", a Human Right has rightly said that, "water is a basic human need for health—indeed, for survival—and therefore it is not an exaggeration to call it one of the basic human rights. Without safe water and sanitation, there is no real development. A community ravaged by diarrhoal diseases, dracunculiasis or schistosomiasis cannot look beyond its immediate problems towards social and economic welfare. Safe water is the doorway to health and health is the prerequisite for progress, social equity and human divinity.

Infectious diseases resulting from water pollution can be classified into four groups, depending upon the ways in which their incidence can be lessened by improvements in water supply. (See Chart 4.2).

1. "Water-borne" diseases are those in which infectious agent remains alive in drinking water e.g., typhoid, paratyphoid, gastroenterities, etc. The incidence of these diseases can be reduced by the purification of water.
2. "Water-washed" diseases include infection of the outer body surface, e.g. trachoma, skin ulcers, scabies and typhus, bacillary and amoebic dysentery and gastro enterities. The incidence can be reduced by augmenting water quantity.
3. "Water-based" infections, i.e., schistosomiasis, guinea worms. The infection occurs when the skin is in contact with water or through drinking water.
4. "Water breeding" or water promixity diseases are caused by mosquitoes or flies living near aquatic conditions.

There is probably no single factor that has a greater effect on the health, well-being and development of a community than the provision of ample and convenient supply of wholesome and good quality water. In towns and cities water supply is recognised as a basic necessity for industrial and commercial purposes; it is vital for the maintenance of public health and the prevention of epidemics.

"The provision of ample supplies of safe water and the sanitary disposal of excreta have a direct and far-reaching effect upon the health and well-being of rural populations. Indeed, it is believed that no other single measure can make a comparable contribution to the improvement of their health and standard of living. The choice of an appropriate technology depends on local conditions." One hospital bed out of four in the world is occupied by a patient who is ill because of polluted water. Provisions of a

CHART 4.2

Diseased Adjusted Live Years (DALY) Lost due to Adverse Environmental Factors

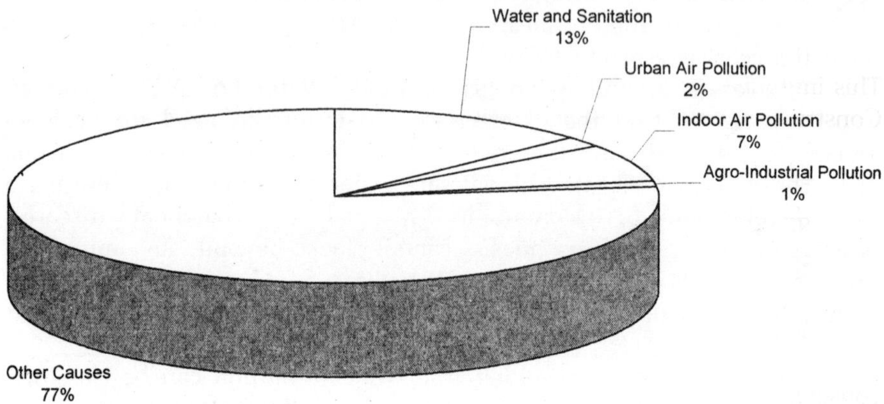

safe and convenient water supply is the single most important activity that could be undertaken to improve the health of people living in rural areas of the developing world."

Drinking water and sanitation improvements could reduce the overall incidence of infant and child diarrhoea by one quarter and cut total infant and child mortality by more than one-half. Country programmes are increasingly taking measures to improve water supply and sanitation within their primary healthcare programmes. Guinea worm disease can be effectively prevented by providing safe drinking water and its global eradication is clearly possible within the next few years. As for schistosomiasis, some 60% reduction could be achieved by improving water supplies. Building latrines, giving health education and introducing selected drug therapy could reduce the prevalence even more.

A great surge in the population of India's big cities, poses huge problems for safeguarding water supplied.

We suggest here the methods of conserving water supply:

- Integration of water and waste water management, coupled with health education for cost-effectiveness and promotion of preventive measures for health;
- Prospecting for water resources through state of the art techniques of remote sensing and geophysical surveys;
- Protection of water sources against pollution;
- Decentralization of water supply matching the required quality and quantity through waste recycle and reuse;
- Maintenance of the water distribution system, which can prevent up to 50% of the purified waste water from being lost; and

- Application of mathematical programming techniques with exact fluid flow relationships in the design of water and waste water systems, so as to ensure functionality and to conserve material and financial resources.

(b) *Construction of storage tanks, wells, etc. were considered auspicious.* This importance was clearly realized by the authors of Dharmsastra works. Construction of tanks, wells, lakes, etc. came under Purtadharama.

इष्टापूर्तौ स्मृतौ धर्मौ श्रुतौ तौ शिष्टसम्मतौ ।
प्रतिष्ठाद्यं तयोः पूर्त्मिष्टं यज्ञादिलक्षणम् ॥
भुक्तिमुक्तिप्रदं पूर्तमिष्टं भोगार्थसाधनम् ॥

Kalika Purana quoted in Krtyaratnakara

Many Grhya Sutras have prescribed regular ritual for the consereation of tanks, well, etc. Chapter 58 of the Matsya Purana and Chapter 64 of the Agni Purana give details about the dedication of waterpales. The parasaragrhyasutra has particularly recommended that acquatic animals like fish, tortoise, etc. should be introduced in the lakes. This clearly reveals the anxiety of the author for the purity of water. The procedure is described in various Puranas, which should be followed strictly. The purity of water was highly praised by the Dharmasastra authors who quote Puranic verses. The Nirnayasindhu III, p. 334, has quoted the following verses from Bhavisya Purana:

सदा जलं पवित्रं स्यादपवित्रमसंस्कृतम् ।
कुशाग्रेणापि राजेन्द्र न स्प्रष्टव्यमसंस्कृतम् ।
वापीकूपतडागादौ यज्जलं स्यादसंस्कृतम् ।
अपेयं तद् भवेत्सर्वं पीत्वा चान्द्रायणं चरेत् ॥

Even the Samkalpa, at the time of some rituals is significant:

सामान्यं सर्वसत्त्वेभयो मया दत्तमिंद जलम् ।
धर्मार्थकाममोक्षेषु साधनं स्यादहर्निशम् ॥

—Quoted in Rajadharmakaustubha, pp. 179, 216.

Reservoirs of water which are constructed by man (i.e. which are not natural) are of four types.[7]

In order to keep these places clean, Taithriya Arnayak (16.6.77) prohibits the urinating, execration and even nude bath in water to avoid pollution of water.

(c) *Water Management*. Water management has been provided in Kautilya Arthasastra whereby water was preserved carefully, used cautiously and supplemented as and when necessary.

Ancient people in India have developed unique methods to store rain water for drinking purposes and was kept carefully so that it remains fit for drinking purposes and is not polluted.

Manu Smriti (6.4.46-48) prescribes the use of some herbs and plants to purify water.

However, the condition of water is highly poor. Kirti S. Parikh in his Article, "Social Infrastructure: As Important as Physical Infrastructure's states:

The relatively high mortality in the country is not just due to inadequate public health measures alone, poor quality of water is also a major cause. A large fraction of deaths are due to infectious and water-related diseases. A rather rough estimate by the Indira Gandhi Institute for Development Research (IGIDR) in terms of World Bank's disability adjusted life years (DALY) suggests that the country loses about Rs. 36,600 crores a year (1995 prices) due to water-related diseases (see Chart 4.1).

The quality of water in most of our rivers is unsatisfactory. Over large stretches it is not fit for even bathing, let alone drinking. Attempts to provide clean drinking water to our people are bound to fail if we don't take care of the pollution of our water bodies. The task of providing clean water is made difficult by a rapidly increasing number of habitations (defined as where 50 to 100 people live but not a revenue village). It is difficult for the government to provide safe drinking water to these growing number of habitations. One has to rely on cleaning up the rivers and water bodies. We see that only 7.5 percent of the rural and 9.8 per cent of the urban population has no access to drinking water. These numbers may vary due to natural causes (droughts) or how we define water availability (currently, a problem village is that where drinking water is not available within a radius of 1.6 km, or, in hilly regions, water is not available within 100 mt. Elevation difference).

Lack of access to drinking water in urban areas is mainly a problem of inadequate resources to invest in water supply and faulty urban development that attracts people where it is difficult to provide water. The lack of resources for improving water supply is the result of not charging appropriately for water. As a consequence, water supply in urban areas deteriorates and has become unreliable. Thus, large amount of private expenses are incurred on aquaguards and bottled water by the relatively rich. Others also pay for unreliable water through infections and sicknesses. Surveys have shown the willingness of people to pay for clean water. We must increase water charges and improve coverage, supply and quality of water.[8]

Need of making use of Old Technology

R. Radhakrishna Rao in his article, "Indigenous Water Technology" in the *Sunday Tribune*, October 6, 2002 clearly stated that:

- Many community managed water distribution projects centering round the traditional water harvesting system are being tried out in various parts of the country with a certain degree of success.

- With the revival of the age-old Johad system in 650 villages of perpetually drought prone Alwar district of Rajasthan, drinking water problem has become a thing of the past and crops are grown round the year.
- Johads are the simple mud and stone barriers built across the contours of a slope to arrest rain water. They have high embankments on three sides while the fourth is left open for the rain water to enter.
- In the opinion of Magsaysay award recipient Rajendra Singh, "There is not a single village in the country which cannot quench its thirst and that of its fields though the revival of traditional water harvesting techniques."
- In the tribal dominated Chhotanagpur belt of Jharkhand, the traditional system of conserving water is a ahar or surface gravity irrigation tank which continues to be a popular mode to end water shortage. It is essentially a hill technology but has been extended to the gently sloping plains with the help of fun-off diversion called pynes.
- An ahar involves building earth fill check dams across the natural drainage joining the uplands for harvesting the runoff water.

The earth's Six Billion People already overtax its supply of accessible freshwater. What happens when the planet gets a few billion more hands.

Ten Montaigne

The answer is the use of technology and precautions as prescribed in Ancient Sanskrit Literature.

EARTH AND SANITATION

God will not seek thy race,
Nor will he ask thy Birth,
Alone he will demand of thee,
What hast thou done on earth.

The earth is one of the five elements and is an evolute from water. That part of earth becomes holy. Where the praises of Lord are sung. It is very important to note, as mentioned in Ancient Sanskrit Literature, that on the one hand, we are the guest and on the other offspring. The earth is mother to earth as he is dependent on all the products that come from earth.

Earth provides all vegetation, minerals, medicines and many other organic and inorganic materials. It is our sacred duty to keep it clean and

TABLE 4.3

Types of Output in Illustrative Environmental Health Programmes

Programmes	Direct Outputs	*Intermediate Effects or Impacts*	*Ultimate Effects or Benefits*
Water supply	Safe water provided to households in adequate amounts and used efficiently	Reduced disease from water borne pathogens; support to hygiene, nutrition and economic activity	Longer survival
Water Pollution Control	Reduced contamination of (used water returned to)watercourses, seas, soil and food	Improved water resources for human use; reduced damage to marine life; improved aesthetics	Less disability, suffering impairment and pain
Solid Wastes Management	Wastes confined, removed and disposed of (treated recycled)	Reduced disease from vector borne pathogens and from pathogens and chemicals transferred to air, water and land; economic gains; improved aesthetics	More efficient personal and social performance
Air Pollution Control	Reduced introduction of toxic, irritant and nuisance elements into ambient air	Reduced death, disease and discomfort; reduced economic losses; improved aesthetics	Improved quality of life
Occupational Health	Reduced physical/ chemical hazards in work environment, through primary and secondary disease prevention services	Reduced illness, trauma and poisoning; safer work environment; improved working conditions and productivity	Socio-economic development
Food Sanitation	Food safeguarded against contamination in production, processing, delivery, preparation and consumption	Reduced disease and death from pathogens and toxins in food; enlarged markets; improved aesthetics	

Source: WHO: Public Health Paper, No. 59, p. 113.

provide due respect as it is known in Ancient Sanskrit literture as Mother Earth.

समुवक्सने देवि पर्वतस्तनमण्डले ।
विष्णुपत्नि नमस्तुभ्यं पादस्पर्शं क्षमस्व मे ।।

Soil provides us with innumerable types of food.

Kalidasa in his raghuvansa illustrates with the example of Atithi's who showed great to respect to mother earth who in return filled his kingdom with riches.

खनिभिः सुषुवे रत्नं क्षेत्रैः सस्यं वनैर्गजान् ।
दिदेश वेतनं तस्मै रक्षासदृशमेव भूः ।। (रघु 17-64)

The Mother Earth gave to Atithi jewels from her mines, crops from her fields, elephants from her forests, by way of her price for the protection received from him. The earth yields her riches to man as long as he judiciously protects and nourishes her riches. Once he begins to misuse her riches out of greed, he would render her barren and meet with his own disastrous end. This is the message that we can derive from the above instance.

Earth provides all types of food:

यस्यां समुद्र उत सिन्धुरापो यस्यामन्नं कृष्टयः संबभूवुः । यस्यामिदं जिन्वति प्राणदेजत्
सा नो भूमिः पूर्वपेये दुधातु ।। S.Y. 12-1-3 and

त्वज्जातात्वयि चरन्ति मर्त्यास्त्वं बिभर्षि द्विपदस्त्वं चतुष्पदः । तवेमे पृथिवि पञ्चच
मानवा येभ्यो ज्योतिरमृतं मर्त्येभ्य उद्यन्तसूर्यो रश्मिभिरातनोति ।। *Ibid.* 12-1-15

To keep the earth/soil purified, we should follow the instructions given in Vishnu Smriti

ब्राह्मे मुहूर्ते चोत्थाय मूत्रपुरिषोत्सर्गं कुर्यात् । --न अप्रच्छादितायां भूमौ । न
फालकृष्टांयाम् न चोषरे न शाब्दले । न पथि । न रथ्यायां न उद्याने । न
उद्यानोदकसमीपयोः - न गोव्रजे । न आकाशे । नोदके ।

One should get up early in the morning for Bowl movement and should not do it on an uncovered land, not in the field, not on the ploughed ground, not on the lawn, not in the street, not on a small road, not in the garden, not near the garden or water—reservoir, not in the cowpen, not in the open air or space, and not in water reservoir.

In one hymn of the Atharva Veda the "mighty mystery" to be known is that Heaven and Earth are the universal Father and Mother. In another it is the sun, the vivifier and generator, who brings to birth both heave and Earth.

The origins of the earth come first. When she was as yet hidden in a fluid state in the bosom of the primeval waters, the seers were already seeking to discern her by means of sacrifice.[9]

A geographical description, or, as we could equally aptly call it, a highly poetical vision of nature, follows. The earth is composed of hills and plains, of snow-clad peaks, of deserts, oceans, and rivers, of lakes and streams, trees and plants, rocks and stones. The seasons appear with unfailing regularity and bring to her their own gradations of climate. Even included in an account of her fragrance, which is described distinctively according to whether it emanates from plants or from water, from the lotus, from animals, from human beings, or even from the Gods. We are also told to her underground treasures of jewels and gold.

Third, earth is the dwelling place of people. It is upon her that in the beginning the first humans were scattered abroad. It is upon her that they sing and dance and find their happiness. It is she who diversifies Men's speech into different languages. It is upon her many paths that men and women pass to and fro and it is her highways that men use for their wagons and chariots.

Further, the earth is protected by the Gods; she is the conveyer of Agni, Universal Fire, and the place where men offer ritual sacrifice. It is upon her breast that men build their altars and construct their tabernacles and shelters and ritual posts. It is she in whose praise priests chant their hymns. The earth points beyond herself by means of the cultic acts of Gods and Men.

She is, furthermore, the dwelling place of all living creatures, mention of whom is not omitted. She is the home of cattle and horses, of the beasts, of the forest, of deer and birds, reptiles and two-legged creatures.

She is, finally, a cosmic giant, a cosmic power, the receiver of prayers and the bestower of blessings, the protector and the inscrutable judge. Ecology was a sacred science for Vedic Man.

Pritivi Mahini
R.V.V. 84

The Might Earth

The mighty burden of the mountains bulk
Rests, Earth, upon your shoulders; rich in torrents,
You germinate the seed with quickening power,

Our hymns of praise resounding now invoke you,
O far-flung Earth, the bright one.
Like a neighing steed you drive abroad your storm clouds.

You in your sturdy strength hold fast the forests,
Clamping the trees all firmly to the ground
When rains and lightning issue from your clouds.

Bhumi Sukta
A.V. XII-1

The Vedic attitude towards the earth springs from mankind's primordial experience of being on the one hand a guest, and on the other an offspring, of Earth. The earth is undoubtedly mother, is close to Man, but at the same time she is also alien, other and aloof. The earth is the foundation, the basis out of which emerges all that exists and on which everything rests. The earth is the basis of life and, when considered as a divine being, she always occupies a special place among the Gods.

Man is the earth and earthly, but the earth is not simply nature, is not merely geographical or material; it is part of Man himself, so that Man can no more live without the earth then he can live without a body. At the same time, though he stands on the earth, he also stands above her. Man is more than earth. The earth is the mother of Man, but Man is also lord over the earth.[10]

Today, we need a communion, that our heart be wide enough so that no one is excluded as all of them have a well defined subtle role to build up ecological capital and to maintain the balance in nature.

In the 21st century the Deep Ecologists begin to feel a sense of oneness with nature and as a part of Natural order of life, the very same philosophy our ancestors practices, propagated and insisted to adopt to maintain peace in the planet.

They had respect to nature, which is the fastest, cleanest and most refined level of inter-species communication and communion.

In the last, we can say that Ancient Sanskrit Literature has many solutions to solve problems of Air and Water pollution. We must make use of them in our programmes. Scientists today are engaged merely with pollutions of Air, Water, Earth, etc. while ancient Sanskrit literature contains not only the need and methods of removing pollution of water and Air but also the medicinal use of Water, Air and Earth. The Naturopathy which is now coming up as a system of medicine is mostly based on treatment with air, water and earth. The Sanskrit literature also contains the impact of heavenly bodies, beyond our planets, on the Air and Water. What is needed is the expert collaboration of scientists and Sanskrit to solve the problem arising out of Air, Water and Earth pollution as well as take their positive benefits.

Land is a finite resource and put to many competing uses. It comprises soils, minerals, water and biota. In India land is a source of livelihoot for 60% of the population through agriculture and related activities. Population growth and the consequent demand for land, water and biological resources has put tremendous pressure on land.

The marine environment, which includes the adjacent coastal areas supports productive and protective habitats such as mangroves, coral reefs and sand dune. The marine environment is facing a number of pressures, arising out of need of people, and the multiple uses that coastal and marine area can be put to. These pressures contribute to the depletion of marine resources and degradation of the marine environment. In the absence of good management, these pressures may result in severe stress. A healthier marine environment needs integrated policy approaches, which involve scientific disciplines to address the complexity of the interaction between the social and natural systems in the coastal and marine environment. The need for a single administration to deal with governmental responsibilities for policy implementation is recognized and the GOI is taking steps to initiate programmes which involves inter-departmental collaboration.

Mountains are an important source of water, energy and biological diversity. Furthermore, they are source of such key resources as minerals, forest products and agricultural products of recreation. As a major ecosystem representing the complex and interrelated ecology of our planet, mountain environments are essential to the survival of the global ecosystem. Mountain ecosystems are, however, rapidly changing. They are susceptible to accelerated soil erosion, landslides and rapid loss of habitat and loss of indigenous knowledge. As a student, most global mountain areas are experiencing environmental degradation. Hence, the proper management of mountain resources and socio-economic development of the people deserves immediate action.

Land degradation is the most important environmental problems affecting extensive areas of land in both developed and developing countries. The problem of soil erosion is particularly acute in developing countries, while problems of sailiniation, waterlogging, soil pollution and loss of soil fertility are increasing in all countries. Land degradation is serious because the productivity of huge areas of land is declining just when populations are increasing rapidly and the demand on the land is growing to produce more food, fibre and fuel. Efforts to control land degradation, particularly in developing countries, have had limited success to date. Well planned, long-term national and regional land conservation and rehabilitation programmes, with strong political support and adequate funding, are now needed. While land-use planning and land zoning, combined with better land management, should provide long-term solutions, it is urgent to arrest land degradation and launch conservation and rehabilitation programmes in the most critically affected and vulnerable areas.[11]

The approach Paper to the Tenth Five Year Plan assigns high priorities to area-specific programmes such as watersheds, river valleys, arid areas and wastelands.

It is imperative to ensure the full participation of and a sense of ownership amongst the beneficiaries of land development programmes in order to make these sustainable. There is a need to involve the stakeholders from the planning stage onwards and address other socio-economic and poverty issues in land development programmes.[12]

CONCLUSION

It would be unrealistic, however, to suppose that the damage that has been done, and still continues to be done, can be arrested and undone in the short-term. Rather, long-term global policies must be envisaged and, if they are to be successful, they will require changes in our perceptions of man in nature. If our global physical environment is not to be further degraded, we must change our conceptual environment, our ways of thinking and behaving. Perhaps the worst environment pollution is pollution of the mind, and the greatest need is for well thought out principles of environment ethics.

All spheres of human conduct private and public, are subject to ethical principles or rules. When governments or other corporate bodies despoil the environment in the name of development or political dominance or national security, when government adopt *laissez faire* policies that permit the exploitation of nature for narrow, short-term gains, they contravene the basic ethical principle of the greatest good for the greatest number of people.

In reviewing all these environmental effect of water, earth and air and their possible dangers, we should however reach too gloomy a conclusion. A comforting finding, which may be extended to many other aspects, is the recent discovery that fish caught in the last century and preserved in museums have been found to have similar mercury levels as those found in fish today. And after all, the human race with its great adaptability has survived the innumerable disasters and environmental hazards it has encountered for several million years. Modern replacing old ones, and there is no reason to doubt that man's ingenuity and intelligence will prevail as far as environment problems are concerned.

(a) Faecal-borne diseases can be prevented by using a latrine.
(b) Pathogenic microbes survive from days to years in the moist soil and may become wind borne.
(c) Social status and prestige can be attained by having a latrine.
(d) Constipation, particularly among rural women, can be eliminated.
(e) Privacy can be achieved.
(f) Low cost sanitation options are available, and these can be maintained in an eco-friendly way.

Lack of sanitation causes many diseases related to human excreta, sewerage disposal, garbage and the use of pesticides and the industrial and radio active wastes, (see Chart 4.3). Following the suspected plague outbreak in the country during 1994 the planning commission constituted a high power committee on urban solid waste management in India under the chairmanship of member (health). This committee undertook a comprehensive review of current situation of urban solid waste

CHART 4.3

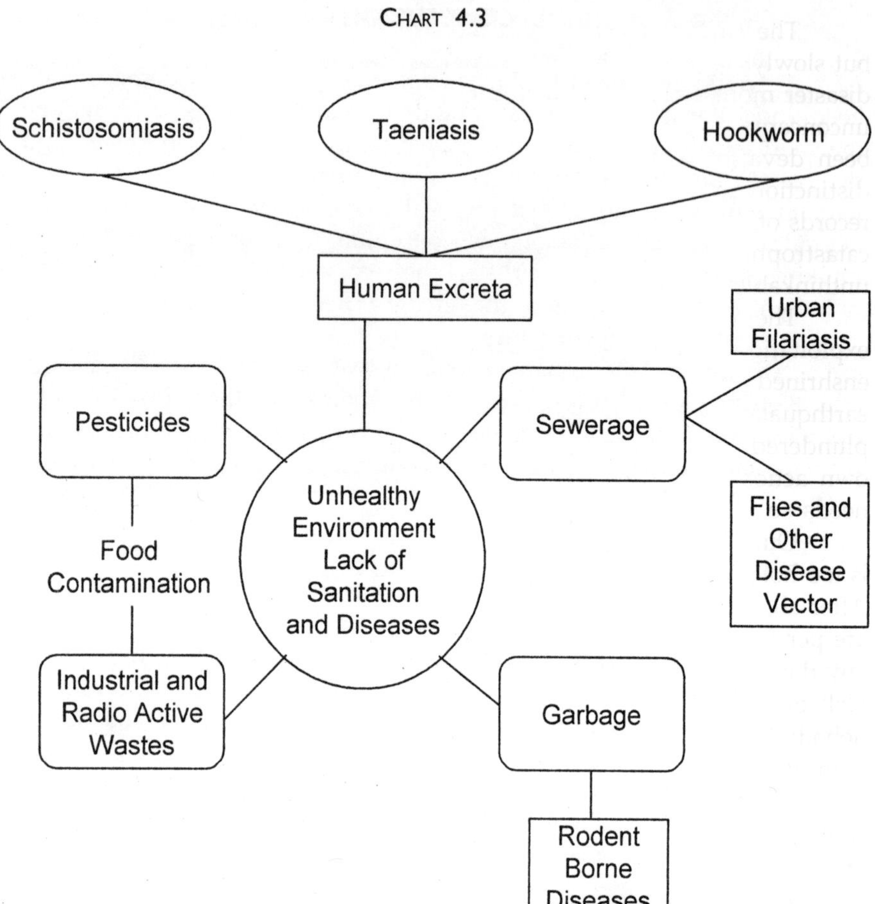

management, specially in cities with one million or more inhabitants and made recommendations for safe methods for collection, transportation of waste and suitable cost-effective, environmentally friendly methods for disposal of these wastes. Pilot projects exploring the dimensions of the problem and aimed at seeking realistic solutions were initiated during the eighth plan period.

Historically, sanitation has been provided a lower priority by the planners. Most of our cities and towns are not in sanitary conditions due to inadequate facilities of toilets and wastewater disposal and solid waste management facilities. Over the years, if anything, the quality urbanization and rapid population growth, mounting costs, growing gap between the needs of these services and the resources of the municipal bodies has increased managerial problems. In the rural areas, even elementary sanitary services are non-existent in most villages.

Carl Sagan in his magnificent, awe inspiring work Cosmos has described human predicament and dilemmas that surround us in the most thought provoking manner:

The earth is a lovely and more or less placid place. Things change, but slowly. We can lead a full life and never personally encounter a natural disaster more violent than a storm. And so we become complacent, relaxed unconcerned. But in the history of Nature, the record is clear. Worlds have been devastated. Even we humans have achieved the dubious technical distinction of being able to make our own disasters, planets where the records of the past have been preserved there is abundant evidence of major catastrophes. It is all a matter of time scale. An event that would be unthinkable in a hundred years may be inevitable in a hundred million.

The greed, lust and material urges in modern times have led to the exploitation of the mother earth ignoring all the valuable principles enshrined in Ancient Sanskrit Literature leading to disastrous results—earthquake, cyclone, floods, deforestation, etc. The mother earth has been plundered and has become unsafe place to live. This is the result of our own actions. What is required is to make use of earth only to meet the needs so that earth and human beings can live in perfect harmony.

Our lovely blue planet, the earth, is the only home we know. Venus is too hot. Mars is too cold. But the earth is just right, a heaven for humans. After all, we evolved here. But our congenial climate may be unstable. We are per furlong our poor planet in serious and contradictory ways. Is there any danger of driving the environment of the earth towards the planetary Hell of Venus or the global ice age of Mars? The simple answer is that nobody knows. The study of the global climate, the comparison of the earth with other worlds, are subjects in their earliest stage of development. They are fields that are poorly and grudgingly funded. In our ignorance, we continue to push and pull to pollute the atmosphere and brighten the land, oblivious of the fact that the long-term consequences are largely unknown.

A few million years ago, when human beings first evolved on Earth, it was already a middle aged world, 4.6 billion years along from the catastrophes and impetuosities of its youth. But we humans now represent a new and perhaps decisive factor. Our intelligence and our technology have given us the power of affect the climate. How will we use this power? Are we willing to tolerate ignorance and complacency in matters that affect the entire human family? Do we value short-term advantages above the welfare of the Earth? Or will we think on longer time scales, with concern for our children and our grandchildren, to understand and protect the complex life-support system of our planet. The earth is a tiny and fragile world. It needs to be cherished.

Bearer of all things, hoard of treasures rare, sustaining, Mother Earth. What of thee I dig out, let that quickly grow over. Let me not hurt thy vitals, or the heart.

—Atarva Veda (c 1200 BC)

"O Mother Earth! Sacred are the hills, snowing mountains, and deep forests, be kind to us and bestow upon us happiness. May you continue supporting people of all races and nations."

—Atharva Veda (c 1200 B.C.)

NOTES AND REFERENCES

1. Gurcharn Singh, Pollution to Purity of Environment, New Delhi, Deep & Deep, 2000, p. 42.
2. B. Sudhakara Reddy, The Urban challenge, in India Development Report, 2002, Indira Gandhi Institute of Development Research, Oxford University Press, New Delhi, *op. cit.*, pp. 134-35.
3. Air Act, Section 2(a).
4. S. Murty, Economic Growth and Environment: Some Issues in Environmental challenges of the 21st century, Editors S. Radha, Amar Singh Sankhyan, New Delhi, Deep & Deep, 2000, pp. 58-59.
5. GOI: Planning Commission, Ninth Five Year Plan, pp. 930-32.
6. V.H. Date, Upanisads Retold, Vol. I, 1999, Delhi, Munshiram Manoharlal, p. 267.
7. Tushar R. Hathi, Water Crisis and Indigenous Approach Towards Resource Utilisation in G.S. Monga, (Ed.) *Environment and Development*, Deep & Deep, New Delhi, 2000, pp. 270-71.
8. WHO: *World Health*, January, 1979, p. 3.
9. UN: Report on the World Social Situation, New York, 1971, pp. 167-68.
10. B. Sudhakara Reddy, *op. cit.*, pp. 135-36
11. Madhusudan Mishra, "Apah in Vedic Literature: An Environment Approach", in V.N. Jha (ed.), *op. cit.*, p. 36.
12. *Ibid.*, 2.24; p. 149.

CHAPTER 5

CONSERVATION OF BIO-DIVERSITY AND HEALTH EDUCATION

> Biodiversity is the basis for life support systems and hence it should be preserved and managed for a sustainable future.
>
> —*Author*

Conservation of Bio-diversity and Health Education

Biodiversity is defined as variability and variety in life forms including genes, species and ecosystems. Biodiversity conservation seeks to maintain life support systems provided by nature. Adding to the impact of natural processes, human intervention has had an adverse effect on these life support systems and thereby on biodiversity. Much attention therefore has been focused internationally on formulating policies towards the conservation of biodiversity over the past decade.

The idea of conservation is not a new one for India. References are scattered in Indian literature emphasizing the conservation of fauna and flora. Ashoka's Pillar Edicts are a glowing example. The descriptions of fauna and flora of the area also occur very often in the ancient Indian literature. These references and descriptions are not surprising and go well with India's cultural heritage which in essence has been conservational in approach. The Indian region (8°-38° N and 60°-47.5° E) with a total area of 328 million hectares is indeed very rich in biological diversity. It is estimated that about 45,000 species of plants occur in this country. The vascular flora, which forms the conspicuous vegetation cover, itself comprises 15,000 species, of which more than 60 per cent are endemic and have so far not been reported from anywhere else in the world. The total plant wealth of the country includes not out the usually large, showy-flowered vascular plants, but a large number of non-flowering plants, viz. ferns, liverworts, algae and fungi. The region is equally rich in fauna. More than 50,000 species of insects, 4,000 of moll uses, 6,500 of other invertebrates, 2,000 of fish, 140 of amphibians, 420 of reptiles, 1200 of birds and 340 of mammals (i.e. more than 65,000 species of animals) are recorded from this country.

The wild relatives of the crop plants together with related species constitute gene pools which are rich source of many important and desirable traits. Such spices are distributed in centers of diversity/origin of crop plants. Over 150 species of economic plants have their genetic diversities in the Hindustan Center of Aversity (Zeven and Zhukovsky, 1975) in the Indian subcontinent and most of these species do grow in some of the proposed Biosphere Reserves. Besides, there is a vast number of other economic plants which are utilized only from their wild populations which have their home in the proposed biosphere reserves.

Parallel to such an enormous diversity in plants, there is also considerable diversity in domesticated animals and their wild and semi-wild relatives such as buffalo, goat, sheep, pig, poultry, camel, ass, ýak, horse, etc. The productivity of these animals by the standards of developed countries is very low. However, having undergone periods of rigorous selection, races are adaptable to heat and parasitic stresses, and can survive on very poor roughage. These are very important characteristics, now in great demand in Australia, the USA and the Latin America. Obviously, such genetic treasure at present existing in the wild or with tribal populations also needs to be conserved.

Plants and animals are part and parcel of human being in Sanskrit literature. It cannot be imagined that they can live independently. That is why people in India used to give proper respect to plants and animals. Most of the houses must contain one plant or the other for worship, e.g. Tulsi, Pipal, Banana, etc. People celebrate many festivals in the name of animals like Nag-Panchmi, Goverdhan, etc. There were in-built ethical principles which promoted the growth of plants and animals. At the time of death, donation of a cow, was considered to be a good omen as the donor would get place in heaven. Whether, it may be a birth ceremony or marriage ceremony or death ceremony, these could not be performed without the leaves or fruits of plants. Desi-ghee which is the product of cow milk is needed on all ceremonies. Even, the poets, philosophers, lovers, etc. would bring in flowers of plants to depict their feelings. Even daily puja to God requires some leaves/flowers. Thus human being cannot live without plant/animals.

Our planets' essential goods and service depend on the variety and variability of genes, species, populations and ecosystems. Biological resources feed and clothe us and provide housing, medicines and spiritual nourishment. The natural eco-systems of forests, savannahs, pastures and rangelands, deserts, tundras, rivers, lakes, and seas contain most of the Earth's biodiversity. Farmers' fields and gardens are also of great importance as repositories, while gene banks, botanical gardens, zoons and other germplasm repositories make a small but significant contributions. The current decline in biodiversity is largely the result of human activity and represents a serious threat to human development.

Out of eight good qualities of the soul, the first one is compassion on all creatures, others are forbearance, freedom from anger, purity, quietism auspiousness, freedom from avarice and freedom from covetousness.

—Gautmadharma Sutra

Plants, gardens, forests have been benefiting human life and animal life since the evolution of life on this earth. We cannot imagine human life without plants. We need them in all seasons as different plants fructify in different seasons. Ancient Sanskrit literature is full of the knowledge about their origin, classification, development, utility, and medicinal properties.

The entire universe is in motion under certain rules. These are accepted as unchangeable natural laws which are known as RITA. All sentient and insentient objects are tied with this rule. The sun, the moon, the planets, the stars, the nights and days, the seasons—winter and summer, growth of vegetation, flowering and bearing of fruits by trees and then perishing, birth and childhood, old-age and death—all are the different aspects of one eternal law. Indians are believers in these eternal laws. Therefore, they pray to live for hundred years. They always made effort to strike balance with nature, not to conquer it. Therefore, they not only respect vegetation but also worship it. They neither desired the immortality of the body nor made prayer for this because they have been having abiding faith in natural laws. They don't believe that by breaking the laws of nature, they will spend their lives in peace and prosperity.

We all, human beings and animals depend upon plants which came into existence first than human and animal life. Life is impossible without plants. (Manusmriti 46-48)

To quote Manusmriti

उद्भिजाः स्थावरास्सर्व्रे बीजकाण्डप्ररोहिणः
ओषध्यः फलपाकान्ताः बहुपुष्पफलोपगाः ।। 46 ।।
पुष्पाः फलवन्तो ये ते वनस्पतयः स्मृताः ।
पुष्पिणः फलितश्चैव वृक्षास्तूभयतः स्मृताः ।। 47।।
गुच्छगुल्मं तु विविधं तथैव तृणजातयः ।
बीजकाण्डरुहाण्येव प्रताना वल्क एव च ।। 48 ।।
तमसा बहुरुपेणा वेष्टिताः कर्महेतुना ।
अन्तःसज्ञा भवन्त्येते सुखदुःखसमन्विताः ।। 49।।

The plants were put to different uses as contained in Sanskrit Literature and these have positive effects on environment. Life without plants is impossible to imagine.

सस्नेहानामथोष्णेन तिलकल्केन चाविकम् ।
कार्पासिकानों वस्त्राणां शुद्धिः स्याद्बहिरम्बुना ।। 14-63।।
तत्किमर्थमपास्यैतालन लकारान् जटा धृताः ।
चीनांशुकं परित्यज्य किं त्वं वल्कलधारिणी ।। 51-59।।
बटूरूपं समाधाय आषाढी मुन्ज्मेखली ।। 51-45 ।।

–वामन पुराण

Let us discuss the role of plants in maintaining environmental equilibrium.

1. Supply of Oxygen

Plants absorb carbon dioxide produced by human and animal life continuously and through photosynthesis emit oxygen, vital for the survival of human and animal life. If the plants are cut or their number decreases, the result would be depletion of oxygen supply causing many health hazards. Therefore, our ancient Sanskrit literature prohibits cutting of trees or their parts without any purpose. It was considered to be a sin to cut trees as trees were like their own children.

2. Medicinal

In India, the Vedas, written in circa 11500 BC contained substantial material on herbs. Lord Brahma is known as the profounder of Ayurveda "The science of life." The knowledge passed on different persons. The work of Agnivesa has come to us as "Charak a Samheta" written by Charaka in 700 BC. This medical treatise includes about 350 herbs. The human body responds better with herbal remedies as herbs act both as medicine and nutrient. Now herbs and plants extracts are being used world over.

The Ayurveda system of medicine which took birth in India uses different parts of plants for restoring health of the people. Even today, advanced countries where allopathic system originated, use Ayurvedic system. This is based purely on the flora and fauna of the area.

Patanjali's Mahabhasya rules p. 4.1.71, 1.2.45, 4.3.55, 8.4.6, 6.1.157 pertain to medicinal use of plants as plants were the only source of life saving qualities.

As stated in Rigveda and Yajurveda, plants have medicinal value.

ओषधीः प्राचुच्यवुर्यत् किं च तन्वोरपः - ऋक् 10-97-10
ओषधीर्हस्त आददे आत्मा यक्ष्मस्य नश्यति - ऋक् 10-97-11
इष्टकृतिर्नाम वो माता । - यजुं 12-83

In Vayu Purana, it has been stated that one can live upto 10,000 years by taking Panasajuice

तत्र दिव्यो महावृक्षः पनसः षड्रसाश्रयः ।
ईश्वरो ब्रह्मणः पुत्र कामचारी मनोजव : ।।
तस्य पीत्वा फलरसं जीवन्ति हि समायुतम् ।।

- पूर्वार्ध 43-4

Matsya Purana lists 85 plants which are of great medicinal value (De, 218 Muees 22-34).

1. Vandhya, 2. Karkotaki, 3. Visnukranta, 4. Utkata, 5. Satamuli, 6. Sitananda, 7. Bala, 8. Moca, 9. Patolika, 10. Somapinda, 11. Nisa,

12. Dagdharuha, 13. Kamalini, 14. Visali, 15. Sankhamulika, 16. Candali, 17. Hastimagadha, 18. Goparni, 19. Ajaparni, 20. Karambhika, 21. Rakta, 22. Maharakta, 23. Barhisikha, 24. Kosataki, 25. Naktamala, 26. Priyala, 27. Sulocani, 28. Varuni, 29. Vasugandha, 30. Shyamala, 31. Iswari, 32. Shivagandha, 33. Shyamala. 34. Vamshanalika, 35. Jatukali, 36. Mahasweta, 37. Sweta, 38. Madhuyastika, 39. Vajraka, 40. Paribhadra, 41. Sindhu Varaka, 42. Jeevananda, 43. Vasuchhidra, 44. Nata nagara Kantaka, 45. Nala, 46. Jalee, 47. Jaati, 48. Vata patrika, 49. Kartaswara, 50. Mahaneela, 51. Kunduru, 52. Hansapadika, 53. Mandukaparni, 54. Varahi, 55. Tanduliyaka, 56. Sarpaksi, 57. Lavali, 58. Brahmi, 59. Vaswarpa, 60. Sukhakara 61. Rujapaha, 62. Vriddhikari, 63. Salyada, 64. Patrika, 65. Rohini, 66. Raktamala, 67. Mahousadhi, 68. Amalaka, 69. Vandaka, 70. Syama, 71. Chitraphala, 72. Kakali, 73. Ksrakakoli, 74. Pluparni, 75. Kesini, 76. Vrscikali, 77. Mahanaga, 78. Satavari, 79. Garudi, 80. Vega, 81. Kumudini, 82. Utpalini 83. Mahabhamilata, 84. Unmadini 85. Somaraji.[1]

Ancient Sanskrit literature has not only listed the names of medicinal plants but also mentions their properties, method of use, quantity to be taken. All this knowledge is contained in different branches of Ayurveda.

Sanskrit literature contains the list of plants for food, for ceremonial purposes, cleansing material, plants in furniture, etc.

3. Natural Calamities

Vayu Purana in Chapter 8 explains the occurrence of calamities and disturbing of eco-system when the plants are cut in mass through a story. We are witnessing today increase in calamities like earthquake, floods, deforestation, cyclones, etc. due to cutting of trees. The whole of the ecology has been disturbed and is out of control. It needs to be reversed other wise we may have to face disastrous consequences.

Felling of trees is considered to be a sin and person doing such activity will go to hell as felling of trees result in disasters.

छेदनं वृक्षजातीनां द्वितीयं नरकं स्मृतम् ।

-वामन पु० अध्याय 61.2

फलदानां तु वृक्षाणां छेदने जप्यं ऋक्शतम् ।। 36 ।।
गुल्मवल्लीलतानां तु पुष्पितानां च वीरुधाम् ।
अण्डजानां च सर्वेषां स्वेदजानां च सर्वश: ।। 37 ।।
फलपुष्पोद्भवानांश्च घृतप्राशो विशोधनम् ।

कूर्मपुराण उत्तरार्ध अ० 33

This chapter also warns those who cut trees unnecessarily and in the process suffer from bad health. To give some original sloka as an example.

CHART 5.1

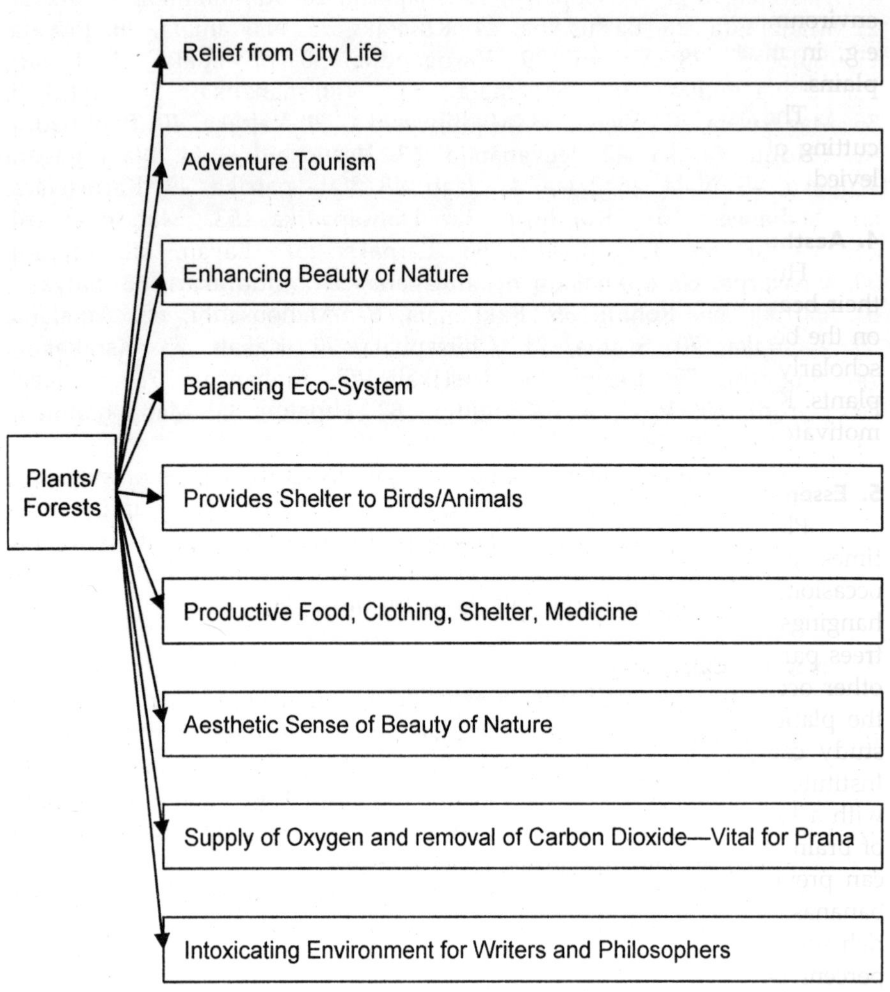

वृक्षच्छेत्ता वृथा यस्तु स नाडीव्रणवान् भेवत् ।
वक्ष्यामि तत्प्रतीकारं सर्वलोकहिताय तु ।।
दशकूपसमा वापी दशवापीसमो द्रुमः ।।
दशद्रुमसमः पुत्रः दशपुत्रसमो टुमः ।।
पुत्रैर्विना शुभफलं न भवेन्नराणाम्
दुष्पुत्रकैरपि तथोभयलोकनाशः ।।
एतद्विचार्य सुधिया परिपाल्य वृक्षान् ।
यत्नेन वेदविधिना परिकल्पनीयाः ।।

13th Chapter of Dhankhanda

Plant Ecology is the study of the relationship of plants with their environment. The structure of plants would depend upon the ecology, e.g. in mountains plants will be different as compared to deserts and plains.

The Manusmriti and the Arthasastra have taken a serious view of cutting of trees. This is considered as an offence for which punishment is levied.

4. Aesthetic Value

Human beings in the company of plants enjoyed the beauty of plants, their beautiful aroma and fragrance. Wordsworth has written many poems on the beauty of flowers. Many Indian writers like Kalidas, published many scholarly works depicting the beauty, splendour and enchanting quality of plants. King Dusyant when he sees Shakuntla in the midst of flowers, got motivated to love her and ultimately marry her.

5. Essentials for Sacred Occasions

Plants have been held in high esteems in Sanskrit Literature from times immemorial. The plants are considered auspicious on sacred occasions. For example, leaves of mango trees are put in the form of hangings on the upper side of doors to welcome the birth of child. Banana trees parts are put while doing puja at the time of marriage ceremony and other occasions. A recent research study proves the reason of worshiping the plants which are of great use directly and indirectly. According to a study carried out by Dr. Deborah M. Green, MD of the Neuroscience Institute at the Queen's Medical Center in Honolulu, Hawaii, USA, people with a low amount of potassium in their diet may have an increased risk of brain stroke. Bananas are rich in potassium. Therefore, a banana a day can prevent the deficiency of potassium. Rich in vitamins A, C and B-6, bananas also contain high levels of calcium and phosphorus. They are a rich source of nutrition with 16 percent fibre, 15 percent Vitamin C and 11 percent potassium, we need every day. A banana is low in calories and contains no fat or sodium. It has enough energy to keep us on our feet all day.

People worship different trees especially Tulsi, pipal trees whose medicinal values have been proved. In Ramayana, Hanuman brings Sanjeevani herb to save Laxman from Coma. There are references in Sanskrit literature when plants have been used for food, clothing, shelter, medicine, fuel, to protect soil, erosion, beauty, etc.

6. Status of Plants is Equated with God

Plant in Sanskrit is known as Vrska and the growth of plants is the development of environment. Trees are devatas, gods. Tulsi is a goddess, Rudraksha is a diety. We have rudrakasha trees. Rudraksha is Shiva's favourite.

7. Plants Provide Space for Meditation and True Knowledge

Mahatma were enlightened and attained jnanam, wisdom, under the trees. Lord Buddha was enlightened under the banyan tree and became a jnani. Dattatreya, who was the embodiment of the trinity, Brahma, Vishnu and Mahesh, were enlightened under the gular tree. He attained jnana and samadhi under a tree. Neem tree is being used in large number of medicines, and products as its anti-septic potentiality is being recognized now by foreign and Indian scientist. This was already available in Ancient Sanskrit Literature.

8. Need of Developing Equilibrium and Integration with Eco-System Especially Plants

Let us illustrate the role of Sanskrit Literature in promoting good eco-system. Agamashastra concentrates on principles to protect and develop forest wealth. Yajurveda deals with biological functions to ensure ecological equilibrium. Dharamshastras point out details of using resources without disturbing eco-system. Vrksa Ayurveda, Gaja Ayurveda, Ashva Ayurveda, etc. deal with Biotechnology and Genetic engineering to ensure better yield of good quality. We can quote hundreds of source which deal with eco-system directly or indirectly.

Man is advised in Mahabharata to develop equilibrium and integration with all existent beings. Human beings should utilise all the fruits of nature with rationality and gratitude.

सर्वभूतहित is the watch word of Mahabharata.

हितं यत्सर्वभूतानामात्मनश्च सुखावहम् ।
तत्कुर्यादीश्वरे होतत् मूला सर्वार्थसिद्धये ।। (उद्योग—Ch. 37.)
भूतानां हि यथा धर्मो रक्षणं परमा दया । (Ch. 73)
सुभाषी प्रिकृत् शान्त: सर्वसत्त्वाविहिंसक: (अनुशासन—Ch 163)
अद्रोहेणैव भूतानां यो धर्मस्स सतां मत: (शान्ति—Ch. 21)
सर्वभूतहिते तिष्ठ धर्मं चैव प्रतिस्मरन् (*Ibid.*—Ch. 151)

Bhishma's final advice before his स्वर्गारोहण to one and all born in the lineage of Bharata also mentions the same.

आनृशंसपरैर्भाव्यं सदैव नियतात्मभि:
ब्रह्मण्यैधर्मशीलैश्च तपोनित्यैश्च भारता: ।। (अनुशासन—Ch. 163)

Control over one's senses and a good and healthy management of one's life is at the root of a good society and a good physical environment according to Vyāsa. He poses a fundamental question. How can a man who can not organise his own life properly ever contribute towards the welfare of the community? The physical environment is of great significance.

आत्मानं योऽत्रिसंधत्ते सोऽन्यस्य स्यात्कथं हित: ? (शान्ति—Ch. 143)

Self-contentments and internal harmoney among the members of a community is at the root of a healthy environment according to Vyasa. One who is disorganised within cannot promote balance and harmony around.[2]

The new priority for environmental sustainability that has emerged in the 1990s does not negate the need for agriculture to continue contributing to growth, poverty alleviation, and increased food security. It is just that agriculture is now required to do this in ways that do not degrade the environment. Hazell argues that two fundamentally different types of environmental problems are associated with agriculture. The first type arises in intensive farming systems and is associated with the misuse of modern inputs (irrigation water, fertilizers, and pesticides). The second type arises in extensive farming systems and is associated with rapid population growth, poverty, and growth in agricultural productivity insufficient to meet the increasing need for food and livelihood.

A general finding of the past on policy perspectives is that significant strides can be made toward sustainability. But clearly, appropriate policies and institutions are a precondition. These are important for growth, equity, and environmental reasons; they are also needed to find appropriate technical solutions.

Agriculture in developing countries has been remarkably successful during the past few decades in enabling food production to keep pace with the growing population. This success has been achieved in part at the cost of placing more stress on natural resources and the environment. As we look to the future, the need to continue increasing food production, while at the same time minimizing environmental damages, conserving the resource base, and reducing poverty, hunger, and malnutrition, poses an enormous challenge.

The challenges for the rural sector loom large, and the constraints are serious, but with good governance and a real commitment to environmentally and socially sustainable rural development at all levels, much can be achieved. We at the World Bank and those of us involved with CGIAR will do everything we can to alleviate rural poverty and hunger and to assist with participatory rural development, while safeguarding natural resources and the environment.[3]

9. Plants are Living Entities and thus Needs Care, Protection and Affection

Plants have all the faculties like seeing, smelling, fasting, touching. This has been proved even by modern science. It has been proved that the music near the plants make them grow faster and better. Bharadvaja and Bhrugu have gone deep in their study.

उष्मतो म्लायते पर्णं त्वक्फलं पुष्पमेव च ।
म्लायते शीर्यते चापि स्पर्शस्तेनाद्य विद्यते ।।
वाय्वग्न्यशनि निर्घोषैः फलं पुष्पं विशीर्यते ।
श्रोत्रेण गृह्यते शब्दः तस्मात् शृण्वन्तिपादपाः ।।
वल्ली वेष्टयते वृक्षं सर्वतश्चैव गच्छति ।
न ह्यद्ष्टेश्च र्मोगॅस्ति तस्मात्पश्यन्तिपादपा : ।।
पुण्यापुण्यैस्तथा गन्धैः धूपैश्चविविधैरपि ।
आरोगाः पुष्पितास्सन्ति तस्माज्जिधन्ति पादपा : ।
पादै : सलिलपानाच व्याधीनां चापि दर्शनात् ।
व्याधिप्रतिक्रियत्वाच्च विद्यते रसनं द्रमें ।
वक्त्रेणोत्पलनालेव यर्थोर्ध्वं जलमाददेत ।
तथा पवन संयुक्त पादैः पिबति पादपः ।।

Finally

सुखदुः खयोश्च ग्रहणाच्छिन्नस्य च विरोहणात् ।
जीवं पश्यामि वृक्षाणां अचैतन्यं न विद्यते ।। (शान्ति—Ch. 184)[4]

Some times the mantras that are uttered at particular times depict the feelings in their mind effectively. Look at this verse from the nirnayasindhu:

बिल्ववृक्ष महाभाग सदा त्वं शङ्क्करप्रिय ।।
गश्हीत्वा तव शाखां च देवीपूजां करोम्यहम् ।।
शाखाच्छेदोद्भवं दुःख न च कार्यं त्वया प्रभो ।
गृहीत्वा तव शाखां च पूज्या दुर्ग्रेति च स्मृतिः ।।

Oh Sir, Bilva tree, you are always dear to the Lord Samkara. Taking your branch I now worship the goddess (Parvati). Please bear the pains of cutting your branch.

It is obvious from this that he is fully aware of the pains he is causing to the tree by cutting its branch. It is also noteworthy that the tree is addressed as lord.[5]

13th Chapter of Danakhanda even goes to the extent to say that tending of trees is like bringing up one's son. Hemadri has quoted many verses from above source.[6]

अतीतानागतौ चोभौ पितृवंशौ च भारत ।
तरायेद्वक्षरोपी च तस्माद्धक्षांश्च रोपयेत् ।।
पुष्पैः सुरगणान् वृक्षाः फलैश्चापि तथा पितृन् ।
छायया चातिर्थास्तात पूजयन्ति महीरुहाः ।।
पुष्पिता : फलवन्तश्चः तारयन्ति परत्र च ।।
पुत्रवत् परियाल्याश्च पुत्रास्ते धर्मतः स्मृताः ।।

10. Human beings Need to Imbibe the Qualities of Self-sacrifice and Devotion to Duty from Plants

A poet bows down to Tree, the supreme preceptor who preaches to the world by its own example the lesson of self-sacrifice for the sake of serving others:

धत्ते भरं कुसुमपत्रफलावलीनां धर्मव्यथां वहति शीतभवां रुजं च ।
यो देहमर्पयति चान्यसुखस्य हेतोस्तस्मै वदान्यगुरवे तरवे नमस्ते ।।

247/14, Anyoktis

The tree bears the burden of rich foliage of blooming flowers and of juicy fruits; it forbears the formenting heat and also the agony caused by cold. Still it submits its body for the happiness of others. Salutations to such a tree, the preceptor of the benevolent.

If we cannot be such a devotee and offer salutation with a bent head, let us at least be thankful like the following poet:

भुक्तं स्वादुफलं कृतं च शयनं शाखाग्रजैः पल्लवैस्त्वच्छायापरिशीतलं सुसलिल पीतं व्यपनेश्रमैः
विश्रान्ताः सुचिरं परं सुमनसः प्रीतिः किमत्रोच्यते त्वं सन्मार्गतरुर्वयं च पथिका यामः पुनर्दर्शनम्

(248/20)

"O Tree, we enjoyed your sweet fruits; we rested on the bed made from your tender leaves; thus getting rid of our fatigue, we drank the water which was quite cool due to your shade. We relaxed under you for a long time. Still, what can be said about the love and affection of good people? You are after all a benevolent tree on the road-side and we are travellers moving from one place to another. Hence, we bid good-bye to you; see you again."

Hence the present age demands urgently and unavoidably that man should imbibe fully and perfectly environmental awareness and follow the age-old rule of "Live and Let Live." He should allow the surrounding Nature to grow and spread fragrance leading to his own progress and prosperity. Let him repeat 'सह वीर्यं करवावहै' and enjoy the conditions of ॐ शान्तिः शान्तिः शान्तिः

11. Forests Provide Socio-economic Development

Forests play a vital role in the economy of developing countries. A large segment of India's population depends on forests for energy, housing, fodder and small timber. The demands for forest products and services is increasing with the growth in population and economy whereas the forest cover in the country is deteriorating. The increasing demand of forest produce, land hunger by the increasing population and poverty are among the main causes of deterioration in forest cover. Environment friendly agriculture is the path way to sustainable food and livelihood security. It is based on the non-exploitative use of natural resources. It is based on

Gandhiji's advice, "Nature provides for everyone's needs but not everyone's greed." It is the spread of a greed revolution that causes harm to our life support systems. An ever-green revolution based on harnessing solar energy through green plants and adopting environment friendly agricultural practices can alone ensure opportunities for a productive and healthy life for all.[7]

Environment friendly agriculture is the pathway to sustainable food and livelihood security. It is based on the non-exploitative use of natural resources. It is based on Gandhiji's advice. "Nature provides for everyone's needs but not everyone's greed." It is the spread of a greed revolution that causes harm to our life support systems. An ever-green revolution based on harnessing solar energy through green plants and adopting environment friendly agricultural practices can alone ensure opportunities for a productive and healthy life for all.[8]

Past agricultural growth has been associated with a variety of environmental and resource problems including excessive deforestation and forest degradation, water depletion, water logging and salinization, fish stock depletion, soil degradation, health effects, and biodiversity losses.

In the last 8,000 years, world forest cover declined more than 40 percent, from 62 million to 33 million square kilometers (Bryant, Nielsen, and Tingley, 1997). Contemporary concern about deforestation focuses on tropical countries because that is where the majority of forest cover is being removed. In the period 1980-90, an estimated 137.3 million hectares of tropical forests were cleared, about 7.2 percent of the total that existed in 1980 (FAO, 1996). Any claims regarding the magnitude of global deforestation must be made with caution, however, because there are serious problems with the data and definitions used.

Regardless of the exact magnitude and location of tropical deforestation, it is clear that deforestation often implies:

- The loss of livelihoods for forest-dependent people, many of whom may not wish to be able to find other sources of employment.
- Decreasing stocks of fuel wood and no timber forest products as well as industrial timber.
- Greater soil erosion and river siltation.
- Substantial species and gene loss, in view of tropical forests high level of endemic biodiversity
- Substantial emission of carbon dioxide, which contributes to global warming.
- Other types of local and regional climate change.

We follow the Food and Agriculture Organization of the United Nations (FAO) In defining deforestation as "the sum of all . . . transitions from natural forest classes (continuous and fragmented) to all other classes.[9]

Forests cover about 8% of earth surface and sustain thousands of varieties of flora and fauna. These forests are being cut down by man both for wood as well as for farm land. The process of deforestation results in less photosynthesis and release of millions of tons of carbon dioxide into the atmosphere every year thus aggravating green-house effect, i.e. warming up. Trees generate oxygen, increase soil fertility, control soil erosion, control air-pollution and provide shelter to birds and animals besides providing fruits and flowers, shade preventing desertification. Thus, deforestation can cause the destruction of world's entire ecological balance. In this century alone we have destroyed 50% of the forests. Deforestation will lead to famine, drought, flooding and extinction of many plant and animal species. This may also lead to the extinction of remaining primitive tribes—Guajas in South America almost extinct, and the two tribes Parakana and Xikrin (now exist only in photographs or the slums of Rio-de-Janeiro).[10]

Vandana Shiva States that although, it is always local people who are held responsible for deforestation, it is commercial demands that have more frequently resulted in large-scale forest destruction. In the Himalaya region, there is evidence that it were the needs of the Empire and not of the local people that led to rapid forest denudation. According to Atkinson Gazetteer:

The forests were denuded of good trees in all places leading to deforestation. The destruction of trees of all species appears to have continued steadily and reached its climax between 1855 and 1861, when the demands of the Railway authorities induced numerous speculators to enter into contracts for sleepers, and these men were allowed, unchecked, to cut down old trees very far in excess of what they could possibly export, so that for some years after the regular forest operations commenced, the department was chiefly busy cutting up and bringing to the depot the timber left behind by the contractors.[11]

Deforestation often implies:

- The loss of livelihoods for forest-dependent people, many of whom may not wish or be able to find other sources of employment.
- Decreasing stocks of fuel wood and no timber forest products as well as of industrial timber.
- Greater soil erosion and river siltation
- Substantial loss of species and genes, in view of the high level of endemic biodiversity in tropical forests.
- Substantial emission of carbon dioxide, which contributes to global warming.
- Other types of local and regional climate change.

The concern is not only with deforestation but also with forest degradation, which can be defined as a decrease of density or increase of disturbance in forest classes. In the long-run, this may be just as important as deforestation itself.[12]

CHART 5.2

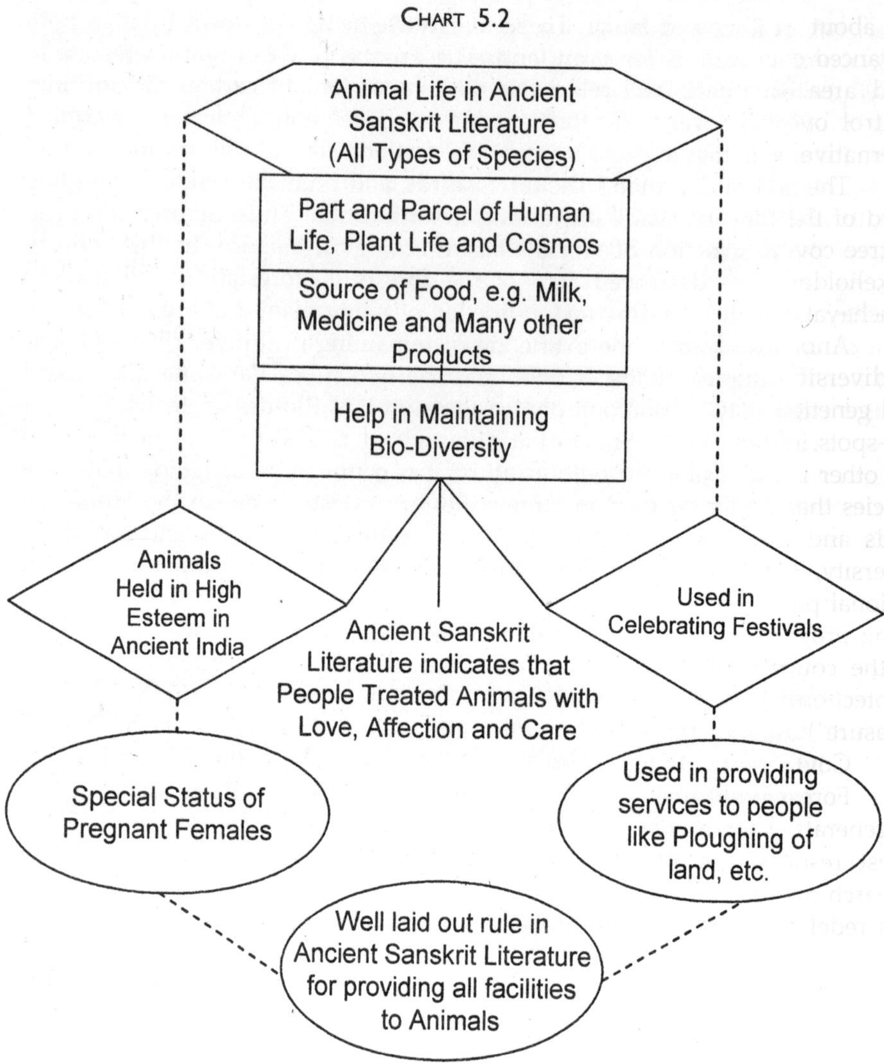

Forests are important for maintaining ecological balance and preserving the life supporting system of the earth. They are essential for food production, health and other aspects of human survival and sustainable development.

Indian forests constitute 2% of the world's forest area but are forced to support 12% of the world's human population and 14% of world's livestock population. This is sufficient to indicate the tremendous biotic pressure they face.

Forests in India have been shrinking for several decades owing to the pressure of population on land for competing uses, such as agriculture, irrigation and power projects, industry, roads, etc. In India, forests account for about 19.27 per cent of the total land area. On the other hand, in advanced countries, the area under forests is often about a third of the total land area. There is a need to have massive reforestation programmes, control over hacking and grazing and provision of cheap fuel through alternative technologies.

The National Forest Policy (1988) stipulates that a minimum of one-third of the total land area of the country should be brought under forest or tree cover. It is envisaged that this will be achieved by involving local stakeholders like the farmers, the tribals, the women , the NGOs and the Panchayat Raj Institutions (PRIs).

Another concern relating to the state of forest resources is that of biodiversity and extinction of species. India has a rich heritage of species and genetic strains of flora and fauna. Out of the total eighteen bio-diversity hot-spots in the world, India has two, one is the north-east Himalayas and the other is the Western Ghats. At present, India is home to several animal species that are threatened, including over 77 mammal, 22 reptiles and 55 birds and one amphibian species. For *in-situ* conservation of biological diversity, India has developed a network of protected areas including national parks, sanctuaries and biosphere reserves. This network, which is being progressively expanded, now covers about 4% of the total land area of the country. As a result of the amendments in 1991 to the Wildlife (Protection) Act, hunting of all species of wild life for commerce or for pleasure has been banned.

Govt. of India is keen to develop and monitor functioning of forestry.

Forest Survey of India (FSI), an organization of Ministry is engaged in generating information and database development on forest cover and forest resources in the country besides providing services of training, research and extension. The mandate of the FSI, established in June, 1981 was redefined in 1986 with the following objectives:

- To prepare a comprehensive State of Forest Report (SFR) including National Vegetation Map (NVM) once every two years. To prepare thematic maps through use of remote sensing data (aerial photographs) with minimum essential ground truth verification.
- To undertake work in regard to preparation of forest inventory in the country.
- To collect, store and retrieve necessary forestry and forestry-related data for national and state level planning and to create a computer-based National Basic Forestry Inventory System (NBFIS).
- To design methodologies relating to forest surveys and subsequent processing and updating.
- To impart training in modern forest survey techniques to foresters at various levels.
- To undertake special studies and consultancies.

The Forest Survey of India with its head quarter at Dehra Dun and four zones located at Shimla (Noth Zone), Kolkata (East Zone), Nagpur (Central Zone) and Bangalore (South Zone) are largely carrying out inventory of forest resources inside and outside forest areas. During the year, infrastructure of these offices have been strengthened for carrying out digital image processing activities.[13]

The constitution specifically prescribes:

The state shall endeavour to protect and improve the environment and to safeguard the forests and wildlife of the country. Artilce 48 of the Constitution (Forty-Second Amandment) Act. 1977.

It shall be the duty of every citizen of India . . . to protect and improve the natural environment including forests, lake, rivers, and wildlife, and to have compassion for living creatures. (Article 51A)

Forests and planting of trees became secrace. This was realized when most of the trees were cut and people were facing environmental problems. Then the Government realised and started planting trees and developing forests to control pollution and hence forests need not be destroyed.[14]

Ancient Sanskrit literature is full of literature dealing about the importance of forests.

द्यौर्वनां गिरयो वृक्षकेशा: । - ऋक् 5-41-11.
न वा अरण्यानि हन्त्यश्चेन्नाभिगच्छन्ति । ऋक् 10-146-5.
मा काकंबीरमुद् वृहो वनस्पतिमशस्तीर्विहि नीनश: -- ऋक् 6-48-17.

The earth destroys the person who destroys the forests

मृगसड्घातसम्पन्नं क्रूरसत्त्वैर्विवर्जितम् ।
वनमात्मविहारार्थं पालयेत्पुरपाश्चर्वत: ।। 42 ।।
प्रत्यन्तदेशसम्भूतं वनं गिरिदरीयुतम् ।
सर्वेषां गोपनार्थं तु पार्थिव: परिपालयेत् ।। 43 ।। -शिवतत्त्वरत्नाकर

On the other hand plantation of trees was considered sacred and pure.

यस्यां वृक्षा वानस्पत्या ध्रुवास्तिष्ठन्ति विश्वहा ।
पृथिवीं विश्वधायसं धृतामच्छावदामति ।। -- अथ् 12-1-27

Moksa can be attained through planting trees for others' benefit.

अश्वत्थमेकं पिचुमन्दमेकं न्यग्रोधमेकं दश चिश्रिणीभि: ।
षट्चम्पकांस्तालशतत्रयं च नवाम्रवृक्षैर्नरंक न पश्येत् ।। 1 ।।
यावन्ति खादन्ति फलानि वश्क्षाद् क्षुद्वहिन्दग्धा: तनुभृन्नराद्या: ।
वर्षाणि तावन्ति वसन्ति नाके वृक्षैकवापास्त्वमरौघसेव्या: ।। 2 ।।

यावन्ति पुष्पाणि महीरुहाणां दिवौकसां मूर्धनि भूतले वा ।
पतन्ति तावन्ति च वत्सराणां शतानि नाके रमतेऽग्रवापी ॥ 3 ॥ बृहत्पारशर

We may take a clue from Sanskrit literature and plant the trees and maintain forests and treat them:

(a) like our own progeny.
(b) Not plucking any part until and unless essential.
(c) Understand the feelings and emotions of plants.
(d) Understand their importance in the overall cosmos.
(e) All people should be educated based upon our Sanskrit literature.
(f) Leaflets from different sources about the inevitability of plants based on our heritage need be publicised.
(g) Planting of a tree is like giving birth to a child.

The World Community is Aware of Plants/Forests Significance

The National Forest Policy, 1988 envisages people's involvement in the development and protection of degraded forests as a permanent resource base to fulfil the requirements of fuel wood, fodder and small timber to local communities as well as to develop the forests for improving the environment. In order to implement the policy prescription, the Ministry issued guideline on 1.6.1990 to involve the village communities in the development and protection of degraded forests on the basis of their taking a share of the product from such areas. The concept of the Joint Forest Management was accordingly initiated by developing appropriate mechanism.

National Forest Policy, 1988 laid down basic objections which need to followed to maintain eco-system.

- Maintenance of environmental stability through preservation and, where necessary, restoration of the ecological balance that has been adversely disturbed by serious depletion of the forests of the country. Conserving the natural heritage of the country preserving the remaining natural forests with the vast variety of flora and fauna, which represent the remarkable biological diversity and genetic resources of the country.
- Checking soil erosion and denudation in the catchment area of rivers, lakes, reservoirs in the interest of the soil and water conservation, for mitigating floods and droughts and for the retardation of situation of reservoirs.
- Checking the extension of sand-dunes in the desert areas of Rajasthan and along the coastal tracts.
- Increasing substantially the forest/tree cover in the country through massive afforestation and social forestly programmes, especially on all denuded, degraded and unproductive lands.

Meeting the requirements of fuelwood, fodder, minor forest produce and small timber of the rural and tribal populations.
- Increasing the productivity of forests to meet essential national needs.
- Encouraging efficient utilization of forest produce and maximizing substitution of wood.
- Creating a massive people's movement with the involvement of women, for achieving these objectives and to minimize pressure on existing forests.
- Creating a massive people's movement with the involvement of women, for achieving these objectives and to minimize pressure on existing forests.

The principal aim of Forest Policy must be to ensure environmental stability and maintenance of ecological balance including atmospheric equilibrium which are vital for sustenance of all life forms, human, animal and plant. The derivation of direct economic benefit must be subordinated to this principal aim.

Thus, the principal reforms that could reduce inappropriate tropical deforestation are likely to be a combination of the following government policies:

- Eliminate subsidies to agricultural and pastoral industries that encourage deforestation.
- Eliminate legal and institutional incentives or requirements to clear forests as a basis for gaining recognized land tenure.
- Reform forest industry concessions and licenses to provide incentives for long-term sustainable management.
- Develop innovative institutional arrangements for devolving more decision-making authority and responsibility to those whose livelihoods and quality of life are directly linked to the extent and quality of tropical forests.
- Encourage voluntary market differentiation by consumers that discriminates positively toward products that have been sustainably produced from forests.
- Facilitate the recognition of and compensation for environmental services provided by forests and ensure that transfer payments are received by the persons making the decisions at the forest frontiers.

Most of the major environmental problems in developing countries are due ot to the pursuit of economic development, but rather to incorrect economic policies: poorly defined property rights, under pricing of resources, state allocations and subsidies, and neglect of non-marketed social benefits. Instead of devising new policies to stop further resource and environmental deterioration while promoting development, one should first try to eliminate those (legal, social, political, and institutional) factors that cause or exacerbate the problems.[15]

ANIMALS AND WILD LIFE VIS-À-VIS ENVIRONMENT

Animal bioethics is a constitution of integrated ethical principles aimed at not only making the animal's life comfortable, productive, painless but also environmentally sustainable for the present and future generations. It also should aim at the protection of mankind from the ill-effects of the sick and unproductive animals. Animal is the dominant partner of our ecosystem deserving due attention for its existence, productivity and growth.

1. Impact of Animals on Eco-system to Ensure Positive Impact

Since, animal is an integral and most important part of our ecosystem, we have to understand its impact on the society and the environment and *vice-versa*.[16]

Livestock can damage global natural resources in a number of ways, but there are also many examples of environmental balance and positive contributions. Livestock interact on a global scale with land, water, air, and plant and animal biodiversity. About 34 million square kilometers, or 26 percent of the world's land area, are used for grazing livestock. In addition, million kilometers, or about 21 percent of the world's arable area, are used for cereal production for livestock feed. Livestock produce 13 billion tons of waste a year. A large part of this is recycled, but where animal concentrations are high, waste poses an enormous environmental hazard. Livestock and livestock waste cause gaseous emissions that have important local and global impact on the environment. Livestock grazing can affect the water balance in certain areas. Water is needed to produce fodder and feed concentrate, to provide drinking water for animals, and to drain surplus waste and chemicals. Livestock interact directly and indirectly with biodiversity; although biodiversity often is compromised, there are also examples of mutual benefits.[17]

2. Animals were held in High Esteem in Ancient India

Animals and wild life were held in high esteem in ancient India. Even the pictures of God have been grafted on some animals. Lord Krishna was associated with cows and these cows were named as (गौ माता) Mother cows. All waste matter is toxic, wherever it comes from, be it human, chemical, industrial or nuclear waste. The only waste matter that is not toxic is the waste from a cow. There are no bacteria, infections or worms in a cow's waste matter that could harm you. All other living beings excrete waste matter that is highly toxic. Everything in the world creates waste matter which is poisonous and hazardous to health. No waste matter in the world is safe except that of the cow. There is only one living being whose stool and urine are edible and drinkable. Therefore, when a cow's waste matter or excreta is so pure, can you imagine how pure and clean that creature must be? The cow is the most holy of animals; she is called, 'holy cow'.

Farmers decorate their animals on particular occasions. Even some festivals are named after animals like Nag Panchmi (नाग पंचमी). Position of a person was equated with the number of animals he possessed. This is prevalent in North-East even today particularly Arunachal Pradesh.

Bioethics in livestock industry is concerned with our role and responsibilities and consequences of our lifestyles, our attitudes and values, policies, activities, processes, products, in much wider sense than the other ethical systems. It should be remembered by every one that equality of consideration is the basic right of every animal.

3. Need of Love and Kindness to Animals

Ancient Indian Sanskrit literature is the first to recognize the importance bioethics in veterinary practice and education. Love and kindness towards dumb animals is the inherent character of ancient Indian culture, where Cow, Bullock, Elephant, Tiger, Lion, Monkey and even Cobra and a number of other animals are considered very sacred.

When man expresses positive attitude towards his animal and when the animal is not afraid of man, and when there is better social bond between man and animal, sows will have more piglets, hens lay more eggs, work animal show better performance, cows produce more milk, meat animals produce more meat with better quality and pets show more affection and faithfulness, thus fulfiling the universal motto "Health and Wealth for all."[18]

4. Need to Preserve Animal Species

Environment and ecology are under tremendous strain. Every essential item of life support system—energy, water, land, forest is experiencing an exponential growth in demand due to its profligate use by the rich and for meeting the basic necessities of the poor whose number is ever increasing. Environment is an issue which concerns generations yet unborn. An inch of top soil takes, 10,000 years to form. Erosion has removed this vegetable cover/base. Scores of animal and plant species have disappeared and more are facing extinction. This is tragic as it means the loss of genetic stock and up-sets the final balance in nature that ensures the existence of life itself on earth. The death of plants and animals these days is caused not so much by physical extermination—hunting, fishing, etc. as by the chemical and other industrial pollution of the bio-sphere and because of deforestation. It is said that out of 9,6000 species of birds known world-wide, 6,000 are on the decline.

5. Special Importance of Cow in Ancient India

In Vedic literature quoted above animals are part and parcel of our environment. Cow has been given the supreme importance. Let us quote from Athurveda and Rigveda.[19]

एतद् वै विश्वरुरूपं सर्वरूपं गोरूपम् । - अथ 9-7-25

All deities reside in a cow. It is omnipresent.

गावो भगो गाव इन्द्रो मे अच्छान् गावः सोमस्य प्रथमस्य भक्ष : ।
इमा या गावः स जनाम इन्द्र इच्छासीद्धृदा मनसा चिदिन्द्रम् ।।
ऋ 6-28-5

Cow is a great source of wealth and have positive impact on environment—

गवो ममाग्रतो नित्यं गावः पृष्ठत एव च ।
गावश्च सर्वगात्रेषु गवां मध्ये वसाम्यहम् ।।
इतयाचम्य जपेन्मन्त्रं सायं प्रातरिदं शुचिः
सर्वपापक्षयस्तस्य स्वर्लोकं पूजितो भवेत् ।।
यथा गौश्च तथा विप्रो यथा विप्रस्तथा हरिः ।
हरिर्यथा तथा गड़ाग एते न ह्ययवृषाः स्मृतः ।।
गावो बन्धुर्मनुष्याणां मनुष्या बान्धवा गवाम् ।
गौश्च यस्मिन् गश्हे नास्ति तद्बन्धुरहितं गृहम् ।।
पद्मपुराण सृष्टिखण्ड 57-152-156

It is prayed that we should live amongst cows. Cows are our real relatives and well wishers. Without cows house will not look auspicious and prosperous.

Ancient people were aware of the fact that balance in nature is necessary for the happiness of human beings. Look at the following verses which depict the feeling of gratitude towards the dumb animals for their service to the mankind.[20]

उत्पाद्य सस्यानि तृणं चरन्ति तदेव भूयः सकलं वहन्ति ।
न भारखिन्नाः प्रवदन्ति किञ्चित अहो वृषैर्जीवति जीवलोकः ।।

(Skandhapurana quoted by Hemadri in the 7th chapter of Danakhanda)

6. Necessary for many Rituals

Animals serve as a factory for releasing carbon-dioxide for plants and getting oxygen from plants. Hence, their presence keep the eco-system in equilibrium. Government of India has been promoting for the Conservation of wild animals to maintain Eco-System.

Some specifications in the Grhya-sutra appear conducive towards the birds and animals which were not necessarily domestic. The bali materials offered in the rite of baliharana, a rite prescribed for the performer as a part of his daily routine, were actually partaken by the birds and animals of outside. In sarpabali milk and food articles were offered for the snakes. The GGS IV.4.30 mentions that the king of moles in the mole-hill was offered sacrificial food cooked in the ceremony for ploughing. The Dharma-sutras and the Smrtis add that the flesh of a number of birds like cock, heron, sparrow, crow, cuckoo, pigeon, dove, cakravaka, vulture, crane peacock, swan, maina, tittibha were prohibited for food. (cf. Gau. Dh. Su. XVII.15, MS IV. 209, Yajsm 1.161).[21]

INDIAN BOARD FOR WILDLIFE (IBWL)[22]

7. Administration of Wild Life

The IBWL is the apex advisory body in the field of Wildlife Conservtion in the country and is headed by the Honourable Prime Minister of India. It has been reconstituted w.e.f. 7.12.2001. The XXI meting of the IBWL was held on 21.1.2002 under the Chairmanship of the Honourable Prime Minister at New Delhi and the following resolutions were adopted:

- Wildlife and forest shall be declared priority sector at the national level for which funds should be earmarked.
- Law enforcement agencies must ensure that those engaged in poaching, illicit trade in wildlife and wildlife products, destruction of their habitat, and such other illegal activities are given quick and deterrent punishment.
- We should fully tap the potential in wildlife tourism and at the same time take care that it does not have adverse impact on wildlife and protected areas. The revenue earned from increased tourism should be used entirely to augment available resources for conservation.
- Protecting interests of the poor and tribals living around protected areas should be handled with sensitivity and with maximum participation of the affected people. They should have access to the minor forest produce, in the forests outside of national park and sanctuaries. Employment and means generation for these people is crucial for maintaining symbiosis between the forests, wildlife and the people. People should be encouraged to take up aforestation and conservation in new areas.
- While strengthening protective measures against traditional threats to wildlife, we should also respond to newer threats such as toxic chemicals and pesticides.
- There should be greater government as well as societal

recognition and support for the many non-governmental organizations engaged in wildlife conservation. Mainstream media to better highlight their activities as also successes of governmental initiatives that have worked.

- Creatively produced Television Programmes on wildlife and ecology are widely appreciated by young and old as seen from the popularity of dedicated T.V. channels like discovery, National Geographic and Animal Planet. It is proposed that Prasar Bharati and other private channels alongwith the agencies like WWF for nature should collaborate and increase original Indian content in different languages on our television.
- No diversion of forest land for non-forest purposes from critical and ecologically fragile wildlife habitat shall be allowed.

NATIONAL WILDLIFE ACTION PLAN[23]

Objective

Establish a network of scientifically managed protected areas such as national parks, sanctuaries and biosphere reserves, to cover representative and viable samples of all significant biographic sub-divisions within the country. Such protected areas should have an adequate geographic distribution.

Action Required

Review classification of protected areas in India and establish agreed biographic classification. Review location, size, ecological composition and viability of all existing protected areas in relation to the biographic zones, protected areas to ensure adequate representation of all zones and institute a periodic review of the overall situation.

Priority Projects

- Establish agreed bio-geographical classification for India;
- Review status of existing protected areas in relation to biographic zones of the country;
- Draw up proposals for adding more areas under protected status in order to rectify present deficiencies;
- Draw up detailed recommendations for improvement of the management of presently poorly managed protected areas;
- Bring above recommendations to the attention of States/Union Territories for appropriate action regarding gazettement and management of protected areas, etc.; and
- Institute periodic review (every five years) of protected areas within the country.

What wildlife conservation needs is a long-term and pragmatic development and management policy, which is appreciative of the needs of other land-use agencies. Plans should be able to cope with the situation today and with the long-term future.

Policy requires us to ensure a network of protected areas covering the full range of India's biodiversity. Conservationists must set priorities and decide on the implementation of this network now. Protected areas to be viable have to be large, conservation science now has capability to determine just how big. But there are limits. Planning must be a rational compromise between biological needs and people's requirements. Conservation cannot successfully be imposed on people, there must be some degree of acceptance if conservation is to work.

The eco-system in the environment is an inter-depending phenomenon. Nature has certain set rules and conditions to maintain the cycles of each component of the environment, i.e. animals, plants, human beings, air, water, etc. To maintain the balance, all the species created by the creator and the destruction of these will lead the destruction of environment. Every species is important and a role to play in the purification of environment. Patanjali's examples in this context give such ideas. The example Pl. 4.24 (Vr.1) quoted with reference to how people were protecting and preserving their crops, fields, food grains and forest, etc. amply clarify that since that time environmental awareness was known to all. And the role of these were undoubtedly the major one for the development of the environment and maintenance of eco-system was also ingrained in their mind. This has been revealed in very clear terms in our ancient literature.

8. Kautilaya's Arthasastra and Animal Protection

There is extensive evidence in the Arthashastra on Kautiliya's concern for the welfare of animals. Regulations for the protection of wild life, a long list of punishment for cruelty to animals, rations for animals, regulations on gazing and the responsibilities of veterinary doctors are some of the major topics.

As a part of the creation of infrastructure of a settled and prosperous kingdom, an animal sanctuary, 'where all animals were welcomed as guests', was established {2.2.4.}. Live birds and deer received as tax were set free. A list of protected animals and fish is given. Killing or injuring protected species and animals in reserved parks and sanctuaries was prohibited. Even animals which had turned dangerous were not to be killed within the sanctuary but had to be caught and taken outside and then killed {2.26.1.4-6.14}.

Village headmasters were responsible for preventing cruelty to animals. If protected animals or those from reserved forests strayed and were found grazing where they should not, they were to be driven away without hurting them; anyone who let such animals stray were to be warned to prevent a recurrence. Stray cattle were to be driven off with a rope or a whip without harming them. Any means could be used to restrain a person found to be treating an animal cruelly {3.10.30-34}.

Some animals, like deer, were given special treatment {4.10.5}. Temple bulls, stud bulls and cows for up to ten days after calving were exempt from payment of grazing charge {3.10.24}, riding or driving a temple animal, a stud bull or a pregnant cow was prohibited {4.13.20}. Animals fights between horned or tusked animals was also prohibited {4.13.19}.

Special regulations applied to animals in Crown herds, horses and elephants, since the latter two were important for war. The possibility of herdsmen starving calves of their mother's milk is foreseen; milking cows twice in seasons when they should be milked only once was punished by cutting off the thumb of the culprit; killing or inducing someone to kill animals in crown herds was punishable by death {2.29.3.16.32}. Special provision were made for looking after non-productive cattle {2.29.6}. Rations are laid down for horses and elephants, including special rations for tired horses. Attendant who ill-treated elephant or kept them in dirty stalls were punished {2.32.19}. Horses unfit for use in war were used to breed animals for the benefit of the people {2.30.28}.

Veterinary doctors were fined if the condition of sick animal became worse; they had to repay the cost of animal if it died {2.30.43.47.48}

In newly conquered territory, animal slaughter was prohibited for four days around full moon day and during one fortnight in each of the four month of devotion (chaturmasya). Slaughter of female and young animals and castration of males was prohibited {13.5.12.13}.[24]

Ancient Sanskrit Literature is full of readings which describe the beauty of nature, e.g. Ramayana, Mahabharta, Atharvaveda, Rgveda, Vedic literature, Kalidasa's books Rtusamhara, Meghaduta, Kumarasmbhava, Abhijnancoskuntala describe nature in all its aspects establishing intimate relationship between the human beings and nature. It is impossible to think of human beings without plants and animals. Poets, Philosophers, writers have described the beautiful nature surrounded by plants, animals and human beings. Valmiki in Ramayana observes that Ram enjoyed the pleasures of nature more than the kingdom of Ayodhya. Ram's stay at Chitrakoot is described as a memorable period. Even today, Chitrakoot is very soothing with plants and animals around. All the busy people become dull after sometimes with the unnatural environment and that is why they take pleasure for some days in natural settings which acts as a charging agent of their life. They come back with vigour, vitality and freshness.

Let us illustrate the role of Sanskrit Literature in promoting good eco-system. Agamashastra concenterates on principles to protect and develop forest wealth. Yajurveda deals with biological functions to ensure ecological equilibrium. Dharmshastras point out details of using resources without disturbing eco-system. Vrksa Ayurveda, Gaja Ayurveda, Ashva Ayurveda, etc. deal with Biotechnology and Genetic engineering to ensure better yield of good quality. We can quote hundreds of source which deal with eco-system directly or indirectly.

We are sure that the present day generations would take advantage of Ancient Sanskrit literature in improving the present day degradation of environment.

9. Role of UN System in Promoting and Protecting Animal Life

The Declaration of the UN Conference on the Human Environment held in June 16, 1972, followed what is already contained in Ancinet Sanskrit Literature. To quote briefly:

The natural resources of the earth, including the air, water, land, flora and fauna and, especially, representative samples of natural ecosystems, were to be safeguarded for the benefit of present and future generations through careful planning or management, as appropriate.

The state should take all possible steps to prevent pollution of seas by substances that are liable to create hazards to human health, to harm living resources and marine life, to damage amenities or to interfere with other legitimate uses of the seas. The man and his environment must be spared against the nuclear weapons and all other means of mass destruction.[25]

After the United Nations Conference on Human Environment held in Stockholm in 1972, in 1976, 42nd Constitutional Amendment was done in the Indian Constitution committed to the protection of environment. In the Chapter of Directive Principles of State Policy, Article 48A was included:

'The state shall endeavor to protect and improve the environment and safeguard the forests and wild-life of the country.'

By the same amendment is created a fundamental duty of every citizen under Article 51-A(g).[26]

"To protect and improve the natural environment including forests, lakes, rivers and wildlife, and have compassion for living creatures."

Besides Parliament and Judiciary also become active. Parliament enacted Water Prevention and Control of Pollution Act, 1974, Air (Prevention and Control of Pollution) Act, 1981, and the Environment (Protection) Act, 1986.

International Union for Conservation of Nature and Natural Resources (ICUCN) in 1980 devised the World Conservation Strategy as to maintain essential ecological processes and life-support systems (such as soil regernation and protection, the recycling of nutrients, and the cleansing of waters) on which human survival and development depend; to preserve genetic diversity (the range of genetic material found in the world's organisms), on which depend the functioning of many of the above processes and life-support systems, the breeding programmes necessary for the protection and improvement of cultivated plants, domesticated animals and micro-organisms, as well as much scientific and medical advance, technical innovation, and the security of the many industries that use living resources; and to ensure the sustainable utilization of species and ecosystems (notably fish and other wildlife, forests and grazing lands) which support millions of rural communities as well as major industries.

Indian National Man and Biosphere Committee (M.A.B.) and Department of Environment, Govt. of India, in their paper presented at the First International Biosphere Reserve Conference at Mink (USSR), Sept. 26-October 2, 1983, appreciated the role of ancient Sanskrit Literature in developing (Forests/Plants) Wild/Domestic Animal life. To quote:

The idea of conservation is not a new one for India. References are scattered in ancient Indian literature emphasizing the conservation of fauna and flora. Ashoka's Pillar Edicts are a glowing example. The descriptions of fauna and flora of the area also occur very often in the ancient Indian literature. These references and descriptions are not surprising and go well with India's cultural heritage which in essence has been conservational in approach. The Indian region (8°-38° N and 60°-97.5° E) with a total area of 328 million hectares is indeed very rich in biological diversity. It is estimated that about 45,000 species of plants occur in this country. The vascular flora, which forms the conspicuous vegetation cover, itself comprises 15,000 species, of which more than 60 per cent are endemic and have so far not been reported from anywhere else in the world. The total plant wealth of the country includes not out the usually large, showy-flowered vascular plants, but a large number of non-flowering plants, viz. ferns, liverworts, algae and fungi.

The region is equally rich in fauna. More than 50,000 species of insects, 4,000 of moll uses, 6,500 of other invertebrates, 2,000 of fish, 140 of amphibians, 420 of reptiles, 1200 of birds and 340 of mammals, (i.e. more than 65,000 species of animals) are recorded from this country.

The wild relatives of the crop plants together with related species constitute gene pools which are rich source of many important and desirable traits. Such spices are distributed in centers of diversity/origin of crop plants.

Over 150 species of economic plants have their genetic diversities in the Hindustan Center of Diversity (Zeven and Zhukovsky, 1975)[27] in the Indian subcontinent and most of these species do grow in some of the proposed Biosphere Reserves. Besides, there is a vast number of other economic plants which are utilized only from their wild populations which have their home in the proposed biosphere reserves.

Parallel to such an enormous diversity in plants, there is also considerable diversity in domesticated animals and their wild and semi-wild relatives such as buffalo, goat, sheep, pig, poultry, camel, ass, yak, horse, etc. The productivity of these animals by the standards of developed countries is very low. However, having undergone periods of rigorous selection, races are hardly adaptable to heat and parasitic stresses, and can survive on very poor roughage. These are very important characteristics, now in great demand in Australia; the USA and the Latin America. Obviously, such genetic treasure at present existing in the wild or with tribal populations also needs to be conserved.

Under the inspiration of various disciples of Gandhiji and Sarvodaya workers, the process of educating the masses through folk songs, foot-marches, etc. began and the following slogan was popularized:

What do the forests bear?
Soil, water and pure air,
Soil, water and pure air,
Are the basis of life.

Policies need to be designed to correct the environmental effects of livestock production, which are not reflected in product and input prices. These policies should address the causes of environmental degradation and must be flexible, site-specific, and well targeted. Instruments to enhance positive and mitigate negative environmental impacts include pricing, regulations, and institutional development. The collective purpose of these instruments is to establish feed-back mechanisms that ensure that livestock's use is consistent with overall social objectives.

Improved management is essential if the world's natural resources are to continue to provide the basis for life support and human well-being. Only with improved management can be dual objectives of sustainable agricultural production be fulfiled—to feed the world's growing population, while sustaining its natural resource base. Livestock production is the largest user of land and is about to become the most important agricultural activity in terms of economic output. Left to uncontrolled growth, the environment will suffer, compromising human welfare. However, this is unlikely to happen. The opportunities not only to mitigate environmental damage but also to tap the immense development potential offered by livestock are large: awareness, political will, and readiness to act are growing among all those involved and ensure that the problems will be tackled effective.[28]

Man must recognize the necessity of cooperating with nature. He must temper his demands and use and conserve the natural living resources of this earth in a manner that alone can provide for the continuation of this civilization. The final answer is to be found only through comprehension of the enduring process of nature.

The theory of consumerism is an ism based on maximum utilization and utmost consumption of available resources—material physical, geo-biological, etc. It is a state of temperament and mental inclination. It gives maximum emphasis on optimum utilization of available resources both natural and man-made. It is a craze against preservation or gradual use of available resources. We know that natural resources such as—air, water, soil, minerals are scare. They are not to last for all the time to come. But in consumerism, this hard reality is not kept into account. Due to unsatiable desire to have more and more, hard realities of the prevailing environment is ignored. This negligence, in a long-run, proves to be hazardous for the human beings residing on this planet. Scientists, economists and other specialists are warning us against the rapidly diminishing reserves of minerals, decreasing areas of forests, flora and fauna and many endangered species, global warning, depletion of ozone layer, increasing temperature of earth and other alarming dangers.

Gandhi observed, "Our ancestors, therefore, set a limit to our indulgence . . . our fore-fathers knew that, if we set our hearts after such things, we would become slaves and lose our moral fibre. They, therefore, after due deliberation decided that we should only do what we could without hands and feet. They saw that our real happiness and health consisted in a proper use of our hands and feet.

Sh. T.N. Chaturvedi in his editorial to *IJPA* July-Sept. 1989 (Special Number on Environment and Administration) rightly sees the intimate relationship between human beings and nature since times immemorial. To quote: Man, since his origin, has lived in harmony with Nature through the ages, holding Nature in awe and reverence. The Vedas, folklore, and scriptures of different religions, faiths and beliefs also speak of the need for harmony with the universe, which is the habitat not only of man but also of all animals, birds, insects, plants and vegetation. The mutually supportive role of all living things is often mentioned as a crucial factor for a balanced social and harmonious existence. The ecological balance is inherent in the very process of creation. Every where, the seers, poets and thinkers, through the ages, have referred to the need for living in harmony with environment. In fact, the Taitariyopanished looks at the relationship between man and his environment in its totality and stresses complete harmony and inter-dependence between them in order to attain real prosperity.

The basic purpose of plants and animals and human life is not to appear a cluster but should seem to be in perfect rhythm and harmony. A.N. Yellapa Reddy in his article, "Role of Sanskrit Literature in Preservation of Wild Life Biodiversity and Environment rightly stresses: Eminent scientist like Einstein strongly believed in nature's inherent harmony. This concern throughout was to find a unified foundation of physics. According to our Seers and Sages as well as Einstein's observations were that "nature is like a vibrating veena'" with perfect rhythm with live wave. They were also aware of the vital functions of non-living entities such as clouds which move and brake down, rivers grow, air gains strength and speed, etc.

Today, we need a communion, that our heart be wide enough so that no one is excluded as all of them have a well defined subtle role to build up ecological galance and to maintain the balance in nature.

In the 21st century the Deep Ecologists begin to feel a sense of oneness with nature and as a part of Natural order of life, the very same philosophy our ancestors practiced, propagated and insisted to adopt to maintain peace in the planet.

They had respect to nature, which is the safest, cleanest and most refined level of inter-species communication and communion.

Our planners, policy-makers, scientists, etc. are appreciating the knowledge contained in our Sanskrit Literature about Eco-system and especially about Forests and animals, Air, Water, etc.

The Supreme Court's decision in *M.C. Mehta* v. *Kamal Nath and others*,[29] published in July 2002 issue of the All India Reporter, awarding exemplary damages to the tune of ten lakh of rupees against a private commercial enterprise—M/s Span Motels Pvt. Ltd. at Manali (Himachal Pradesh). This award was in addition to the damages to be paid on the principle of polluter pays, because it was found as a fact the said Motel enterprise, by constructing stone-walls and bunds on the river banks and in the riverbed across the channel, interfered with the natural flow of the river Beas, resulting in the degradation of the environment. This has been so conclusively determined on the basis of the patent breach of the doctrine of public trust—a doctrine which is held to have become, by following the decisions of the American courts, a part of the law of the land.

In India, it is the constitutional obligation of the State to protect and improve the environment and to safeguard the natural resources like the forest and wildlife of the country. It is also one of the fundamental duties of every citizen under the constitution of India to protect and improve the natural environment including forests, lakes, rivers and wildlife and to show compassion for living creatures. The conjoint consideration of both the duty of citizens and the obligation of the State in the light of the provisions of Article 21 of our constitution, any destructive disturbance of the environment and ecology that affects the guaranteed fundamental right to life and personal liberty either directly or indirectly is forbidden.

The lessons to be learnt in environmental protection may be identified and crystallized as under:

(a) the state is a trustee of all such natural resources as seashores, running waters, airs, forests, and ecologically fragile lands that are by reason of their very intrinsic value and character meant for the enjoyment of all.

(b) As a trustee, the state is under an affirmative duty to preserve and protect the natural resources, which are the people's common heritage.

(c) The natural resources meant for public use cannot allowed to be converted by the state into private ownership or commercial interests.

(d) As a part of planning and allocation of natural resources, if the State may have to approve their appropriation, the same has to be consistent with the purposes of public trust. If allocated, the State is empowered to rescind the allocation if there occurred harm to public interest uses despite the anticipation of that harm.

The public trust doctrine expounded in the context of preservation and protection of environment and ecology is essentially and truly global in character, environmental degradation knows no barrier drawn by man. This doctrine, therefore, needs to be perceived and practiced from that perspective. In the Indian jurisprudential thought, this is the perspective which is so eloquently expressed by our sages when they ordain us to treat all the inhabitants of this earth as members of one big family and direct that all human activities must be anchored in the welfare of all the raison deter of our social existence.[30]

BIOLOGICAL DIVERSITY BILL, 2000

A National Biodiversity Bill for the conservation of biodiversity is under consideration. The bill proposed by the Government of India envisages setting up of a National Biodiversity Authority (NBA) to regulate the movement of bio-resources in the country. The bill not only includes a framework for protecting traditional knowledge, but also provides mechanisms by which important bioresources and related traditional knowledge can be utilized sustainability with fair benefits for the communities.

Approach Paper for the Tenth Five Year Plan: Forests

The Approach Paper sum up the main concerns in the factory as follows. The problems and constraints in the forestry development include lack of awareness about multiple roles and benefits of forests, especially its role in drought proofing and prevention of soil and water run-off, no linkage between management and livelihood security of the people, low level of technology, inadequate research and extension, weak planning capability, wastage in harvesting and processing, market imperfections, overemphasis on government involvement and control, low level of people's participation and NGO's involvement, lack of private sector participation, unwanted restrictions on felling, transport and marketing of forests produce grown by people, lack of inter-sectoral coordination and weakness and conflicting roles of public forests administration:

The following strategies are proposed to address these concerns:.

- Strengthening farm forestry and tree plantation in marginal and wastelands belonging to the poor.
- Integrated land-use planning.
- Measures to sustain, JFM beyond the project period.
- Protecting women's unsufruct lights and enabling women groups to collect and market non-timber forest products.
- Upgradation of forests technology such as to promote more gatherable biomass.
- Conservation and promoting of bamboo by *inter alia* classifying it as an NTFP.
- Prevention and control of forest fires.
- Priority to agroforestry, mountain, watershed development, river valleys, arid areas, wastelands afforestation programmes.
- Conservation and development of medicinal plants.
- Research and technological development to increase productivity and production of new products alongwith focus on value addition, improved marketing, export and productive employment generation.
- Promotion of coastal shelter belt plantations for prevention of natural calamities.

It is also proposed that the government gradually withdraw from some segments and tap the potential of the local communities or an efficient market such as in the areas of marketing NTFP's or retail sale of fuelwood and bamboo.

Notes and References

1. Quoted in A.R. Panchmukhi, Socio-economic Ideas in Ancient Indian Literature, New Delhi, Rashtriya Sanskrit Sansthan, 1998, pp. 285-86.
2. Ramaswamy Iyengar, Environmental Awareness in the Mahabharata, V.N. Jha (ed.), *op. cit.,* p. 67.
3. World Bank, Agriculture and Environment , edited by Ernst Lutz Development, 1999, Washington DC, pp. 7, ix, x.
4. Quoted in Ramaswamy Iyengar, *op. cit.,* pp. 69-70.
5. Ujjawala Panse, Attitude and Feeling of Man, Towards nature as reflected in Dharmagranthas, in V.N. Jha, *op. cit.,* pp. 82-83.
6. *Ibid.,* pp. 84-86.
7. C.P. Oberoi, Sustained Afforestation: Key to Sustainable Development, In Environment Management and Audit P. Passi Bhushana Rao and P. Mohana Rao (ed.), New Delhi, Deep & Deep, 2002, p. 147.
8. M.S. Swaminathan Environment, Friendly Agriculture, In *Ibid.,* p. 164.
9. World Bank, Agriculture and Environment, 1999 Washington DC, Editor Ernst Lutz, pp. 302, 345.
10. Ram Parshad Gupta, Food for Thought, New Delhi, 1996, pp. 12-13.
11. Vandana Shiva, Conserving India's Forests Protecting India's People, in *IJPA,* July-Sept., 1989, p. 380.
12. Ernest Lutz, *op. cit.,* p. 211.
13. GOI, Ministry of Environment and Forests, Annual Report, 2001-02, pp. 37-38.
14. A.R. Panchmukhi, *op. cit.,* pp. 319-22.
15. Ernest Lutz, *op. cit.,* p. 213.
16. M.V.G. Ahobala Rao, Bioethical Issues in Livestock Industry, In Environment Management and Audit, Editors P. Pasi Bhushana Rao and P. Mohana Rao, New Delhi, Deep & Deep, 2000, pp. 52-53.
17. Ernest Lutz, *op. cit.,* p. 283.
18. M.V.G. Ahobala Rao, *op. cit.,* p. 54.
19. Quoted in A.R. Panchmukhi, *op. cit.,* pp. 154-57.
20. Ujjwala Panse, Attitude and Feelings of Man towards Nature as reflected in Dharmagrant has, in V.N. Jha (ed), *op. cit.,* p. 80.
21. Sulok Sundar Mohanty, Ecological Awareness and the Grhyasutras, in V.N. Jha, Ed., *op. cit.,* p. 29.
22. GOI, Ministry of Environment and Forests, Annual Report, 2001-02, pp. 63-64.
23. National Wildlife Action Plan, Document in *IJPA,* July-Sept., 1989, p. 710. (Reproduced from Samar Singh, "Conservation of India's Wild Life Heritage."
24. L.N. Rangarajan, Kautilya, The Arthashastra, Penguin Books, 1987, pp. 96-97.
25. Mathurs (Ed.), ETMA, p. 523.
26. Constitution of India Articles 48A and 51A(g).
27. A.C. Zeen and P.M. Zhukovsky, Dictionary of Cultivated Plants and their centres of Diversity, the Netherlands Wageningen, 1975.
28. Ernest Lutz, *op. cit.,* pp. 294, 299.
29. M.K. Gandhi, *Hind Swaraj, op. cit.,* pp. 61-62.
30. Virendra Kumar, Breach of the Doctrine of Public Trust: Lessons to be learnt in Environmental Protection in Chartered Secretary, Sept. 2002, A 406, 1297.

CHAPTER 6

VALUE EDUCATION AND HEALTH EDUCATION

"Devoid of Sathya, Dharma, Santhi, Prema and Ahimsa"
All Education is a zero
Bereft of Sathya, Dharma, Santhi, Prema and Ahimsa
The value of all meritorious deeds is a zero.

—*Ministry of HRD*

Value Education and Health Education

> "Our power of life lies in thoughts. Thought is the secret key of our mental software. Human Resource Development should take us from negative thoughts (darkness) to positive thought (light), from Untruth to Truth, from Immortality to Mortality."
>
> —*Ministry of HRD*

Swami Visharananda in his book, "Human Values" beautifully states that to be happy is the universal urge of all beings and at all times. One has to be at peace with oneself to be happy. There can be no peace for a turbulent mind. Vasanas, desires, take away the peace of mind. It is only when we follow a value system that we can have a serene, contemplative mind. When mind is calm, we can turn it within to 'see' the treasure of pure consciousness. No treasure on earth is equal to a slice of that tattva. Mind has to be loosened from durvyapara (misdeeds and engaged in acquiring sadgunas (virtues). In Gita, Krsna talks about the developing human values and says that a mind which has daivisampatti (divine qualities) has shanti (PEACE). These values make us introspective and correct our personality.

Education institutes today are engulfed by materialistic values. Teachers have become salesmen while the students indulge in indiscipline, take drugs, alcohol, and smoking. This scene has emerged as teachers in higher education do not take interest in the development of the personality of the students. (See Chart 6.1)

R.T. Deopurkar in his article, "Values in the Modern Indian Education Thought" rightly observes: Plain living and high thinking is becoming a out-dated notion. Increase of one's needs and desires and the efforts to fulfil them all has become the philosophy of life and education in the modern world. Control of one's own sensual desires is considered to be out of date. The number of desires cherished increases in proportion to the

CHART 6.1

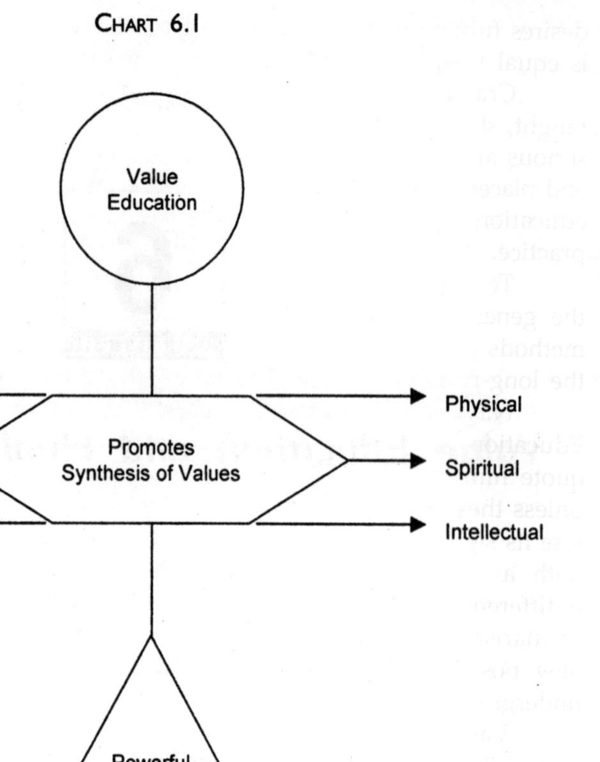
Value
Education
Emotional
Moral
Aesthetic
Promotes
Synthesis of Values
Physical
Spiritual
Intellectual

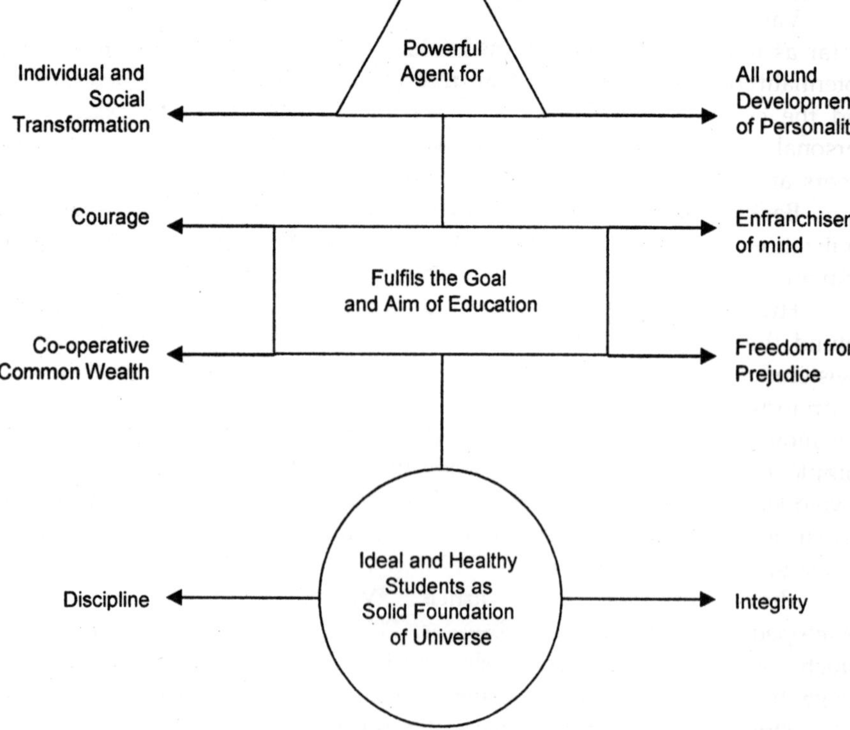
Powerful
Agent for
Individual and
Social
Transformation
All round
Development
of Personality
Courage
Enfranchisement
of mind
Fulfils the Goal
and Aim of Education
Co-operative
Common Wealth
Freedom from
Prejudice
Ideal and Healthy
Students as
Solid Foundation
of Universe
Discipline
Integrity

desires fulfiled, and so the sum total of happiness is the same as happiness is equal to the desires fulfiled upon desires cherished.

Craving for cheap popularity on the part of the teachers and the taught, short cuts in study, a longing of easy life, guide books—all need a serious attention on the part of the modern Indian educators. Their values and places must be fixed once and for ever and the decisions taken by great educationists in the interest of the nation should be strictly put into actual practice.

To get through the annual examination in a higher class has become the general immediate goal of education in India and it tells upon the methods of learning and teaching and on the national character as such in the long-run. The whole attitude to education needs revision.

N.N. Prahallada in his Article, "Contemporary Significance of Higher Education" beautifully explains the role of Moral Values in Education. To quote him, "Indian Culture is rooted deeply in her spiritual values and unless these values find their way into the life of students, education will lose its significance and will not fulfil its function of endowing the students with a vision to life and by and with ideals to work for, therefore indifference to the cherished goals of democracy, socialism, humanism and secularism, it is very essential that our education system should evolve a new positive morality which could effectively be built into the school, undergraduate/Post-graduate curriculum.

Value education involves social education but extends beyond it in so far as it covers the way the individual deals with his own powers and potentialities as well how he behaves in his relationship with other people and the community at large. It is as much concerned with striving for personal wholeness as with generating a responsible attitude towards others and an understanding of right and wrong behaviour.

Background papers New Delhi conference on Dialogue among civilizations "Quest for New Perspectives" held on July 9-10, 2003, Vigyan Bhavan, New Delhi spells out the need for values . To quote:

Humankind is passing today through an acute crisis, and the reason behind this crisis is a disequilibrium between the progress that has been registered in recent times in the externalities of life and the progress or lack of progress in the inner realms of life. The human mind has achieved an enormous development in the building of a structure of hugeness and complexity. On the other hand, the contemporary human being has not developed enough spiritual and moral capacity to manage the hugeness of structure and its complexity. Inwardly, man has remained too small to utilize and manage the complex political, social, administrative, economic and cultural machinery. The world has become global, but man has not developed yet the required global consciousness. It is this disequilibrium, which is reflected in the great challenges that the contemporary civilizations of the world are confronting.

The necessity to develop quality education is paramount. The notion of quality education does not merely encompass aspects of educational attainment, but especially the aspects of curricula and their content focusing on peace, shared values, human rights, democracy, tolerance and mutual understanding. Educational institutions and educational materials should serve as a vehicle for peace, dialogue and intercultural understanding, but not be instrumentalized for and used as vehicles to spread misunderstanding, intolerance and hate. For its part, UNESCO has deliberately placed programmes related to education for peace and human rights within the area of quality of education, emphasizing the importance of addressing these issues in any long-term education strategy.

Quality education for peace and security should focus in particular on:

- Improving knowledge of cultures, civilizations, religions and traditions;
- Developing an understanding of universally shared values; and
- Encouraging the development of key competencies for peace and the prevention and resolution of conflict.

There is a widespread feeling among a cross section of the people in India today that, all is not well with our body politic and that education must contribute actively and positively to find a part of the solution. The growing malaise in modern education is that it is seen and practised merely or mainly as a means of acquiring techno-informative knowledge and skills, with little or no anchoring in cultural roots of the country and its perspectives. Unless education helps the students to develop not only a personal identity (which essentially means a set of value perspectives and world views, linked to ones cultural traditions) education cannot be said to have fulfiled its essential role.

Leaders, not only in the field of education but also in other fields have tried to enhance the quality of life. Various kinds of remedies have been applied or tried but, of late, it has become, the united voice of all that Moral, Social and Human Values are the ultimate and the much-needed remedy.[1]

G. Chandrarlekka Rao in an Article; "Value Education for College Students" rightly feels that realizing this need our curriculum needs to insist on educating the young students in the art of living with values. If learning remains detached from value judgements, scholarship runs the risk of degenerating into indifference. Value judgements actually enhance the accuracy of learning, teachers, therefore, should be aware of the important role they are called upon to play as professionals and citizens, as agents of development and change. They must make an effort to light a candle instead of cursing the darkness and sow the seeds of value education with a fond hope that they would diffuse their own fragrance towards the creation of a just and new society as they sprout and blossom. Can we be good role models if we are not ethical ourselves.

University education which is worthwhile should lead to the

development of integrated personality and inculcate values like patriotism, spirit of national unity and a healthy appreciation of the rich variety of cultural expressions and promote a humanistic outlook. It is only in the highest education stage that the students can be enabled to acquire intellectual, democratic and aesthetic values and a deeply felt concern for the environment.

The content of value-oriented postgraduate education should include: (a) a yearning for knowledge and capacity to utilize it for the good of the society, (b) Democratic education, (c) Aesthetic education, (d) a course in ethics, (e) spiritual education, and (f) provision for activities involving values.[2]

R. Satya Raju in his Article, "Human Values in University Management" suggests the following:

(a) Value education means a positive effort for bringing about a synthesis of physical, intellectual, emotional, aesthetic, moral and spiritual values in a human being;
(b) Due to total neglect in the last five decades after independence, the present focus is on revival of moral and spiritual values in education; and
(c) The government should have no reservation in introducing and funding universal religion of human values in the form, in the contents and in the methodology of education at all levels.

Let us understand three areas of education and our values; viz.:

(a) 'Truth" seeking through scientific and objective processes which are followed by the scientists;
(b) "beauty" creates appreciation through the processes of artistic and unique expression followed by artists; and
(c) "goodness" constructed through the processes of subjective and meaningful contracting followed by social scientists. There is danger in trespassing the boundaries of sciences to arts-to-social sciences without transforming our own respective perspective and amending the tools of analysis used by our own discipline areas. This has implications of prioritizing values in various disciplines and their scholars. These scholars in turn influence the value substance and methodology prescribed for institutions in a centralized model of education.[3]

All these three aspects if practiced would make students value conscious. The need for value education has been stressed by all the commissions set-up for educational development from time to time.

Radhakrishnan Commission (1948)

"If we exclude spiritual training in our institutions we would be untrue to our whole historical development."

Sri Prakasa Committee on Religious and Moral Instruction

"Every effort must, therefore, be made to teach students true moral values from the earliest stages of their educational life."

Kothari Commission (1964-66)

"A serious defect in the education system is the absence of provision for education in social, moral and spiritual values. A national system of education that is related to life, needs and aspirations of the people cannot afford to ignore this purposeful force."

National Policy on Education (1986)

"The growing concern over the erosion of essential values and an increasing cynicism in society has brought to focus the need for readjustments in the curriculum in order to make education a forceful tool for the cultivation of social and moral values."

Programme of Action NPE (1992)

"The framework emphasized value education as an integral part of school curriculum. It highlighted the values drawn from national goals, universal perception, ethical considerations and character building. It stressed the role of education in combating obscurantism, religious fanaticism, exploitation and injustice as well as the inculcation of values."[4]

In addition to the emphasis of commissions on moral education, persons of eminence have also advocated the cause of moral education for all round development of the youth.

Education is a powerful and pervasive agent for all round development, individual and social transformation. This alone can sustain culture and civilization. A balanced development of mind and body in harmony with the spirit is the key to the enrichment of human personality and also the key to 'true education,' which must in the ultimate analysis help humanity to rise to a higher level of consciousness. Gandhiji said: "Unless the development of mind and body goes hand in hand with a corresponding awakening of the soul, the former alone would prove to be a poor lopsided affair. By spiritual training, I mean education of the heart. A proper and all round development of the mind, therefore, can take place only when it proceeds *paripassu* with the education of the physical and spiritual faculties of the child. . . . Our children must from their infancy be taught the 'dignity of labour'. Thus, the true meaning of education is harmonious development of head, heart and hand, i.e. enlighment of mind, compassion and dignity of labour." Such qualities would automatically promote the development of youth.

Sarvepalli Radhakrishnan said: "The three things—vital dynamism, intellectual efficiency and spiritual direction together constitute the proper aim of education. Moral and spiritual training is an essential part of education. Enfranchisement of the mind, freedom from prejudice and fanaticism, and courage are essential. What we need today is the education of the whole man—physical, vital, mental, intellectual and spiritual..... If education is to help us to meet the moral challenge of the age and play its part in the life of the community, it should be liberating and life giving. It must give a basic meaning to personality and existence and equip us with the power to overcome spiritual inertia and foster spiritual sensitivity. . . . Seat of learning should produce men and women who will move together to develop common ideals and purposes, love each other and co-exist to create a co-operative common wealth."

Swami Vivekananda had proclaimed: "We must have life-building, man-making, character-building education." Shanker Dayal Sharma, former President of India, the scholar-educationalist had said, "The aim and objective of all education is to maintain, sustain and develop a healthy mind in a healthy body. Co-curricular and extra-curricular activities have as much place in our system as the curriculum and the syllabus. The lack of such activities is the reason for the growing evils of habitual smoking, drinking and drug-addiction fast growing amidst our student community. . . . Education is not injection or injunction. It is not indoctrination of views and ideas or just an imposition of one's views upon others. In short, education should not be an infliction. The moment education becomes such an infliction, the consequence will be student indiscipline, strikes and agitations within the campus." Pandit Nehru rightly said: "A vast responsibility . . . rests on our universities and educational institutions and those who guide their destinies. They have to keep their lights burning and must not stray from the right path even when passion convulses the multitude and blinds many amongst those whose duty is to set an example to others."

Gurudev Rabindranath Tagore had a vision for such an education: "Education must aim at the development of moral, spiritual and ethical values and we should seek them in our own heritage as well as in other cultures and civilizations. . . . It should be such that Indians do not lose sight of their rich heritage—their thought must be rooted to the ideals set forth in the great writings and works of our sages, poets and philosophers. The noble goals and high values set forth in our precious culture must be adhered to."

Shanker Dayal Sharma had said: "Thus a teacher must succeed in conveying the larger ideals of service to the community, virtues of tolerance and respect for all faiths, the importance of character, integrity and discipline and the value of humanism to his pupils. They should also be made aware of our heritage and culture." He was a great advocate of 'developing a mature attitude towards religion'. To quote him again: "Acquaintance with prayers of different religion and hymns and songs of various faiths could also, surely, help our youth to recognize the intrinsic purity, beauty and practical usefulness of different religious thoughts."[5]

Value is a "conception explicit or implicit, distinctive of an individual or characteristic of a group of those desirable traits which influence the selection from available modes and ends of action."

(Wuchohn, 1957). (Rokeach 1973) defined values as "enduring belief, a specific mode of conduct and state existence along a continuum of relative importance." Values are the criteria for determining levels of goodness, worth or beauty.

Values in our education is a hotly debated subject nowadays. This is because of the chaotic conditions observed in almost all spheres of our national life. It is conjectured, not without reason, that this chaos is mainly due to *lack of values* in the education being imparted in India. This was formulated, as is well-known, by Macaulay in 1836 more to enslave the Indian mind than to liberate it, so that Indians would remain loyal to British Raj, being alienated from their native Vedic culture, education and Sanskrit language. As planned, this gradually weaned our intellectuals away from our classical heritage and from the Sanskrit language, in which lay all our spiritual, cultural, social, and political traditions. We lost our indigenous system of education in which hearing, chanting and memorizing played a great part, assimilation of ideas took place through a well-planned life of service to teacher, contemplation and meditation, all under his guidance. Thus the educated ones in that system were men who had not only knowledge but also character. Knowledge had become a part of their life, influencing their thoughts, emotions and actions.

The Sanskrit for values is dharma or Sadâcâra. Dharma is described as 'the set of values that sustains the creation without which the very existence of it would be threatened.' Sankaracharya defined dharma as the values that sustained human beings and helped them to enjoy happiness both in this as well as in the spiritual world.

Thus education in India meant not merely intellectual cramming of information into the brain but the application of them into one's life so that life became better at individual, social, secular, spiritual levels. Education was a life-transformer. That is real education which liberates.[6]

Eminent Journalist, Mr. V.N. Narayanan, Editor, *The Hindustan Times*, delivered the Convocation Address at the XV and XVI convocation of the Nagarjuna University. He said, "When we face problems of ethics, we tend to solve them by research, by statistics, by the use of instruments and resources rather than by moral energy. The Victorian society in Britain, the pre-Independence Congress party under Mahatma Gandhi, Abraham Lincoln's era in U.S. politics displayed this moral energy. This is not to be confused with excessive Puritanism or moralism. All it demanded of the people was the feeling that they were put on this earth in order to leave it a better place than you found it."[7]

RATIONALE AND PHILOSOPHY OF VALUES

A recent conference, "Dialogue among civilizations quest for new perspectives", July 9-10, 2000 elaborated the concept of values as:

Values may be defined as those desirable ideals and goals which are intrinsic in themselves and which, when achieved or attempted to be achieved, evoke a deep sense of fulfilment to one or many or all parts of what we consider to be the highest elements of our nature. Values are norms, which hold and sustain life and society and establish a symbiotic and interdependent relationship between humankind and ecosystem. Values denote a fundamental category; in a common understanding they correspond to what we mean when it is said that Truth, Beauty and Goodness are the Supreme value of life. They occur to us whenever we try to conceive all those states of our being or becoming in which we are likely to find some kind of ultimate fulfilment.

There are, indeed, values of physical life, values of emotional life, values of mental life, but these values constantly point towards certain basic and ultimate values, which are moral and spiritual in character.

Moral and spiritual values are the foundations of the highest peaks of civilization, and since they emancipate humanity from narrow grooves of thought, they deserve to be understood more and more clearly and more and more meaningfully. Moral and spiritual values appear to be the common elements of various religions promoting everlasting peace and universal harmony; we look up to the ethical and spiritual values in our effort to rise above differences among religions. In recent times, a vast effort has been made to discover the pursuit of those values—moral and spiritual—which are to be found among all religions. And it has been rightly argued that what is most important in religions is the pursuit of ethical and spiritual values, which transcend the externalities of religious institutions.

Science, morality and spirituality are intimately intertwined and they should not be viewed as antagonistic to each other. Indeed, the survival of human race at the present critical juncture of human history will depend upon the pursuit of ethical and spiritual values. It has been rightly contended that peace is a most desirable objects of the present world and that peace cannot be achieved unless individuals and increasing masses of people contemplate and practice ethical and spiritual values such as those of unity, harmony, mutuality, friendship, faithfulness, sincerity and respect for diversity.

Spirituality is premised on universal consciousness, which can serve as the basis of the unity of humankind, and ethical systems derive their force and sustaining power from spiritual consciousness. In the field of education, ethical and spiritual values need to be encouraged, since they are directly related to the character development of students. In the latest reports of UNESCO, "Learning to Be" and "Learning: Treasure within", the highest ideals have been put forward. The concept of "To Be" is so defined as to mean development of the fullness of personality in all richness. And this fullness of personality involves fullness of ethical and spiritual development. The ideal of "To Be" is distinct from the ideal of "To Acquire" and "To Possess." The ideal of "To Be" refers to that direction of effort which leads the individual to look deeply within oneself and to find in his or her inner being the source and treasure of his or her potentialities and actualities, the source of a harmony of the complexity of personality, and the source of fulfilment in some kind of perfection that transcends egoism and which rests in a vast and integrated self-hood.

The National Policy on Education has laid special stress on value-education. It has said, In our culturally plural society education should foster universal and eternal values, oriented towards the unity and integration of our people. Such value education should help eliminate obscurantism, religious fanaticism, violence, superstition and fatalism. Apart from the combative role, value education has a profound positive context based on our heritage, national goals, universal perceptions. It should lay primary emphasis on this aspect."

R. Natarajan, Chairman AICTE has rightly said in his convocation address at Triputi:

When we say that a person has 'values', we imply that he has certain fundamental beliefs about what is desirable or good, and that he attempts to use these in directing his life. For beliefs of this kind to be called values, two conditions are generally held to apply:

Values are formed as a result of reflection and judgment; this they are different from desires.

- A person's values are beliefs which he sees as applicable not only to himself, but also to others; essential to the idea of value is the function of commanding.
- A person's values are beliefs which he sees as applicable not only to himself, but also to others: essential to the idea of value is the function of commanding.[8]

The Seven Sins, according to Mahatma Gandhi, are:

Politics without Principle.
Wealth without Work.
Pleasure without Conscience.
Knowledge without Character.
Commerce without Morality.
Science without Humanity.
Worship without Sacrifice.

To quote Anita Shetty again;

Values are those standards or codes of conduct conditioned by one's cultural tenets, guided by conscience, according to which one is supposed to conduct himself and shape his life pattern by integrating his benefits, ideas and attitudes to realize the cherished ideals and aims of life. By values we mean the criterion or basis for choosing between alternative courses of action. High values lead to objective, fair, correct decisions and actions and ensure the welfare of all concerned. Low values do exactly the opposite. Therefore, what we need more today is moral leadership focused

CHART 6.2

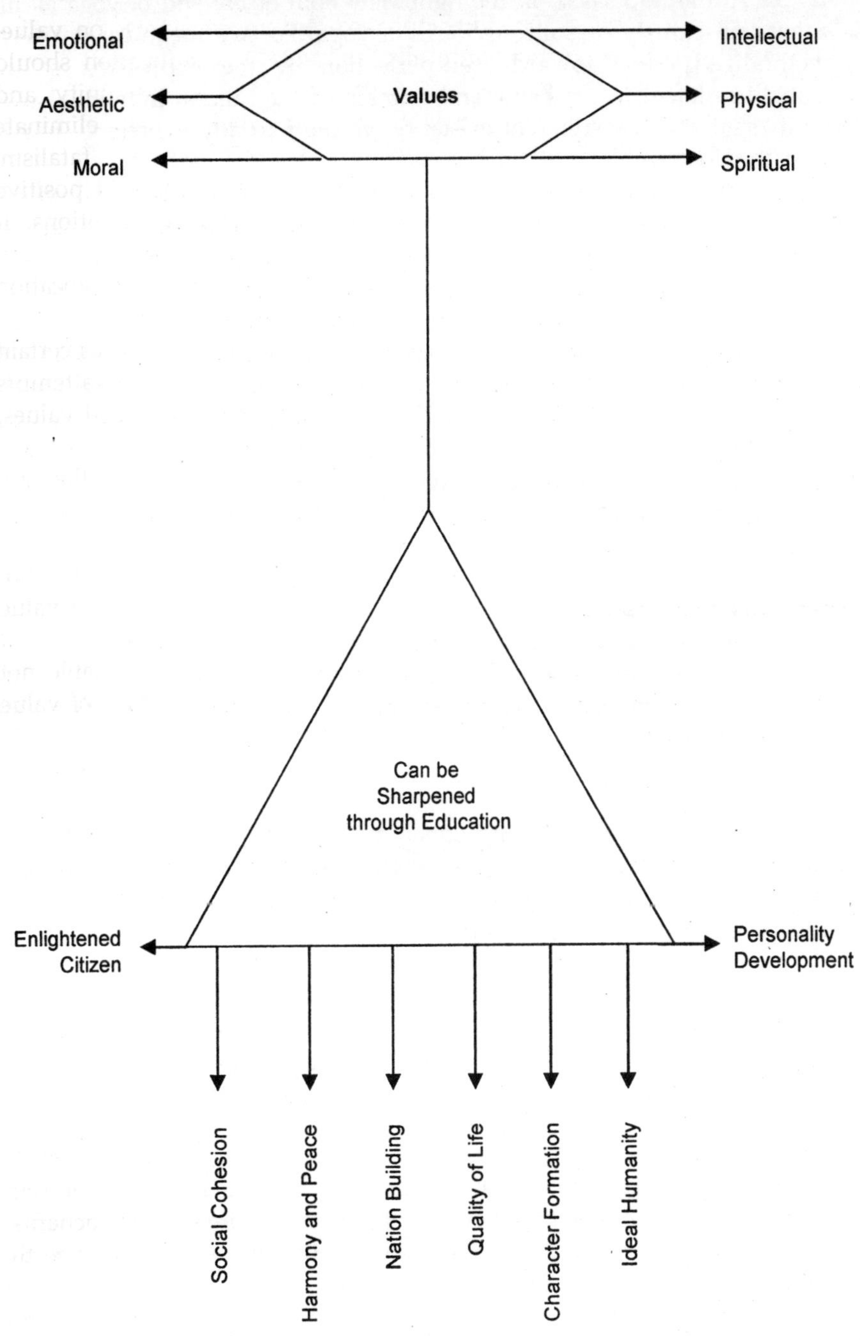
Emotional
Aesthetic
Moral
Values
Intellectual
Physical
Spiritual
Can be
Sharpened
through Education
Enlightened
Citizen
Personality
Development
Social Cohesion
Harmony and Peace
Nation Building
Quality of Life
Character Formation
Ideal Humanity

on courage, intellectual integrity and sense of values. There is no substitute for a sense of value.

Sir Aurobindo says: "In the right view both of life and of yoga all life is either consciously or subconsciously a yoga. For we mean by this term a methodized effort towards self-perfection by the expression of the potentialities latent in the being and a union of the human individual with the universal and transcendent existence we see partially expressed in man and in the cosmos."[9]

To quote Anita Shetty, "Value is a conception, explicit or implicit, distinctive of an individual or characteristics which influences the selection, from available modes and ends of action." Wuchohn (1957), Rokeach (1973) defines values "as an enduring belief, a specific mode of conduct or end state existence along a continuum of relative importance."

Values maybe described as a system of personality traits which are in harmony with the inner nature of an individual and which are in accordance with the values approved by the society. The process of valuing is what we go through when we make judgment about things, events and people that we encounter in our day-to-day life.

Adisankaracarya has given many values which can make life beautiful. Let us mention some of them.

Yogah Karmasukausalam

Yoga is special skill in the performance of activities. The skill consists in maintaining the uniformity of mind in success and failure. The person who maintains this skill performs all the works as his duty. He dedicates his mind to God.

That is Knowledge

Samacittatva is unfailing equanimity—or evenness of mind in all situations—favourable or unfavourable. The person is not elated when good things happen nor gets angry when misfortune betides. This unwavering evenness of mind is true knowledge.

That is Yoga

That is knowledge, understanding of things like the self, acquired from the scriptures and the Preceptors. The single-pointed and striking realization of these truths, by controlling the sense organs is Yoga.

Achieve the Goal

Here in this present human life the self must be known. This is the injunction. How? If the Self is known in this birth the life's goal is achieved. This is the supreme truth. His life is fruitful. If the Self is not known in this life, that would become useless.

Experience True Knowledge

Tapah, the concentration of the physical body, the sense organs and the mind; damah, discontinuance from sense objects, Karma, Agnihotra, etc. rituals. One who attains holiness by means of purification of the heart through these things can get the knowledge of Brahman.

Don't Speak Untruth

Not that there ever was or is in them any falsehood. Contrary to that speaking untruth is the behaviour of bad people. Can any body become free from death? and decrepitude by his falsehood. For which reason (martyah), man (sasyam iva) like corn, (Pacyate), tatters and dies and after death (punah) again; sasyam iva ajavate, (reborns like conr). Thus what one can gain in this impermanent human world by breaking his own words?

CLASSIFICATION OF VALUES

Values have been classified differently by different educationists and philosophers. Mascarendhas classified them as professional values, operational values and dynamic values. National Education Policy (1986) classified all the values into three main categories—Personal values, Social values and National values. All the three supplement one another. Adherence to personal values would promote better social and national values.

Education with Value Focus

Sri Sathya Sai Institute of Higher Learning Prasanthi Nilayam (AP)

Sri Sathya Sai Institute of Higher Learning Prasanthi Nilayam (Andhra Pradesh) found on November 22, 1981, by Bhagavan Sri Sathya Sai Baba which grew out of the Colleges founded earlier by Bhagavan Sri Sathya Sai Baba at Anantapur, Andhra Pradesh, Whitefield (near Bangalore, Karnataka) and Prasanthinilayam, Andhra Pradesh.

Bhagavan, in His Divine Message to the students, announced that the main purpose of establishing the Institute of Higher Learning was to help them cultivate self–knowledge and self-confidence, so that each one of them can learn self-sacrifice and earn self-realization. He defined the goal as spiritual upliftment, self-discovery and social service through love and detachment.

The consistent endeavour of the university since its inception has been to develop core courses bringing out value-orientation in an appropriate manner, blending of science and spirituality, providing interaction between head and heart through self-reliance programmes and co-curricular activities, designing Awareness and Foundation courses and incorporating these as part of the curriculum with credits.

The philosophy of education of the Institute is based on the appreciation of the need to provide full scope for the development of body, mind and heart. Discipline, duty and adherence to basic human values are deeply appreciated as the best qualities of students in the Institute. These are being observed in various situations in the hostel, on the playground and in the Campuses and during the celebration of various festival and organization of festivals and other important functions. It is precisely because of the importance of these activities for the overall development of personality, that the Institute attaches great importance to integral items of education like Yogasanas, games and sports, attendance in morning prayers and meditation, attendance in universal prayers and participation in morning assembly talks, attendance in classes and social work/self-reliance programmes. These are incorporated in the total system of our education offered in the Institute.

A society without values will cease to be human. The more human values are cherished, the better will be the growth of society, the nation and the world. We cannot rest content with an educational system which is confined to academic achievement. It has to promote human virtues simultaneously. The main problem of our education today is how to adapt the spiritual and cultural traditions we have inherited from the past to our present day life.

The Institute believes that teaching of values cannot be confined only to specific programmes such as Awareness Programme under Undergraduate and Postgraduate Courses and foundational courses in Professional Studies. Values will have to be presented as a part and parcel of teaching of the subject. In the process of teaching of various subjects, whether it is physical sciences, biological sciences, social sciences or Commerce and Management, the values are appropriately incorporated in the subjects in order that the students would appreciate and imbibe the practical applications of values in their day-to-day living.

Even research is value-based. For years, the Chemistry department has been focusing on the Chemistry of Natural Products, and in particular on the possible use of various native plants for producing drugs. Many of the Dissertations of the students of M.Tech. [Computer Science] address the needs of the Sri Sathya Sai Institute of Higher Medical Sciences [popularly known as the Super-Specialty Hospital]; and so on.

On the sports field, the stress is less on competition and more on collective enjoyment. Indeed, the events presented on the Institute's Annual Sports and Cultural festival held every year on January 11th are carefully planned to promote such a spirit.

"We do not need today a new faith or creed, nor a new system of education. Nor need we create a new society. All we need are men and women who have pure and loving hearts. Their hearts must be filled with sacred feeling. The transformation has to be effected in the minds of the people."

"Our educational institution (University) is making an endeavour so that in a few years from now we shall have thousands of these students who will scatter themselves to all parts of the world. The uppermost thing for the students is that they should futher this moral aspect of ours." Most of the research studied carried out in the field of value education revealed the following:

Chart 6.3

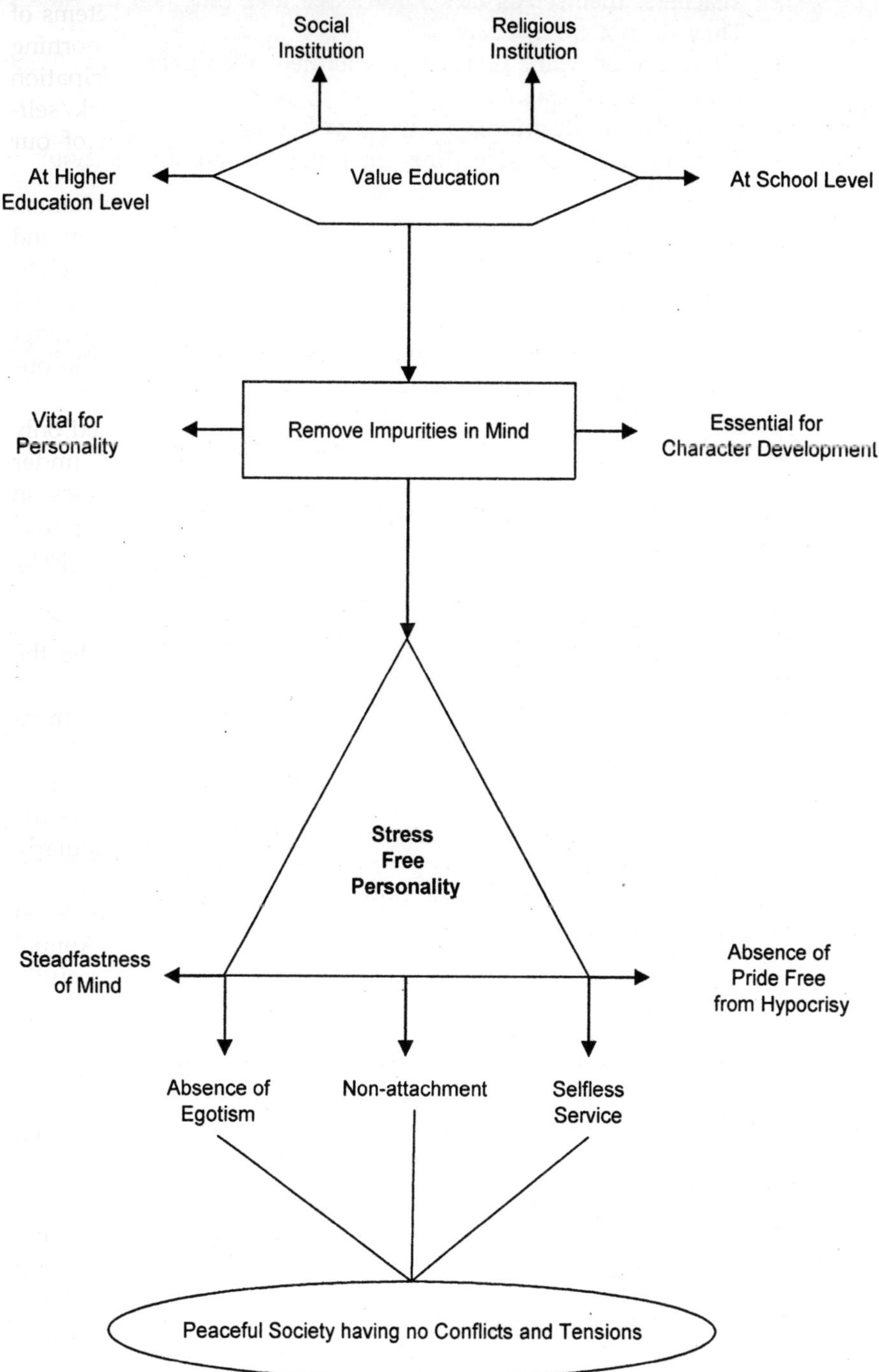
Social Institution
Religious Institution
At Higher Education Level
Value Education
At School Level
Vital for Personality
Remove Impurities in Mind
Essential for Character Development
Stress Free Personality
Steadfastness of Mind
Absence of Pride Free from Hypocrisy
Absence of Egotism
Non-attachment
Selfless Service
Peaceful Society having no Conflicts and Tensions

1. Educational system at present is not congenial to value promotion.
2. Teachers, themselves lack knowledge and rationale of values. They do not follow values.
3. Literature on value education is limited. Whatever is available is not of good quality.
4. Students are murmured by modern fashion.
5. Families are also forgetting their role as the first school of citizenship.
6. Materialism has left no place.
7. Leaders have no values.
8. The aim of students is to pass the examination and not personality development.
9. Negative values like drinking, smoking, gambling are common among teachers and students.

Let us discuss the role of Moral Values in education.

I. Building of Human beings with Strength and Power based upon our Ancient Values

Even during the last century Swami Vivekananda had issued the following warning, "All political and social system and organizations basically depend upon the goodness of man. Men cannot be made virtuous by an Act of Parliament. It cannot be taken for granted that if the Parliament enacts good legislation a nation becomes automatically strong. But if the people of a country become good and great, that country becomes automatically good and great. Of all forms of wealth in the world man is the most valuable.

"Acts of Parliament, Government, political administration, all these are indeed means, but they are not our final goal. Beyond them there is a goal, which is not governed by any of these factors. Christ discovered that moral fervour and purity of heart are true sources of strength. Our sages proclaimed the same truth. It is thus that religion strikes at the root of the problem, it moulds man's character.

"So every improvement in India requires first of all an upheaval in religion. Before flooding India with socialistic or political ideas, first deluge the land with spiritual ideas. The first work that demands our attention is that the most wonderful truths confined in our Upanishads, in our scriptures, in our Puranas must be brought out from the books, brought out from the monasteries, brought out from the forests, brought out from the possession of selected bodies of people, and scattered broadcast all over the land. . . .

"The secret of achieving national spirit in our country lies in regaining our spiritual strength, which seem to have been lost. If we have to lift ourselves up, we should stop quarrelling among ourselves. Keep the motto before you—"Elevation of the masses without injuring their religion."[10]

2. Education for Peace: Values for Co-operation

His Holiness The Dalai Lama in his extension lecture at NCERT spoke of the exceptional intellectual abilities and qualities possessed by human beings, which make them superior to all other species. These qualities could be developed and nurtured through education to help man achieve higher levels of development. He referred to the rich legacy of Indian tradition, its ancient system of education, which promoted spirituality and produced great thinkers, philosophers and spiritual leaders. The inculcation of good human qualities like compassion, respect and sense of truthfulness, caring, etc. have been a part of the Indian way of life. But now when India has achieved tremendous progress, there is a decline in human values. The modern system has no place for spirituality whereas human values are essential for leading a happy life. Human values, therefore, have to be brought in the education system but without attaching them to any religion. Friendly relationships with others according to Him are essential for peace. Modern society is becoming increasingly interdependent hence learning to live together in the family, with neighbours is essential for national and world peace. Children from young age have to be made aware of the interdependence between human beings.[11]

3. Promotes Efficiency through Ethical Values

When the mind is concentrated efficiency is found to happen. Swami Purananda rightly states:[12] The right values step up one's efficiency. In order to manage our own life at home in the world and in our professional field, the higher values are necessary, so that our reaction to the outside world, our judgement of the situation that is around us—all is totally changed. And, we will be able to, not only face the challenges in front of us, but also still discover in our minds a lot of mental energy left, which we can apply for our quantity purpose of planning the future.

Ethical virtues are the intelligent ways of reviving man's exhausted energies and fatigued spirit to live. By living these healthy values of righteous living, the individual unshackles his psychological personality from its self-made entanglements. As a contrast to this, the negative tendencies cultivated by the 'diabolically fallen' are self-made shackles that chain a man to a realm of confusions and sorrows forbidding him to grow into the ampler fields of his own inner possibility.

4. Co-ordial Relations between the Teacher and Students: Values of Respect, Love and Affection

Swami Lokeswarananda observes that according to the Indian tradition, a teacher is like a lighted lamp from which other lamps may be lighted. This underlines the fact that a teacher must himself be a highly educated man, otherwise he is not entitled to teach. Can a blind man lead another blind man?

But it will be a mistake to think that academic qualification is the only criterion of a teacher. He may have encyclopaedic knowledge, but to

CHART 6.4

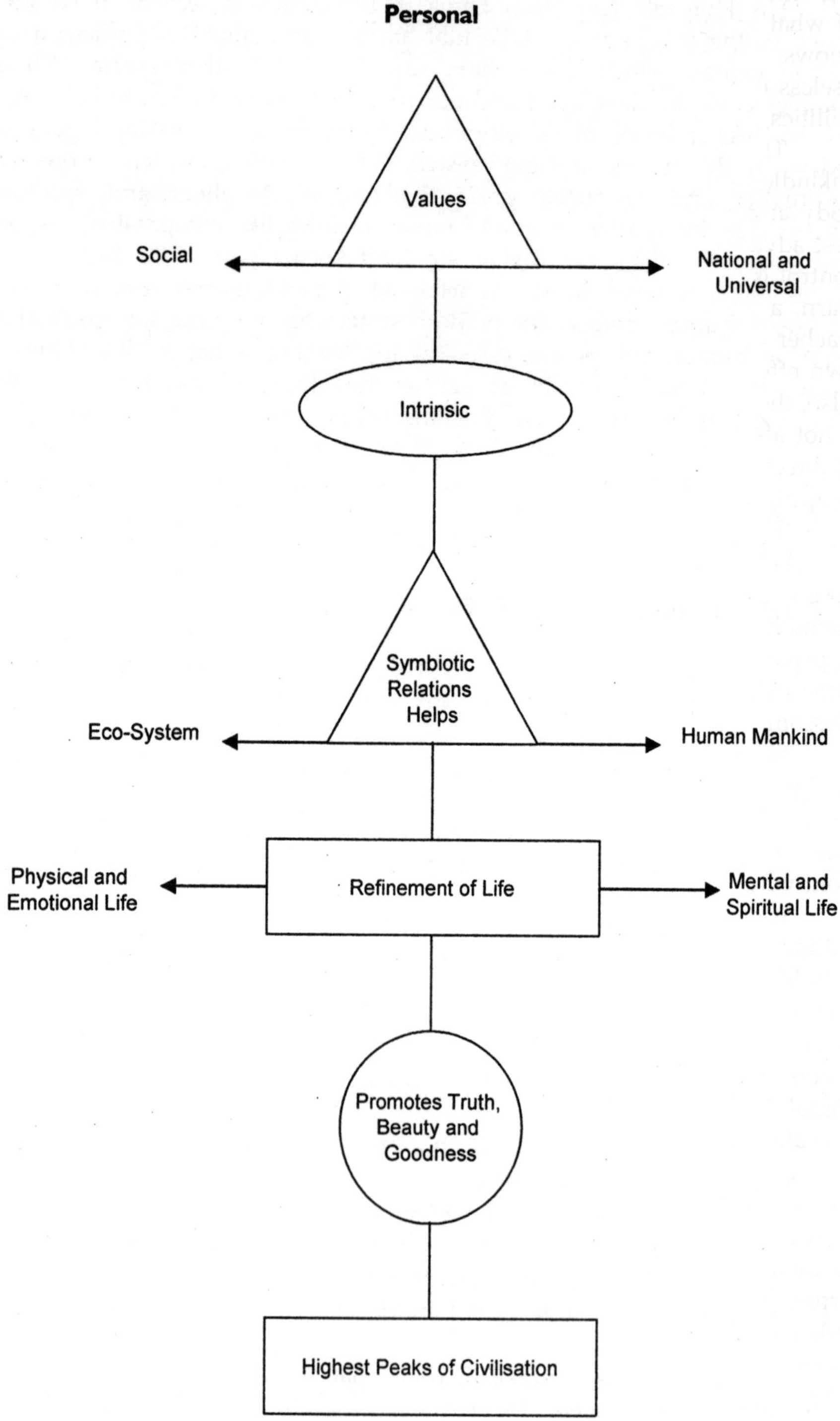

Personal

Values

Social

National and Universal

Intrinsic

Symbiotic Relations Helps

Eco-System

Human Mankind

Physical and Emotional Life

Refinement of Life

Mental and Spiritual Life

Promotes Truth, Beauty and Goodness

Highest Peaks of Civilisation

this must be added moral excellence of the highest order. He need not teach high moral principles, he has to live them. A teacher should be an example of what is best in man. He can inspire by what he is and not by what he knows. 'To know is to be'—runs a popular dictum in India. Knowledge is useless if it does not make a man perfect—perfect not merely in skills and abilities, but also in character.

The teacher's task is to impart knowledge but to do this, he must first enkindle in the pupil a thirst for knowledge. He must also train his pupil's body and mind, train his faculties, so that the pupil can use them to his best advantage. Mind is man's most powerful organ. A healthy mind under control is man's best friend and guide. Given such a mind and a desire to learn, a student can learn by his own efforts, with the assistance of the teacher or even without. In fact, one learns best when one learns by one's own efforts, for how much knowledge can a teacher pass on to his pupil? Also, the knowledge that the teacher imparts may turn out to be outdated, if not also wrong. The most a teacher can do is to give his pupil a sense of direction, that is, tell him what to learn and how to learn it and also how to apply that knowledge for his own good and the good of his community.

The relationship between the teacher and the taught is exactly like the relationship of the gardener and the flowers on the bush. The gardener does not create the flowers from the soil and the manure; the flowers must themselves come from the bush. The gardener can only tend its roots, water it, protect it, see that it has the correct amount of sunlight and shade—all these externals he can provide. But no mere gardener can guarantee the blossom; it can come only from the bush itself.

Similarly, the teacher's job is to nurture the student with right thoughts. The student must be given a conductive and protective environment where he or she need not overstrain to live. But the blossoming—the real fragrance and beauty of the personality—must come from within.[13]

If contemporary education is to be value-based, it can never be done without the teachers themselves understanding, appreciating and upholding the life-sustaining moral values. The teachers cannot have any excuse whatsoever. If one cannot practise these values, one should not dream of teaching as a job. In fact, teaching is not a job. It is a mission and vision for life and for posterity. Swami Vivekananda established the Ramakrishna Mission order in 1897. Now there are a number of educational institutions, administered by Ramakrishna Mission throughout the country. They are transmitting the universal values of austerity, brotherhood, compassion, dedication, empathy, faithfulness, grace, hardwork, integrity, justice, kindness, liberty, mercy, non-violence, obedience, perseverance, fortitude, rationality, selflessness, truth, unity, virtue, wisdom, yoga and zest. A unique enterprise in educational endeavour is Shri Sathya Sai Baba Institute of Higher Learning, a deemed university, for the promotion of value-based education. It is situated at Prasanti Nilayam (AP), the headquarters of Sri Sai Baba mission. There are similar institutions, run by other missions in the country. If these educational institutions can be strengthened further, of course, within the secular framework of the Indian Constitution, India will ably meet the challenges of the twenty-first century.

K. Muralidharan in his article, "Value in Education: A Changing Concept" in *University News*, January 7-13, 2002 strongly feels that:

The Indian culture is deeply rooted in spiritual values and unless these values find their way into the life of students, education will lose its significance and will not fulfil its function of endowing the students with a vision to live by and with the ideals to work for. Therefore, in deference to the cherished goals of democracy, socialism, humanism and secularism, it is very essential that our education system should evolve a new positive morality, which could effectively be built into the school curriculum.

It is essential that, the teachers also should be exposed to the traditional values and ethics of education through training programs from time to time. They should not confine to their job to a mere matter of completing syllabus and following the curriculum. There should be a platform for teachers to deliberate on any sensitive issues or topics as and when the need arises. They should also explore the ideas of accepting modernisation, globalisation and liberalisation from the academic point of view. They should also learn while imparting their duties for which they are meant. By creating a conductive atmosphere for intellectual rigor and freedom of expression and thought, one can practice values in education.[14]

The National Commission on Teachers (1852), also known as Chattopadhyay Commission, observed:

"There has been a feeling of grievance on the part of the teachers that they do not receive the status and respect from society that their profession and role demand. . . . It may be recalled that the Guru never demanded reverence by the Shishya, his parents and the adult community gladly and gratefully proffered it to the teacher. So must the teacher earn status through achievements. The closer the teacher the more he is able to link himself and his vocation with the mission for the nation, the more relevant he will become and more revered by students, parents and society. We underscore that the primary task of the teacher is concerned with man-making namely the making of the Indian of tomorrow. The Universal; the Guru (Teacher) is personal in relationship. The illustrious poet, Kalidasa, speaks of the Guru in the following words: "He converts darkness into light and makes the invisible God visible."

5. Value Education Promotes Personality Development and Social Cohesion

Value education helps oneself and one's relation to society. Value education makes one peaceful and by his personality, he adds peace to the society. Individual and society supplement each other.

Education is a personality building process. It has always been linked with society. It has both a personal and social dimension, and like the two sides of the same coin, these are inseparable. According to Gandhiji, real education did not consist in packing the brain with information, facts and figures, or in passing examinations by reading the prescribed number of books, but by developing the right character. At present, our education system is largely involved in preparing the younger generation for developing their cognitive domain. It is mainly based on the preponderance of public examination and excessive competitive spirit at the cost of developing the more important affective domain. Today, what is being done is to educate the heads and hands and not the hearts. Essential education must lead to internalisation of the obligation on the part of each human being to be value-conscious in word, thought and deed. Lack of value education has been an important factor in the global scenario of growing violence and terrorism, pollution and ecological imbalances. The Education Commission (1964-66) and the National Policy on Education (NPE-1986) stressed the importance of value-oriented education in our country. The Rammurthy Committee Report (1990) recommended that the imparting of value education should be an integral part of the entire educational process.[15]

6. An Integral 'Vision' for National Regeneration: National Values

Value education makes the youth powerful. They contribute a great deal to the national reconstruction and national development.

An old Jewish proverb says that 'a man without a dream and a nation without a vision shall perish'. We need a great vision to build a great nation. In the multi-religious context of India, this vision has to be an inclusive one. It must be deeply rooted in the truth, goodness and beauty of our ancient culture and tradition and at the same time, it must also be in harmony with the scientific developments of the era. We are fortunate that our Constitution has been able to capture and embody this spirit of unity and harmony of cultures and religions and the scientific temperament of the modern world.

I am inspired to present to you here a vision of a great India firmly rooted in her own rich spiritual and cultural heritage and at the same time fully open to the scientific development of humankind. I have termed this great India of our vision Bharatiya Dharma Rajya or Dharma Bharathi in short.

Bharatiya Dharma Rajya is the vision of an India of love, unity and peace built on the integral concept of Dharma and on the ensuring Bharatiya Dharma as embodied in the Preamble and Article 51(A) of the Indian Constitution. This is the vision of an awakened India of political stability, social harmony and economic prosperity built on an integral vision of life and reality. It is the vision of a disciple nation of God on earth where all religions and cultures will be respected for their unique insights into Truth and valuable contributions towards human welfare, an India where all living beings will live in harmony and peace with one another as the fulfilment of our age-old dream of a Vasudhaiva Kutumbakam. This is our vision of the great India of the third millennium that will be a land and light of Dharma in humanity's quest for a culture of life, unity and peace on earth.

'Peace and Value Education for Schools/Colleges' should present and promote this noble and inter-religious vision of Bharatiya Dharma Rajya in our intuitions of learning and among our youth if it is to lead to the much needed national regeneration of India. This is a religious task more than a political task that can only be achieved through interreligious cooperative action. It will be difficult for political parties and governments to take up this task on their own, they can only support and collaborate with religious-minded and peace-loving patriotic citizens of India in this divine mission.[16]

7. Value Education will Build Character

At present, the Government of this country is striving to bring about universal education. In this context, it will be useful to consider what the purpose of education is. Great men of this land have declared that education should foster character, help the acquisition of good qualities, or seela, and eradicate vices, knowledge should also enable us to understand the truth about things. Saivite and Vaishnavite saints have proclaimed that God alone is Truth, and the rest is maya or illusion. These sages and saints endeavoured to realise Truth, that is God. In Him they found their supreme joy. They looked at everything else as the sources of evil and suffering. In the Vedas, the Paramatman is spoken of as Truth. When it is declared that everything connected with this world is mithya, or false, it to so much to condemn the world as to affirm that the Paramatman alone is true.[17]

Right education should make us know that God is the Truth. Knowledge must fill one with good qualities through which alone one can realize the Truth, that is God. Therefore, the goal of knowledge is the understanding of the Ultimate Truth. The first fruit of education must be humility and self-control. Education that does not produce these qualities is useless. We find that people in countries where modern education has spread are not as virtuous as they should be. Unsophisticated illiterates, like those slaving in the tribal areas of South African jungles, are found to be more honest than those who have received the doubtful benefits of modern education. It is sad to note that in our own schools and colleges, indiscipline is rampant now-a-days. Even girls, who are by nature docile, have caught this infection of indiscipline. All these developments give rise to the question whether this kind of education is after all necessary or useful. Such education is the cause of stress among students.

From time immemorial, the necessity to acquire knowledge is being emphasized and he who has had no education is considered an animal. Vidyaa viheenah pasuh says Bhartruhari. But what is the type of education our ancients had in mind when they said. . . . Vidyaa vinaya sampanna? A thing can be done either in the dharmic way or in the adharmic way. Good results will flow when a thing is done in the right way.[18]

8. Study of the Life of Great Men to Learn from their Practice in Life

We must train our people from an early age to study the lives of great men who led an unattached life, free from debasing passions like lust, anger, greed and fear and, following their example, develop faith in God. This will help them to grow up into dutiful and honest citizens, disciplined to lead a moral and ethical life. If the government also takes sufficient interest in making provision for teaching moral and spiritual values to children, it stands to gain much. For one thing, expenditure on police and law courts will get reduced. They will also be free from the troubles arising from strikes and other forms of student indiscipline.

"The Inculcation of moral and spiritual values in the minds of the people from the early years is most desirable that provision should be made for the teaching of moral and spiritual values in educational institutions).[19]

9. Nation-building and Promotion of Peaceful World Order

In the words of Sri Sathya Sai Baba, education is for man-making, nation-building and promotion of peaceful world order. At the dawn of the new millennium and in the changed policy framework of the Government, there is an urgent need among teachers to inculcate values among students so that they develop into integrated personalities blossoming mentally, emotionally, intellectually, ethically and spiritually (Khandelval, 2001). Teachers in higher education have to act as a role model to bring back values among students, educational institutions and in the society as a whole. They have to act as role models in terms of their honesty, sincerity, hard work and determination towards their duties and responsibilities in order to create an example before their students. The students at this stage are at the cross-road of their career and life. At this stage, normally students seek to identify with some role models for their life. Therefore, the role of teacher at this level of education is to create and recreate the values among students, in educational institutions and the society as a whole. They have a greater responsibility in shaping the destiny of future generation and the country as well. They should also come forward catering to the educational needs at primary and secondary levels in the society. They should be conscious about their social responsibilities. No external force should be required to inculcate in them a sense of dedication and responsibility. The role of teacher at the higher level is different from their counterparts at other stages on account of these teachers' greater involvement with activities related to research, publications, training and administrative responsibilities.[20]

10. Core Values Based Education Promotes Ideal Humanity

The Parliamentary Standing Committee on Human Resource Development in its Eighty-first Report on Value Based Education (1999) has highlighted that Truth (Satya), Righteous Conduct (Dharma), Peace (Shanti), Love (Prema) and Non-violence (Ahimsa) as the Core universal values, which need to be identified as the foundation stone on which the value-based education programme can be built up. All the religions of the world have also emphasized that non-violence, tolerance and peace are the fundamental components of humanity. Great philosophers and social thinkers of East as well as West have seen education as a process leading ultimately to spiritual development. UNESCO in the context of peace, refers education not only to general education acquiring cognitive capital but ability to live together.[21]

11. External and Internal Values must Act in Harmony

The wonderful development of science during the past three hundred years concerns the external nature and the world outside. The study of the nature and potentialities of the human mind is of more recent origin—it has a history of about hundred years. It is true that with the help of scientific equipment, like the microscope and telescope, the scientist has understood innumerable minute details of the exterior world. But many of the scientists are realizing, though belatedly, that the nature of the mind, its constant tendency to flow outward, prevents it from getting an insight into many other aspects of the mind which can be achieved only by the practice of meditation.

Scientists have provided us with various kinds of conveniences and comforts by discovering innumerable natural laws and thus uncovering the secrets of nature. It has to be admitted that the human power of investigation has reached an all-time high; man has displayed the peak of his intellectual ability. But is it not within his power to create a beautiful world full of honesty, justice, brotherhood, mutual understanding, cooperation, peace and tolerance? Why has he not succeeded in creating such a world?

The following voice of a poet reflects the present predicament of mankind:

People fear people
Doubt reigns everywhere
Behind the curtain of peace
Martial moves the revolution
Meanness yet unheard of
Devilishness in patriotic garb
Tuskers among nations crush life apace
Not to speak of the bloody flame
Rising high on the West
Bullets are at play
Mad after martial joy

The scientist can make the five elements dance to his tune, he can transverse land, water and space at a marvelous speed, and he can drive away terrible epidemics, which threaten the human race. Can't he instill in the hearts of men, who live and thrive now, but who are liable to decay and die, a sense of brotherhood and friendship? Can't he quench the primordial fire of hatred by pouring forth the ambrosia of love?

The following is the answer to the question:

Progress is to take place in two fields. It relates to the two faces of nature:

The one is the physical nature, the nature of the external world. The other is the inner nature of man. The one is related to the world that we see. The other one is related to the inner-self of man with whose help he is able to see the world outside and investigate.

If man is able to increase his power to free himself from the hold of the surrounding world or environment, if he increases his freedom, if he gains control over nature, we may say that the change we call development leads to progress. In this respect, the innumerable discoveries of scientists have helped us gain control over the outside nature. Undoubtedly, we are moving on the path of outward development and progress. But is there a comparable development in the regions of the mind?[20] Upon this understanding depends the solution of educational problems.

12. Ethical and Moral Values: The Foundation of the Quality of Life

Ethical and moral values are the basis of good life as ethical culture indeed ennobles human life. Ethics, religion and spirituality have become synonymous terms in common parlance as they co-exist in the development of moral culture and of righteous and virtuous life. Moral living starts through dedication to ideal principles, maxims and human values. A righteous and virtuous life and a clear conscience provide the backbone of spiritual as well as a humane material progress of the civilized man and his society.

No ideal, ideology, institution or religion is self-operative. It is through human agency alone that ideals and institutions established for their realization are made operational. History bears witness to perversions, distortions and abuse or misuse of ideals and institutions for the reason that human being is essentially imperfect though he seeks perfection. It is true that perfection is not attainable by imperfect beings, however it is always worthwhile attempting and this depends largely upon a meaningful education of man with a view to fertilizing the soil within so that the vessel may bear rich, juicy and truthful fruits. Sustenance of human values, ethics and morals in human society and spiritual enlightenment of man seem to be decidedly more effective and meaningful goals of educational philosophy to follow. It is principally inadequate appreciation of the essentially spiritual nature of man and prevailing disrespectful attitude towards the role of true religion or spiritualism in protecting and promoting the spiritual core of human beings which accounts for the crisis of our times.

Ever since the dawn of human civilization, conscious efforts have been made by man to cultivate values in order to humanize himself by conquering his animal instincts and ennobling his life by harmonious development of all the faculties. When one realizes that one's actions affect the entire society, the value system that we live by and the choices that we make acquire paramount importance. Living a life based on noble values enables human beings to refine their character which is called culture. The culture of a people or a nation is based upon the values that those constituting it live and uphold in their lives. When the cultural values deteriorate, civilization declines but when these are promoted civilization flourishes. Whenever higher ideals are abandoned and fundamental cultural values of the society are totally ignored, civilizations have disappeared. If perversions of man's desires and natural urges transgress the control and limits set by nature, it results in the loss of culture which is his internal aspect. When his culture declines, it eventually results in withering away of civilization which essentially manifests external aspect of man's social life.

The modern world is marked by a widespread explosion of knowledge and tremendous achievements in Science and Technology, coupled with a general decline and reversal of human values as well as an alarming deterioration of moral and mental health both of individuals and societies. The recent spate of crimes, violence, terrorism, and drug abuse makes us aware of the significance of human values, without which human life loses all meaning. It is also evident that a mere economic prosperity and material wealth cannot result in a lasting well-being of mankind. The inner strength of mankind springs from within, which seems ill-nourished now. To fill up the void regarding human values, the richest resources are available in the texts and scriptures of all the religions of the world which have guided people in their thoughts, feelings and actions for ages. Human virtues have been propounded and preached by many great sages, prophets and teachers who had perceived subtle truths of human life, for the benefit of their adherents and for those who would derive benefits by studying their sayings and advices. Some of their sayings were understood by people in letter and spirit, enriching and elevating them, but some others were not understood well, ending up as mere outward rituals, blind faiths, intolerance with others and hatred for other faiths. More than a century ago, Swami Vivekananda had said: "We want to lead mankind to the place where there is neither the Vedas, nor the Bible, nor the Koran, yet this has to be done by harmonizing the Vedas, the Bible and the Koran. Man ought to be taught that religions are but the varied expression of the religion, which is oneness, so that each may choose the path that suits him best."[23]

13. Growth in Spiritual Values

One of our noblest duties in life is to grow. This is the screaming cry of all evolution. Growth in the biological apparatus was the command in the lower stages of evolution. After having attained manhood, the demand is to grow our moral stature, in our spiritual worth, in our cultural dignity. This is where study of the scriptures, regular and continuous, and sadhana, constant and sincere, come to serve us. The study clearly points out the goal and the way—the sadhana yields to us the energy and vitality to walk the path and explode into the goal. These we must.

14. Harmony and Peace: Values for Tolerance

In the world today, we are living through an age of confusions and tensions, both within and without us. The external challenges persecute us and render our lives unhappy and sorrow ridden. The intelligent philosophy of the Rishis advises man 'to live in harmony' with the situations in life and steadily work on to meet them with discretion and constant application. When we live thus for a period of time, a subjective poise develops, giving us inward peace and tranquillity, which, thereafter, remains unaffected by external threats and onslaughts.

Revered Shri Vethatheri, Maharishi says, 'has beautifully written that Harmony is a precious treasure of human life'. Real success and satisfaction, happiness are the different facets of harmony. If one is to enjoy the benefits of life to the fullest, it is necessary to develop and maintain harmony; and for this understanding the philosophy of nature is required.

Harmony should be maintained in all spheres of life, and these are:

- Between body and life;
- Between wisdom and habits;
- Between self and society;
- Between the purpose of life and the method of living.
- Between will and nature.

The more one understands life, the more one will achieve harmony; and success will be proportionate to that. No doubt, harmonizing life is a difficult task, but it is worth all the striving, for it is the only way to equip oneself to enjoy life to the fullest extent and to reach the goal of life, which is the perfection of consciousness. By the development of knowledge man comes to understand the cause and effect system which is the law of nature.

15. Values of Devotion and Dedication

Of the innumerable techniques prescribed by the rishis for self-development, the most popular ones are the path of selfless dedicated service (karma yoga), the path of discriminative knowledge (jnana yoga), and the mystic path of self-development through disciplined contemplation (raja yoga).

According to Sage Narada, true devotion for the Lord is superior and nobler to all these, because devotion is the final outcome of all other methods of self-development.

This supreme devotion is indeed, as a technique, even superior to the path of action, the path of knowledge, and the path of disciplined contemplation. (Narada Bhakti Sutra II:I:25)

All the other paths are the means that take the seekers to the final goal of spiritual experience, but in devotion there is very little difference in essence between the means and the end, between the way and the goal. Love alone is love's own end and fulfilment. Devotion is both the means and the end. As long as residual vasanas (inherent tendencies) are still lingering in the devotee's personality, so long is devotion only the path. But when, as a result of his love for the Lord, his vasanas disappear totally, a stage comes when his supreme love itself becomes the Lord of love Supreme.

Than all other paths, devotion is the one most readily available and most easily attainable. (Narada Bhakti Sutra VI:1:58)

Having dedicated all activities unto Him, the devotee should turn all desire, anger, pride, and so forth toward Him alone. (Narada Bhakti Sutra VI:2:65)

Having gained this supreme devotion, the devotee attains perfection and immortality and becomes extremely satisfied. (Narada Bhakti Sutra I:1:4)

Acharya Vinoba Bhave says: Knowledge, love, and constant effort are the three legs on which life stands. If one of the legs of a tripod is broken, it cannot stand, since all three legs are needed. This is also the condition of life. Even if we logically distinguish between devotion (bhakti), knowledge (jnana), and action (karma), we cannot divide them in experience. The three together make up one great entity.

CONCLUSION

The worst days of a serious threat to Indian society are over. Under foreign domination and western influence we had developed the foolish notion of degrading everything, morals, ethics and spirituality and were easily swept off our feet by the glamour and glitter of the exotic. The wonderful phenomenon that is taking place now is that we are returning to these things which have lent stability and strength to our culture over the centuries. Because the various educational programmes launched by the NCERT, UGC and other organizations (Such as Sri Sathya Sai Organization) ranging all the way from nursery to post-graduate level, are bringing into proper focus the valuable ingredients of our culture. By far the most important aspect of these programmes is that besides giving a theoretical and conceptual base in the curriculum they also seek to transform the quality of life through inculcation of human values of peace, love, truth, spirituality, right conduct, ahimsa and, above all, national character which, in effect, represent the highest and the noblest in our culture system.[24]

About ethical or approved conduct Apastamba-Dharma-Sutra (22.14) enjoins:

Absence of anger, elation, indignation, avarice, delusion, vanity and enmity; speaking truth; moderation in eating; refraining from exposing others' weak points; freedom from jealousy; sharing one's good things with others; sacrifice; straightforwardness; gentleness; quietude; self-control; friendliness with also beings; absence of cruelty; contentment—these form the approved conduct for men of all stations of life. By observing them duly one becomes universally benevolent.

Suresh Prasad Singh in his Article, "Emerging Values in Modern Education" suggests an integrated vision to promote value education. To quote him:

The power of modern education can be better realized by achieving a happy integration of utility and value, integration of body and mind, emotions and ideas, individual and society, and the world. The vision of progress must not be devoid of human element, the aspect of vision which makes the progress meaningful and purposeful. The progress that is aimed at the desired, is an assertion of the powers of human imagination, and soothe fruits of this progress must be realized with the ends of humanity in mind. The tools of change are powerful but their application must be human and they must be employed for pious purposes.

In the wake of the phenomenal developments on the educational front, re-orientation of values in the post-modernist education assumes special significance. Here are certain concrete recommendations for tempering utilitarian pursuit of together education with desirable ideals and visions of human happiness;

(a) Education must promote rational outlook on life and scientific approach to issues confronting the real life situations;
(b) An imaginatively farmed course in fundamental freedom and human rights must constitute of our degree level curriculum;
(c) Power that education generates must be employed for constructive human purposes;
(d) Education must develop sensitivity to environment and must foster human ethos for the enjoyment of the fruits of progress;
(e) Humanism should be the central concern of education in all circumstances, and it must promote quality concern for corporate behaviour and corporate life; and
(f) Education must be able to develop a working mechanism to fight the evil of consumerism and acquisitive culture so that environment may be protected and development may remain sustainable.

In New Delhi Conference on "Quest for New Perspectives", held on July 9-10, 2003 feels that:

As we reflect today on the theme of dialogue of civilizations, it seems imperative that education should be so developed that a new mentality is created which spontaneously turns to dialogue rather than to conflict, which spontaneously responds to the call of interchange, and which is spontaneously eager to see problems from various points of view and which is capable of synthesizing different points of view without sacrificing uniqueness of various truths that are synthesized. We have to develop particularly a new curriculum that aims at explaining the basic theme of human progress as a mighty expression of an adventure of continuous self-exceeding. This curriculum should inspire students to work for unity even while rejecting uniformity; this curriculum should also encourage students to respect cultural diversity. Finally, this curriculum should develop a new science and art of living together which necessitates adherence to the law of mutuality rather than conflict and the law of variety of expressions rather than any uniform monotone. It may also be urged that since science and technology characterize a large part of modern civilization, we should develop a new curriculum where by a fresh impetus is given to scientific studies that are in harmony with the study of values. There is, today, an increasing awareness that unless science and value are blended together, humanity will have to face a great peril, the peril of inner human suffering even in the midst of increase of knowledge and increase of material comforts. It is in the hands of educationists today to develop a new dimension in education so that education can not only build the defences of peace in the minds and hearts of people but also build bridges between the past and the future, and serve the great ends of the dialogue among civilizations.

What is now needed is a concerted action at the development of a curriculum that can bring home to the students three important lessons, namely, (i) that the entire humanity shares one basic impulse towards progress and by sharing this impulse humanity can be seen as one vast surge of adventure which aims at continuous self-exceeding; (ii) that humanity, in its mature developments, tends to reject uniformity and adopts the law of unity that permits and respects cultural diversities; and (iii) that the future progress of humankind is bound up with the development of a new science and art of living together which necessitates adherence to the law of mutuality rather than conflict and the law of varied expressions rather than any uniform monotone. Education should aim at strengthening democratic and universal human values and respect for human rights. Education is the most powerful instrument for preparing a mind which can promote the culture of dialogue. (See Chart 6.2)

Notes and References

1. Anita Shetty and K. Pushpanadham, Valuing Values, *University News*, Dec. 29, 1997, pp. 7-8.
2. H. Venkataiah, Value Education, Curriculum for Graduates and Postgraduates in *University News*, June 22, 1998.
3. R. Satya Rajiv, Human Values in University Management, in AIU, Value Education in India, New Delhi, 2001, pp. 86-87.
4. Quoted in Annitha Shetty *et. al.*, Value Education: Need of the present generation in *University News*, Oct. 13, 1997, p. 12.
5. Quoted in N.P. Sinha, Towards inculcating values in Education, in *University News*, Oct. 22-28, 2001, pp. 1-2.
6. Swami Gautamananda, Values in our Education, in *Values: The Key to a Meaningful Life*, Ramakrishna Math, Madras, India, pp. 83-85.
7. *University News*, Dec. 9, 1996. p. 22.
8. R. Natarajan, *University News*, July 21-27, 2003, p. 16.

9. Sri Aurobindo, The Synthesis of Yoga, 1976, Sixth Edition, Sri Aurobindo Ashram, Pondicherry, p. 2.
10. Swami Jagadatmananda, Learn to Live Vol. 2, Ramakrishna Math, Chennai; India, 2000: pp. 154-57.
11. H.H. The Dalai Lama,, Education for Peace, in *Journal of Value Education*, Vol. 2, No. 1, January 2002. p. 1.
12. Swami Purnananda, Making Life Valuable by Imbiding Values, in *Journal of Value Education*, Vol. 2, No. 1, Journal 2002, pp. 30-31 (NCERT).
13. *Ibid.*, p. 15.
14. P. Dhannavel, Importance of Value-based Teachers, in *University News*, May 1, 2000, p. 2.
15. Hemanta K. Khandai, Value Oriented Approach from Primary to University Education, *University News*, March 31 to April 06, 2003, pp. 9-10.
16. Swami Sachidananda, Vision and values for National Regeneration, *Journal of Value Education*, Vol. 2, No. 1, January 2002 (NCERT), pp. 70-71.
17. H.H. Jagadguru's Madras Discourse Acharya Call, Part III, Peetam Kanchipuram, 1998, pp. 66-67.
18. *Ibid.*, p. 192.
19. *Ibid*.
20. Nageshwar Rao and R.P. Das, Bringing Values Back: The Role of Teachers in Higher Education in *Journal of Value Education*, Vol. 2, No. 1, January 2002, p. 89.
21. J.S. Rajput, Symphony of Human Values in Education, NCERT, December 2001, New Delhi.
20. Learn to Live, Vol. I, *op. cit.*, pp. 139-41.
23. R.D. Dhokalia, External Human Values and World Religions, NCERT, New Delhi, 2001, pp. 10, 13, 24
24. Girijesh Kunal, How to Inculcate Value Education through Teacher Education, *Journal of Value Education*, *op. cit.*, pp. 118-19.

APPENDIX 6.1

VALUES IN SRIMAD BHAGWAD GITA

Selected Slokas

Given below are the five verses from Bhagavad Gita (Chapter XIII, from 7th to 11th) enumerating the important values. The original Sanskrit test is followed by the transliteration and the meaning:

अमानित्वमदम्भित्वमहिंसा क्षान्तिरार्जवम् ।
आचार्योपासनं शौचं स्थैर्यमात्मविनिग्रह: ।। 13/7 (Srimad Bhagavad Gita)

Amanitvamadambhitvamahimsa ksantirarjavam
Acaryopasanam saucam sthairyamatmavinigrahah.

Absence of pride, freedom from hypocrisy, non-violence, forbearance, straightness of body, speech and mind, devout service of the preceptor, internal and external purity, steadfastness of mind and control of body, mind and the senses.

इन्द्रियार्थेषु वैराग्यमनहंकार एव च ।
जन्ममृत्युजराव्याधिदु:खदोषानुदर्शनम् ।। 13/8 (Srimad Bhagavad Gita)

Indriyarthesu vairagyamanahankara eva ca,
Janmamrtyujaravyadhidukhadosanudarsanam

Dispassion towards the objects of enjoyment of this world and the next, and also absence of egotism, pondering again and again on the pain and evils inherent in birth, death, old-age and disease.

असक्तिरनभिषवङंग: पुत्रदारगृहादिषु ।
नित्य च समचित्ततवमिष्टानि ष्टोपपत्तिषु ।। 13/9 (Srimad Bhagavad Gita)

Asaktiranabhisvangah putradaragrhadisu
Nítyam ca samacittatvamistanistopapattisu

Absence of attachment and the feeling of mineness in respect of son, wife, home, etc. and constant equipoise of mind both in favourable and unfavourable circumstances.

मयि चानन्ययोगेन भक्तिरव्यभिचारिणी ।
विविक्तदेशसेवित्वमरतिर्जनसंसदि ।। 13/10 (Srimad Bhagavad Gita)

Mayi cananyayogena bhaktiravyabhicarini
Viviktadesasevitvamaratirjanasamasadi

Unflinching devotion to Me through exclusive attachement, living in secluded and holy places, and finding no enjoyment in the company of men.

अध्यात्मज्ञाननित्यत्वं तत्त्वज्ञानार्थदर्शनम् ।
एतज्ज्ञानमिति प्रोक्तमज्ञानं यदतोऽन्यथा ॥ 13/11 (Srimad Bhagavad Gita)

Adhyatmajnananityatvam tattvajnanarthadarsanam,
Etajjnanamiti proktamajnanam yadatonatha.

Fixity in self-knowledge and seeing God as the object of true knowledge; all this is declared as knowledge; and what is other than this is called ignorance.

ANNEXURE 6.2

ROLE OF UGC IN HUMAN VALUE IN HIGHER EDUCATION

1. A scheme for Promoting Ethics and Human Values in Higher Education

The National Policy on Education has laid considerable emphasis on Value Education by highlighting the need to make education a forceful tool for cultivation of social and moral values. The policy has stated that in our culturally plural society education should factor universal and eternal values oriented towards the unity and integration of our people.

In the present times of unprecedented changes dislocating traditional values and creating conflict between traditional and new values there is a universal concern in respect of erosion of values, promoting values and culture which fit in with the needs of the modern times. This concern is universal but is more acute for our country which has lead its distinct culture, worked view and a living value tradition. The process of developing into a modern nation. with new social, political and economic institutions, and with emphasis on science and technology has thrown up many new values—challenges in all areas of our national life. It is important that we examine these challenges and prepare our youth to face and resolve them.

2. Objectives of the Scheme

(i) To create awareness, conviction and commitment to values for improving the quality of life through education, and for advancing social and human well-being

(ii) To encouraging universities and colleges to undertake academic and other activities pertaining to teaching, research and extension programmes in respect of values and culture like extramural lectures, seminar, conferences workshops and orientation programmes for teachers and students.

(iii) To encourage universities to undertake preparation and production of requisite material including books, handbooks, journals, teaching materials, video and films relating to values.

3. Eligibility/Target

All eligible Universities and colleges which are included under section 2(f) and 12(b) of the UGC Act are covered under the scheme.

4. Nature of Assistance

The different activities for which support will be provided are as under: (i) Research, (ii) Teaching, (iii) Organisation of Conferences/ Seminars, (iv) Awareness/Sensitization/Programme, (v) Human Enrichment/integrated personality development! Character Building Workshops.

4.1 Research of Assistance

The nature of research projects under this scheme would be different from the usual Ph.D. oriented academic research. They would be aimed at understanding and clarifying value issues of contemporary; concern in the public and professional, and to suggest possible ways of resolving these value problems. The research could be a combination of conceptual and empirical investigations. Some of the likely areas of the research projects could be:

Value Issues in:

(i) Core values of human life with reference to the individual, family Community, nation and Human society.

(ii) Values relating to Democratic polity and the Rule of Law.

(iii) Professional values, like of engineering, medicine, law, teaching, public service, management, business, etc.

(iv) Values of good governance, administration, and of judiciary.

(v) Values relating to environment, science and technology, and sustainable development.

(vi) Strategies of transmission of value through formal/informal/ non-formal/Education.

(vii) The role of the films and the Multi-media in respect of Value transmission and the potentials of multi-media learning to promote awareness and understanding of human values.

The theme should be developed in the light of Indian ethos, aspirations and social realities. The outcome of this research should be in the form of book, monograph, research papers, report, the support provided would be by way of seed money which could be utilized for the purpose of contingency, books and journals, travel, stationary, typing and hiring, etc. The duration of the research project would be ordinarily two years.

4.2 Teaching

Support under this head would be provided for encouraging and facilitating introduction of new courses on value related themes like human values, professional ethics, environmental ethics, science, technology, parliamentary democracy, civil society and the rules of law and human values, etc. Financial assistance would be provided by way of:

(i) grant to teachers teaching such courses for books, preparation of teaching material, travel grant to consult libraries elsewhere, to attend conference lectures themes related to the subject matter, preparation of manuscript for writing books, etc.

(ii) grant to university/college, department for paying honorarium to retired teachers visiting Professors to teach such courses.

4.3 Organisation of Conference/Seminars

These could be of two types:

(i) Aimed at generating new ideas related to themes of ethics and human values.
(ii) To provide a platform to teachers engaged in teaching value-related courses to share ideas and experiences.

The conference should be properly focused and their proceedings should be published.

Financial support would be provided to meet expenses on TA/DA, boarding and lodging expenses, local transport, publication of report, secretarial assistance, etc.

4.4 Awareness/Sensitisation Programmes

These could be in a form of lectures, workshops for a day or two, aimed at specific groups, like teachers, research scholars and students of a particular discipline academic administrators, non-teaching staff, etc.

Support would be provided for meeting expenses of the programme including TA/DA for one or two persons from outside the institution.

Human enrichment/integrated personality—development/character building workshops.

These workshops could be very effective non-formal means of seeking a positive change in the value-temper of students and teachers. They could be organized during vacations or after the working hours. They could include presentations and discussions on different themes like spiritual, moral, aesthetic, societal, cultural, environmental values, values of democracy, scientific temper, communication skills, problems of youth, career choices, etc. Some of these workshops could also be for groups from outside the university, like school teachers, NGOs, government officials, corporate executives, etc. As far as possible these external workshops should be self-financing.

The support provided for this activity would be by way of TA/DA and honorarium for resource persons, contingency amount for preparation of reading material, field trips, postage, office assistance, payment to part time organizing assistants, etc.

One time grant will be provided to take up activities described above, Maximum ceiling of financial support will be Rs. 5.00 lakhs. Maximum ceiling does not mean that each College/University will get this grant. It will depend on type of activities that will be undertaken by them.

CHAPTER 7

YOGA: HOLISTIC VALUES FOR HEALTH DEVELOPMENT EDUCATION

योगश्चित्तवृत्तिनिरोध ।। 2।। Patanjli Yogasutra
Yoga is the control of thought—waves in the mind

Water flows continually into the ocean
But the ocean is never disturbed;
Desire flows into the mind of the seer
But he is never disturbed.
The seer knows peace. . . .
He knows peace who has forgotten desire
He lives without craving;
Free from ego, free from pride.

—*Bhagavad Gita*

Yoga: Holistic Values for Health Development Education

Remain in bliss in this world,
Fearless, pure in heart,
Wake up in bliss every morning,
Carry out all your duties in bliss,
Remain in bliss in weal and woe,
In criticism and insult,
Remain in bliss unaffected,
Remain in bliss pardoning everybody.

—*Rabindranath Tagore*

Yoga helps in the overall development of the personality of people. The concept of positive health and lifelong learning are relatively new concepts which need to be promoted. An overall development of the individual is intended to be achieved through higher education using an affective domain in addition to cognitive skills.[1] Shri Kumar Swamiji in his book Dimension of Yoga strongly feels that Yoga aims at recreating the world. Not the acceptance of the world as it is, but to change it, to mould it in the pattern of the Divine Reality, is the main objective of Yoga. To say this, is to say that evil has no permanent place in the scheme of things. Creation is a complex movement which represents the various notes and rhythms that make up the grand harmony of the spheres. This music that moves the cosmos is magnificent and wonderful and is the glory of God manifest therein. But a doubting voice raises the question, is there not some chaos in this cosmos? Is there not a confusion in this concord? Is there not a walpurgis night in this winning light? Yes, there is. In the order of creation, first, there is the consciousness and division of trenchant separation of good and evil. This is the outlook of individualized consciousness. Next, as the consciousness grows and ecompasses the whole existence, good and evil are both embraced and are found to form a secret harmony. This is the outlook of the cosmic consciousness. There is still a higher status, the status of transcendentce in which evil is not simply embraced but dissolved and even transformed into supreme reality of which it is an aberration, a projection or a lower formulation. In Yoga the total eradication of evil from the world and human nature, with a remoulding of terrestrial life in the pattern of the divine Reality, is viewed not as a mere concept but as a concrete fact.

Yoga deals with the problems of human nature and human psychology through a vast repertory of practical methods which aim towards purification, regulation and awakening of human potential. At present, yoga is passing through a momentous period of growth consolidation and expansion with its rapid integration into modern society. Many institutions dealing with the theory of Yoga and its practice have come up. At many levels we can see changes and new developments as yoga is being applied in different facets of life in a variety of new ways, such as a form of therapy, a technique of health and stress management.

Modern man is all set for a revolution after nearly four centuries of continuous growth. From the era of blind faith and superstitutions he has progressed an era of rational thinking, experimentation, matter-based approach and its fascinating applications to comfort his living. The strides of this growth encompasses all facets of life including education (science and technology-orientated) and the very direction of growth of an individual (economy-based) and a country (measured with the yardstick of GNP). Tremendous growth has been made in understanding the structure of this physical universe and the laws governing them.

The two major challenges of this era of science and technology—viz. stress and pollution have become the true triggers for the new revolution. If pollution is working at the material front to direct man towards better ecological and appropriate technology, the challenge of stress is shaking the very foundations of the matter-based objective approach of science. As we glide through the decades of transition, our understanding is bound to encompass a greater spectrum of the universe—life, mind, psyche, etc.

India, known for its wisdom has given us the Upanisads, the quintessence of the Vedas, and a saga of knowledge. From these books of knowledge—Vedas, Upanisads, Yoga texts—are emerging new rays of hopes which are essential to face the new revolution.[2]

Scientific and technological progress all over the globe has made man highly sensitive, critical and also creative. Sharp to the core, his intellect has gained tremendous power of analysis. The left side of his brain is highly developed, helping him to unravel the subtle mysteries of nature and understand clearly the general law of nature. Technology has helped man reap the benefits of its use. Autonomation and computers have brought great speed and sophistication in all our interactions. In search of happiness we are propelled by a desire to increase our living standards by acquiring more and more comfort giving objects and experiencing sensual pleasures. To satisfy this desire we are always on the lookout to earn more and more. In the process, we have become very active and have overcome our lethargy.

Associated with this growth is the emergence of two basic challenges: pollution and stress. The challenge of pollution is being tackled effectively but not met totally. Strict pollution control measures in the industrial sectors and extensive research leading towards the use of ecologically friendly technologies, have certainly yielded dividends. But on the second front, in spite of extensive research all over the globe, a decreasing quality of life, increasing health hazards, social unrest, student unrest, etc. traits which are all different expressions of stress, have shown no trend of decrease. On the contrary, over the last two decades, it is rather on the path of ascent.

The current mechanistic world-view, the matter-based approach, the increased dependence on science and technology and the associated lifestyle have to undergo basic changes towards embracing a more holistic world view and a healthier and more harmonious lifestyle. Emotion trainings and harnessing of the will-power—the growth of the right side of the brain in general—are then the associated adjuncts for such a holistic understanding and also for a healthier and harmonious living. And that is what Yoga offers.

Today, man is subjected to a large number of stressful situations in the modern fast way of life and his balance is frequently disturbed. The system is constantly kept under sympathetic stimulation without enough time for the parasympathetic to do its job. This repeated sympathetic stimulations lead to intermittent upsurges of heart rate, blood pressure, poor digestion, elevated blood glucose, etc. When this happens over a number of years it become a habit for the heart and the blood vessels to remain in stimulated state and they lose the capacity to come back to the resting levels. This is the main cause for the increasing incidence of high blood pressure and diabetes among people today.[3]

Youth in the system of higher education represents a tremendous potential for society, provided it is channeled in the right direction, the enthusiasm, initiative and idealism of young people can help others, including the elderly, the handicapped, the poor, and in so doing can create a happier and more balanced society.

Unprecedented challenges face the youth of today, said Dr. Hiroshi Nakajima, Director-General of WHO, in a message to the world assembly of Youth. And he added that young people maybe given opportunities "to demonstrate their creativity, energy and commitment to solving their own problems and helping to build a healthy future for the entire community in which they live."

Unwise life-styles pose the biggest threats to students' health. Innovative judgments, a tendency to show off, or the desire to keep up with their fellows—all these incline them towards risk-taking behaviour. This may include experimenting with dangerous substances like alcohol or drugs, driving too fast on the highway, or simply defying adult society.

In many cases, the cigarette is the very first contact young people have with the lifestyles of adulthood. This first encounter often occurs at a very early age: by the time they reach their teens, they may already be unable to break the smoking habit. It is vital that they should be aware of the short-term and long-term risks that smoking represents to their health.

The risk destroying their most important assets; the health and physical fitness through laziness and lack of exercise, rash driving and traffic accidents, suicide or attempts to suicide, slow suicide through the use of alcohol, smoking, drug abuse, excessive intake of tea and coffee, unprotected sexual encounters, sexual misadventures like rape, sexually transmitted diseases, teenager pregnancies and abortions or unwed child births. The ill-effects on their health can extend far into later life. Accidents are estimated to disable permanently three times as many as they kill, smoking and alcohol can store epidemics of respiratory diseases, liver damage and cancer. Teenager pregnancy can kill mother or child or else leave them physically and mentally handicapped. Needless to conclude that in some countries youth is the only age-group in which mortality and morbidity rate is rising, due to these ills of modern society. Alcohol and unemployment is behind alarmingly large number of deaths through accidents and suicide (Jerome, 1980).

Before a dam was constructed on Satluj River, at Bhakra, the water resource was not only wasted but it resulted in floods, leading to loss of life and property. The same is true for youth resource. The idle youth is not only a waste, but also the tide of this unutilized energy can result in negative development wasted in the field of health and economy. The youth can be our best resource if they are healthy and if their joyous energy is channelised for building a better society. The potential energy of youth has to be converted into kinetic energy with understanding, support and technological knowledge and its use should be made to build modern India. Much needs to be done both for and by young people. It is not sufficient merely to have activities directed towards youth. If the aims and objectives of International Youth Year, 1985, and the WHO Global Strategy for Health for All by the year 2000 are to be achieved. Serious efforts of collaborative action by everyone—young and old are needed. The youngsters of today, with their capabilities, energy and commitment, represent a vital resource; they must be partners in the quest for a just future.

Life of students in higher education is becoming more and more artificial and they are travelling more and more away from natural living. In order to return to natural life, they should practice Yoga and learn to live more in consonance with nature and cosmic consciousness.

We see the disinterest and inevitable suffering among many students. It has been realized that every individual contains hidden potential, which when developed allows him to attain pertinent bliss, inner peace and the ultimate goal of our existence.

A brief discussion with students revealed the following problems of students in the system of higher education:

(a) Lack of interest in studies,
(b) Lack of vitality, enthusiasm and eagerness,
(c) Enamored by affluent environment leading to alcoholism, smoking, gambling, etc.
(d) Irregular in food habits,
(e) Not interested in exercises and games,
(f) Drudgery in life,
(g) No aim in life,
(h) Lack of reading habits,
(i) Not following any regular course of life,
(j) Full of tensions, worries and agitations,
(k) Lack of peace—restlessness,
(l) Lack of concentration,
(m) Problematic both at home and in a college,
(n) Bad company, and
(o) Aimless life.

How can we overcome the problems inflicting the personality of students in higher education system? How can we channelise their potential energy into kinetic energy to make them enjoy the bliss of life? How can we stimulate students towards holistic approach? How can we make them develop their personality in totality? How can we check students from indulging in bad habits—alcoholism, smoking, gambling, etc.? How can we educate them to put them on right track? The only answer is the need of imparting yoga education which can solve all the problems simultaneously. It requires understanding and practice of science and practice of yoga. First let us understand the meaning of yoga.

MEANING OF YOGA

Patanjali defines yoga as complete suppression of all mental modes or processes (cittavrttinirodha).[4] Vyasa defines it as absorptive concentration (samadhi). It is a universal attribute of the mind.[5] All persons can attain yoga by repeated practice (abhyasa) and detachment (vairagya).[6]

Swami Satyananda Sanswati in his book, "Asana Pranayama Mudra Bandha," (Bihar School of Yoga, Munger, Bihar, Indium, 1999) comments that, "Yoga is not an ancient myth buried in oblivion. It is the most valuable inheritance of the present. It is the essential need of today and the culture of tomorrow." The Yogic culture of tomorrow is something towards which we have to strive, we have to try to attain. Yoga has been the culture to strive, we have to try to attain. Yoga has been the culture of ancient India and the ancient civilization of the world, and it is going to be the culture of tomorrow. It is the science of today which we have to learn, which we have to accept, and which we have to understand. It is a science which deals with the developments of the human personality and which leads to the awakening of untapped energy sources within the brain and mind. The practice of yoga is not new. Ancient rishis, saints and sages have been talking about it for the last fifty thousand years. They spoke about it, not as a religion or philosophy, but as a way of life which could lead to the development and awakening of our consciousness and energy.

The mother in her Diary for all times: The Great Adventure says, "Yoga means union with the Divine, and the union is effected through offering—it is founded on the offering of yourself to the Divine."

For most people, however, yoga is simply a means of maintaining health and well-being in an increasingly stressful society. Asanas remove the physical discomfort accumulated during a day at the office sitting in a chair, hunched over a desk. Relaxation techniques help maximize the effectiveness of ever-diminishing time off. In an age of mobile phones, beepers and twenty-four hour shopping, yogic practices make great personal and even business sense.

The word yoga is derived from the Sanskrit root 'yuj' meaning 'to unite', 'to combine', and 'to integrate', which means total integration of the physical, mental, intellectual and spiritual aspects of the human personality.[7] Yoga is a way of life, propounded by Patanjali in a systematic form.

Yoga is an exact science. It aims at the harmonious development of the body, the mind and the soul. Yoga is the turning away of the senses from the objective universe and the concentrations of the mind within. Yoga is the turning away of the senses from the objective universe and the concentration of mind are eternal life in the soul of spirit. Yoga aims at controlling the mind and its modifications. The path of Yoga is an inner path whose gateway is your heart. Yoga is harmony between the individual and the cosmos, between thought and action, between soul and God, between Organism and respiration.

Yoga is the discipline of a mind, senses and physical body. Yoga helps in the co-ordination and control of the subtle forces within the body. Yoga brings in perfection, peace and everlasting happiness; one can even have increased energy, vigor, vitality, longevity, resistance, calmness, and good sleep at times by the practice of Yoga. The practice of Yoga will help people to control the emotions and passions and resistance power increases and removes the disturbing elements from mind. It will enable them to keep a balanced mind and remove fatigue and get concentration, self-sufficiency, impertinence, pride, luxury, name, fame, self-assertive nature, abstinence, idea of superiority, evil company, laziness, over eating, meat eating, over work, attachments, too much talking, smoking, drinking are some of the obstacles in the path of Yoga.[8]

Swami Parmahansa Niranjanananda in his book, "Yoga Darshan: Vision of Yoga Upanishads" (1993) Bihar observes that the aim of yoga is to take one from the impure aspect of the mind towards the pure aspect, from a state of scattered desire to a state of balanced desire, where the desire becomes positive, constructive, and self-elevating, where the desire does not limit us to the external environment only, but also encompasses the inner dimensions. By transcending the impure mind and obtaining purity of mind and by awakening the faculties of the pure mind, one attains transcendence or mukti. One must go from the impure to the pure, and awaken the faculties of the pure mind in order to attain transcendence.

ASPECTS OF YOGA (See Chart 7.1)

The science of Yoga has its roots in Upanishads, Veadas, Bhagavad-Gita, Yogavashishta of Vashishta, Hathayoga Pradipika, and the Yoga Sutras of Patanjali. However, a detailed classical work could be found in the Yoga Sutras of Patanjali, which dates back roughly to 300 B.C. The Yoga Sutras serve as the basic text for an in-depth study on this great science. Patanjali called it Ashtanga Yoga, i.e., science having eight limbs or constituents, viz.,

1. Yama
2. Niyama
3. Aasana
4. Praanaayaama
5. Prathyaahaara
6. dhaarana
7. Dhyaana
8. Samaadhi

यम - नियामासन - प्राणायाम - प्रत्याहार, धारणा - ध्यान - समाध्योटण्टावडगनि ।

—Patanjali Yogasutra 2.2.9

(1) Yama

The first discipline of restraint (yama) consists in non-injury (ahimsa), truthfulness in thought and speech (satya), non-stealing (asteya), sexual restraint (brahmacarya), and non-acceptance of unnecessary gifts.[9] These are negative virtues. Non-injury (ahimsa) consists in the absence of cruelty to all creatures in all possible ways and at all times. It is tenderness, good will, and kindness for all living beings.[10]

A truthful person must have valid thoughts in his mind, speak them out correctly, excite similar thoughts in the hearer's mind, and his words must be conducive to the welfare of all creatures.

Yama is based on the principle that above all religions, human religion is the best. (Abstinences) viz., Ahimsa (Non-injury), Sathya (Non-falsehood), Astheya (Non-stealing), Aparigraha (Non-acceptance or non-hoarding of things beyond our bear necessities of life) and Brahmacharya (Non-deviation from one's on personal laws of nature).

Steady intellect is a natural and spontaneous state for a man of

CHART 7.1

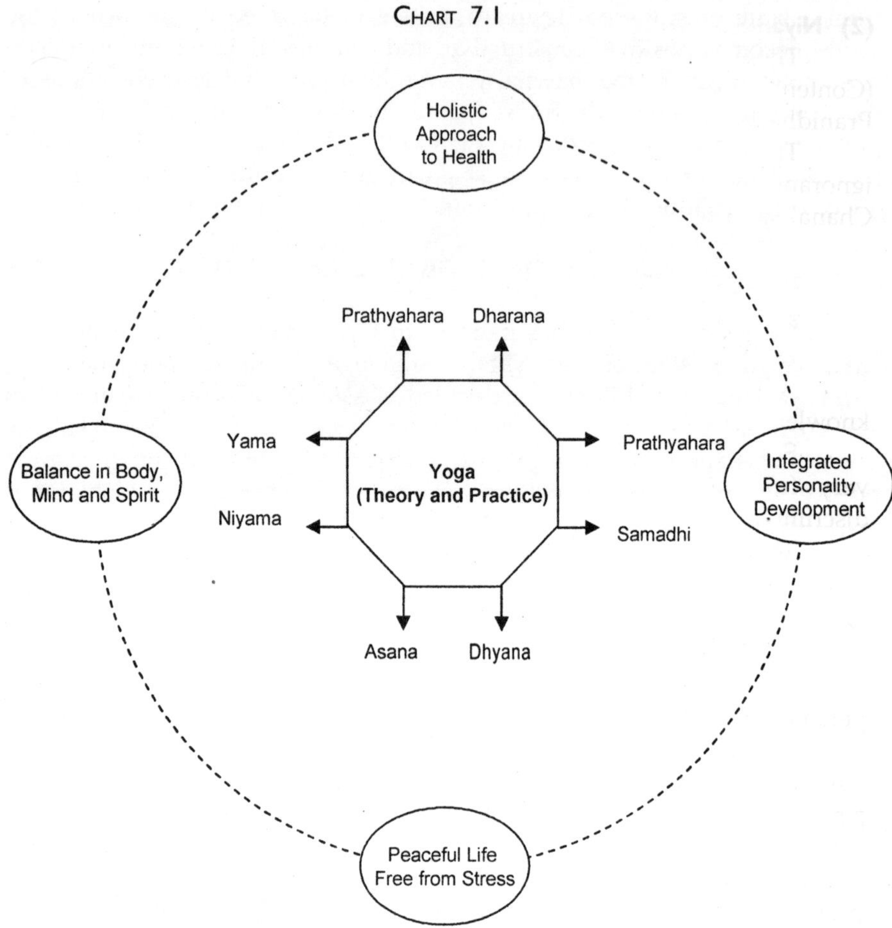

realization. Since he knows the truth, nothing in this world can disturb him. Even ordinary people and spiritual aspirants can derive immense benefit by cultivating a steady intellect. Intellectual, conviction about Reality may help us to develop a steady intellect to a certain extent.

He is a man of steady intellect whose mind is not disturbed by the pair of opposites, namely, happiness and misery, victory and defeat, gain and loss, praise and blame, attachment and hatred, honour and dishonour, heat and cold.[11] Sri Krishna has given a beautiful illustration in the Bhagavad Gita (2.70), of a steady intellect.

आपूर्यमाणमचलप्रतिष्ठं समुद्रमापः प्रविशन्ति यद्वत । शिर्षण

'Water enters into the sea from all directions but the sea remains full and unchanged.'

(2) Niyama

These are the observances viz., Shoucha (Purity), Santhosha (Contentment), Tapas (Austerity), Swadyaaya (Self Study), Eswara Pranidhaana (Total surrender to the Supreme).

Thirst for knowledge is inherent in man and no one likes to be ignorant. Knowledge alone can remove ignorance. A beautiful verse in Chanakya Niti (XVII-17) says:

ज्ञानं नराणामधिको विर्षेशः ।
ज्ञानेन हीनाः पशुभिः समाना ।।

'What distinguishes a man from an animal is his capacity to acquire knowledge. Without knowledge men are equal to animals.'

Spiritual knowledge comes through direct experience of Truth, but very few can reach that state. Others have to follow the path of discrimination, using their intellect.

There is a popular saying:

स्वदेशे पूज्यते राजा विद्वान् सर्वत्र पूज्यते ।

"The king is honoured only in his kingdom whereas a learned person is honoured everywhere.[12]

This is a great psychological truth discovered by the Yoga system long ago. It is a commonplace of modern Ethics. Mackenzie says, "It is generally better to escape from our defects, not by thinking about them and trying to elude them, but by fixing our attention on the opposite excellences. It certainly seems a more effectual method as a rule to expel our evil propensities by developing good ones rather than by seeking directly to crush the evil ones.[13]

(3) Aasana

This Involves practice of physical Postures for correcting any deformities or physical ailments. Hatha Yoga Texts claim that there are as many as 84000000 postures.

The third discipline is bodily posture (asana). It is a steady and pleasant posture of the body. It should not move. It should not be painful. It should not distract the mind. There are many kinds of postures, padmasana, virasana, bhadrasana, svastika, and the like. The various postures of the body are the means of controlling it and keeping it healthy and fit. They tone up the nervous system. They can be learnt from experts. The control of the body is the basis of the yoga discipline.

They are controlled by means of practice and non-attachment. Patanjli Yogasutras-12

Practice is the repeated effort to follow the disciplines which give permanent control of the thought-waves of the mind. Yogasutra-13

Practice becomes firmly grounded when it has been cultivated for a long time, uninterruptedly, with earnest devotion. Yogasutra-14

The practice of yoga prevents psychosomatic disorders/diseases and improves individual's resistance and ability to endure stressful situations. As a primary prevention, yogic exercises should be advised to drive the benefits of prevention of diseases, promotion of health and for therapeutic purposes.[14]

(4) Praanaayaama

This limb deals with practice of breathing exercises involving rechaka, puraka, antara kumbaka and bahya kumbhaka (inhalation, exhalation, internal retention and external retention) thus exercising our lungs—the ventilators of our body.

The fourth discipline is breath control (pranayama). It consists in controlling natural breathing and subjecting it to a definite law. It consists in slow and deep inspiration (puraka), retention of breath (kumbhaka), and slow expiration (recaka).[15] These three functions should be performed for definite periods. The time of inspiration, the time of retention of breath, and the time of expiration should be in the proportion: 1, 4 and 2.

Breath Control is conducive to concentration of mind. It removes the crust of affliction from illumination of the sattava of the mind. It removes the demerit which observes discriminative knowledge. Breath control is the supreme austerity. It purges the mind of impurities and generates illumination of knowledge.[16]

The term pranayama is derived from the Sanskrit term 'prana' which means the 'vital principal'. The vital principle permeates the brain and the nervous system of an individual. It is the source of volition, enthusiasm, spontaneity and happiness in an individual. He spreads the same in the environment which also becomes pure.[17]

Pranayama is the method of rhythmic regulation of breath. It produces stability in the body, and equanimity in the mind of an individual. The subtle physiology of an individual gets purified through regular practice of pranayama. The body of an individual becomes free from leanness, obesity, crookedness, etc. through regular practise of pranayama. Swami Vishnu Devananda states:

Pracchardana-vidharanabhayam va pranasya

It is also achieved by the expulsion and retention of the breath.

This is a reference to the practice of pranayama as a method of purification. Regulation of the breath gives control over the thought waves, for control of breath is directly related to control of mind. There are many pranayama exercises, each of which has a special effect on the autonomic nervous system and the psyche.[18]

We do not pay any serious attention to breathing the most important of all our bodily functions. It has never occurred to us that a great deal of our physical and mental troubles are due to the fact that we do not breathe correctly. Life and breath are synonymous. We live as long as we breathe. We start our life with the first breath and end it with the last breath. We never stop breathing whether we are awake or asleep. We can exist without food for weeks and without water for a few days but without air we cannot exist even for a few minutes. Air is the most important nourishment for our blood. All the activities of body from digestion to creative thinking depend upon the oxygen supply through breathing; yet we treat breathing with utter indifference. If there is a deficiency in the supply of oxygen, the process of ionization will be incomplete and the food is partially assimilated. Nearly 50 percent of delinquency in minors is due to oxygen starvation which is the result of shallow breathing and lack of fresh air.

The habit of shallow breathing is one of many unnatural habits that modern civilization has forced upon us. It has been proved that in the civilized world only babies can breathe in a natural way. Shallow breathing is directly or indirectly responsible for a number of physical and mental diseases ranging from nervous disorders to common colds. To function properly the brain requires three times more oxygen than the rest of the body. If it does not get its due allotment, it exacts it from the body supply. That is why brain workers often possess a poor physic and a bad health. Deep breathing not only nourishes the whole system but also cleanses it.

Prana is not mere breath but it is cosmic energy. It is a life giving principle which pervades the whole atmosphere. It is manifested in every form of existence—organic and inorganic. By breathing exercises it is possible to raise the degree of circulation of Prana in the body. The surplus of Prana is stored in the solar plexus which is the battery of human body.

(5) Prathyaahaara

If the mind is withdrawn from external sensible objects, the external senses are automatically withdrawn from them. They do not follow their objects, but they follow the mind. They are fixed on those objects only on which the mind is fixed. The restraint of the external senses depends upon the restraint of the mind. It can be acquired by repeated practice, resolute will, and sense control.[19]

The five disciplines of restraint (yama), observance (niyama), bodily posture (asana), breath-control (pranayama), and sense-control (pratyahara) are the external aids to yoga (bahirangasadhana). The last three disciplines, fixation of mind (dharana), meditation (dhyana) and absorptive concentration or ecstasy (samadhi) are the internal aids of yoga (antarangasadhana). They directly lead to conscious ecstasy (samprajnatasamadhi).[20]

6. Dhaarana

This involves concentration of mind it is true that the main stumbling block in increasing our knowledge is lack of concentration. The ever-increasing aberrations in the mind with the advent of age would really worsen the situation unless the mind is cultured through yogic techniques. Everything is possible to those who can concentrate, and so we are encouraged to preserve, to break through the barriers of ordinary sense perception and to press forward fearlessly in our search for inner knowledge. The physical strength gained in a gymnasium can be used later for practical purposes. The mental strength gained through these exercises in concentration can be used for the most practical purpose of all; to unite ourselves with the Atman. विशेका वा ज्योतिटठमति ॥ 36 ॥

7. Dhyaana

Dhyaana involves relaxed dwelling of the mind for a longer duration on the object of meditation. Fixation of attention on an object to the exclusion of other objects leads to meditation, if the cognition produced by it continues unbroken for a long time. There is a continuous stream of similar cognitions of the contemplated object undisturbed by dissimilar cognitions.[21]

8. Samaadhi

The meditation involves the continuous flowing of mind energy and steady focusing on the object of meditation effortlessly for a longer and longer time. The very essence of yoga is merger of individual soul with that of universal soul, a state of super consciousness. This essence is achieved through Samaadhi only. Fixation (dharana), meditation (dhyana) and absorptive concenration (samadhi), on the same object together are called samyama. They are the internal aids (antarangasadhana) to conscious ecstasy, while restraint, observance, bodily posture, breath control, and withdrawal of the senses from their objects are the external aids (bahirangasadhana) to it. But they are the external aids to super conscious ecstasy.[22]

Swami Sivananda in his article, "Religious Education and Practice of Yoga" mentions the causes of stresses and strains and suggest meditation as has been laid down in all our ancient Sanskrit scriptures.

"Watch your mind very carefully. Be vigilant. Be on the alert. Do not allow the waves of irritability, jealousy, hatred and lust to disturb you. These dark waves are enemies of peaceful living, meditation and wisdom. To some it is very difficult to keep the mind unruffled and pure, the causes being deep-rooted worldly. Samskaras, unfavourable surroundings, and the predominance of extrovert tendencies. To some, of course, evil thoughts are not a problem at all. They appear occasionally as a passing phase without doing much havoc. The very fact that evil thoughts give you mental suffering is a sign of spiritual progress; for many do not have that much of sensitiveness."

In nutshell Meditation is the process where the mind of a person is attracted towards God without interruption and is always keen to set in prayer from the core of heart. Prayer and Japa always help in supplementing and complementing meditation.

CLASSIFICATION OF YOGA

There are four yogas—Bhakti Yoga, Karma Yoga, Jnana Yoga and Raja Yoga—to realize the Divine, where is the need to practise Buddhi Yoga? The answer is that even to practice the four yogas one has to take the help of Buddhi.

Shri Krishna says in the Bhagavad Gita (18:57):

चेतना सर्वकर्माणि मयि सन्यस्य मत्परः ।
बुद्धियोगमुपाश्रित्य मच्चितः सततं भव ।।

"Resigning mentally all actions to Me, regarding Me as the supreme goal and resorting to Budhhi Yoga, ever fix your mind on Me.

Bhakti Yoga

Devotion mixed with discrimination is an ideal path. Without discrimination devotion ends in mere sentimentalism or emotionalism. Therefore, the place of Buddhi in Bhakti yoga is very significant. When the Lord is pleased with His devotees, he bestows His grace in the form of pure intellect. Sri Krishna himself promises in the Bhagavad Gita (10.10):

तेण सततयुक्तानां भजतां प्रीतिपूर्वकम् ।
ददामि बुद्धियोगं तं येन मापुयान्ति ते ।।

"To those who are ceaselessly devoted to Me and who worship Me with immense love, I grant Buddhi yoga by which they come to Me." A concentrated mind alone is a fit instrument for prolonged and deep meditation on the Divine. Intellect alone can do this since it is superior to the mind and the senses.

Dhyana Yoga

The mind is superior to the senses and the intellect is superior to the mind. Through the constant practice of meditation, we gain control over our senses and mind, which helps us to develop the power of concentration.

शनै शनैः शनैपरमेद्बुद्धया धृतिगृहीतया ।
आत्मसंस्थं मनः कृत्वा न किश्दिपि चिन्तयेत् ।।

Karma Yoga

No one can renounce work but if we learn the skill of performing work, the same work will release us from the bondage of Karma.

Sri Krishna clearly says that even to perform work in the right spirit one must exercise his intellectual faculty. Even a little work, done with the spirit of self-sacrifice and dedication, gives a sense of fulfilment. Therefore, intelligent people always choose the path of selfless work using their discriminative faculty. To work and yet to be free from the effects of work requires subtle understanding of the secret of work and such understanding comes from Buddhi. Sri Krishna says in the Bhagavad Gita (2.39)

नराणामधिको विर्षेश: ।
ज्ञानेन हीना: पशुभि: समाना ।।

"Being endowed with such intellect you will get rid of the bondage of actions, O Pratha."

4. Jnana Yoga

Discrimination between the real and the unreal is called Viveka. Buddhi alone has the capacity to determine the real nature of an object. In the path of knowledge, the aspirant has to realize the Truth by constant reasoning and through Buddhi alone this can be done. Sankaracharya emphasizes this view in the Vivekachudamani (versa: 16):

मेधावी पुरुशे विद्वानूहपोहविचक्षण: ।
अधिकार्यात्मविद्यायामुक्तलक्षणलक्षित: ।।

An intelligent and learned man skilled in arguing in favour of the Scriptures . . . is the recipient of the knowledge of the Atman."[23]

Ordinarily we speak of four Yogas, the royal roads to Reality, viz. Jnana, Bhakti, Raja and Karma Yogas. Strangely enough, the Bhagavata does not recognize Rajayoga as an independent path. It speaks of only three. Sri Krishna says to Uddava: "I have propounded three Yogas for the welfare of mankind. They are Jnana, Karma and Bhakti and there is none other anywhere. Jnana Yoga for those who are disillusioned with the world and have given up Karma ; Karmayoga for those who hanker after worldly pleasures and are attached to Karma; and Bhaktiyoga for those who happen to hear about Me and My sports and are attracted by them, yet are not totally free from worldly pursuits nor are very much attached to them." (Bh. II.10, 6.7.8).[24]

Though the Bhagavata does not accord an independent status to Patanjali's Yoga, it recommends and incorporates all its limbs in the practice of meditation. Yama, Niyama, Asana, Pranayama and the whole host are there, may be in a slightly modified form. (Vide Bhag. 11.14. 32-35; and 11.19.33.35).[25]

According to Aurobindo's Yoga is to want to transform oneself integrally, it is to have a single aim in life, such that nothing else exists any longer, that alone exists. And so one feels it clearly in oneself whether one wants it or not; but if one doesn't one can still have a life of goodwill, a life of service, of understanding; one can labour for the work to be accomplished more easily—all that—one can do many things. But between this and doing yoga there is a great difference. And to do Yoga, you must want it consciously.

Impact of Yoga on Life of People

The ancient literature is full of philosophy, science and techniques of channelising the potential energies of people and their life long journey. But How?

The answer is compulsory education of Yoga from school to university level in graded manner. Let us mention some of the facts which can be developed by Yoga Education to improve the personality of students.

(a) Holistic Development of Personality

Holistic Development of Personality, i.e. physical mental and spiritual. This coincides with the definition adopted by World Health Organization. Health is a state of physical, mental and social well-being and not merely the absence of infirmily. Yoga offers us a holistic lifestyle of bliss, peace, creativeness, emotional balance and physical well-being.

The concept of 'mental equanimity' is more satisfactory than the concept of mental health because the former alone can produce spiritual development in an individual. Swami Vishnu Devananda states:

नदेकवार्यमात्रानिर्भास स्वरुप्शुन्यमिव समाधि ।

When consciousness of subject and object disappears and only the meaning remains, it is called samadhi. Samadhi is a merging of the mind into the essence of the object of meditation. Nothing exists but that pure awareness.[26]

Mind is the most powerful part of the human system. It is a Super Computer. Teachers in the systems of Education don't realize its potential or devise ways and means to harness this most important source. Education system can achieve excellence, provided they know the secret of tapping students mind. We generally notice that most of the students do not mentally position as one or the other problems concerning their education continuously bogs them down. Many of them become mental wrecks and a liability on the Education system. The higher education systems instead of solving their problems, cause further deterioration. 25 percent of students in every higher education system are a liability and the other 75 percent are not contributing as per their potential. Teachers should try to create positive mental attitudes among the students. Positive mental attitude is a state of mind that reflects the strength of students belief in what they do. It generates inner and voluntary emotions which enhances motivation, resulting in positive thoughts. Positive thinking is the key to development and is result-oriented.

The ancient Indian philosophers laid stress on mental equanimity for the general well-being of individuals. The mind of an ordinary person is usually very restless. Myriads of desire produce upheavals in the mind of an individual. Over and above this, the mind of an ordinary person is afflicted by several tensions.

The ancient Indian Philosophers maintained that if the mind of an individual usually remains in a disturbed state, he is very likely to develop pathological symptoms. An individual with pathological mental symptoms quite often develop certain pathological organic symptoms because there is very close relationship between the body and the mind of an individual. The mind of an individual becomes free from anxiety and miseries, if there is peace in his mind."

The mind is a reservoir for numerous powers. By utilizing the resources which are hidden within it, one can attain any height of success in the world. If the mind is trained, made one-pointed and inward, it also has power to penetrate into the deeper levels of our being. It is the finest instrument that a human being can ever have.

Holistic approach to health represents a revisioning of the human endeavour to restore order in the organismic functioning, that has occurred in the past several centuries with the medical profession. The holistic health movement is the reflection of the growing dissatisfaction among the professional as well as lay people about the capacity of modern medicine in delivering the healthcare. A shortcoming of modern medicine is its failure to recognize the interactive nature of the different aspects of human existence, viz. physical, psychological social and spiritual in the etiology of illnesses and in the maintenance of health and well-being.

Since modern medicine is itself a development within the framework of science, many have argued that the change needs to be brought about in the very framework. Thus, holistic movement is viewed as a by-product and manifestation of the contemporary thrust on the revision of the scientific framework. One can find this trend in the works of behavioural, natural and social scientists which are contributing for major change in the worldview. It involves a fundamental shift in cognition leading to radical alterations in the belief and assumptions about the nature of the universe, about the human nature, about organism environment interaction, and about the nature of consciousness. The newly emerging worldview is described as holistic paradigm.

In the final analysis, the physical, social, mental and spiritual balance is the most desirable for holistic health. Unless a person is physically fit and active; he cannot perform at his best level. On the other hand, it is the mind, which accounts for 80 percent of physical and social problems. These are called psychosomatic diseases. Lastly, it is the spirit which ultimately directs the mind and through it to the body. The teachers should devise ways and means to ensure synergy of the physical, social, mental and spiritual capabilities, which would release the infinite potential powers of the students and generate efficiency and happiness in the society.

(b) Control of Negative Thought Waves in the Mind

When Patanjali speaks of "control of thought waves", he does not refer to a momentary or superficial control. Many people believe that the practice of yoga is concerned with "making your mind a blank"—a condition which could, if it were really desirable, be much more easily achieved by asking a friend to hit you over the head with a hammer. No spiritual advantage is ever gained by self-violence. We are not trying to check the thought-waves by smashing the organs which record them. We have to do something much more difficult—to unlearn the false identification of the thought waves with the ego-sense. This process of unlearning involves a complete transformation of character, "revewal of the mind", as St. Paul puts it.

(c) Creation of Positive Attitude

To attain success in life and to reach the desired goal one must have a positive attitude. Faith in oneself and in God, courage, strength and fearlessness are the characteristics of a positive intellect. For a man of intense faith nothing is impossible in this world. That person alone who is ready to undergo any amount of suffering and face any difficulty can reach the goal. One should never harbour negative thoughts, like 'I am only a householder', 'I am a sinner', 'I am good for nothing', I am weak'. Such negative thinking can do tremendous harm to our personality.[27] Swami Vivekananda stressed this idea again and again. He was very particular that our younger generation must cultivate positive ideas. He says, "He is an atheist who does not believe in himself. The old religion said that he was an atheist who did not believe in God. The new religion says that he is an atheist who does not believe in himself.

(d) Vast Intellect

Visala Buddhi is that characteristic of the intellect, which transcends all narrow and selfish ideas and embraces the whole world. When a person lets go his individuality and identifies himself with the whole existence, he is called a man of vast intellect. We bow down to the great sage Vyasa because he possessed this vast intelligence.

नमोस्तु ते व्यास विशलबुद्धें (Gita Dhyana, Sloka 2)

Swami Vivekananda wanted our people to develop such an intellect. In one of his lectures delivered in Madras he said, 'We want that education, by which character is formed, strength of mind is increased, the intellect is expanded and by which one can stand on one's own feet.' Further he said, 'Expansion is life, contraction is death.'

A person who is only interested in himself is like a prisoner. He remains confined within the four walls of his house, without any concern for the outside world. He is quite happy with himself and is not aware of his spiritual dimension. There is no expansion of heart. A little spiritual growth will help us to expand our intellect. The same Divine dwells in the heart of everybody and we are one spiritually. Therefore, we must change our attitude towards others.

Sri Krishna shows us how to develop this vast intellect (6.32):

ज्ञानं आत्मौपम्येन सर्वत्र समं मण्यति योऽर्जन ।
सुखं वा यदि वा दुखे स योगी परमो मत: ।।

'He who judges pleasure and pain everywhere bothersome standard as the one he applies to himself, that yogi is thought to be the highest.

The idea is, the man of vast intellect (Visala Buddhi) empathizes with the joys and sorrows of all beings as his own. He understands the sufferings and shares the happiness and miseries of others. Through this teaching Sri Krishna exhorts us, to love others as we love ourselves. Be full of kindness and compassion, identify yourself with others and partake of their joys and sorrows. Why? Because unity underlies this apparent diversity.

The man of vast intellect breaking all barriers embraces the whole world. A selfish man on the other hand feels miserable when others are happy and feels happy when others are suffering. This is called Bheda Buddhi. He always wants to preserve his separate identity. Such a man does not hesitate to harm others for selfish purposes. Because of his deluded intellect, he divides people into different categories, depending on their caste, creed, religion, sex, social status, just to exploit them for his selfish motives. What happens to such a man?[28]

All the great religions of the world have come out of one Truth. If we follow religion without practicing the Truth, it is like the blind leading the blind. Those who belong to God love all. Love is the religion of the universe. A compassionate one transcends the boundaries of religion and realizes the undivided, absolute Reality.[29]

(e) Decisions-based on Deep Thinking

Our decisions, motives, actions should always be guided by serious and deep thinking and not by mere impulse or emotion. A calm and study mind alone is fit to discriminate between right and wrong. We find a beautiful verse in the Katha Upanishad which can guide our intellect to make the right choices (1.2.2):

श्रेयच्श्र प्रेयच्श्र मनुश्यमेत: तौ सम्परीत्य विविनक्ति धीर: ।
श्रेयो हि धीरोऽभिप्रेयसो वृणीते प्रेयो मन्दो योगक्षेमाद्वृणीते ।।

'Both the good and the pleasant present themselves to a man. The calm soul examines them well and discriminates. He prefers the good to the pleasant; but the fool chooses the pleasant out of greed and avarice.'[30]

(f) Strengthen Spiritual Power

Spiritual strength is the highest strength, the next being intellectual and the last, physical. Those who have made considerable progress in spiritual life alone can experience spiritual strength; till then we have to depend upon intellectual strength. Intellectual conviction is possible only through right understanding. Regular study of the scriptures, teachings of great luminaries and discussions on spiritual matters help us to develop right understanding.

The Taittiriya Upanishad says: (1.19)

स्वाध्याय प्रवचनाभ्यां न प्रमदितव्यमात ।

Do not be careless, about learning and teaching.

Since it is difficult to keep the mind always on the spiritual plane, it is better to engage it in intellectual pursuit, lest it should go down to the physical and sensual level.

Thirst for knowledge is inherent in man and no one likes to be ignorant. Knowledge alone can remove ignorance. A beautiful verse in Chanakya Niti (XVII-17) says:

ज्ञांन नराणामधिको विशेशः ।
ज्ञानेन हीनाः पशुभिः समानाः ॥

What distinguishes a man from an animal is his capacity to acquire knowledge. Without knowledge men are equal to animals.

Spiritual knowledge comes through direct experience of Truth, but very few can reach that state. Others have to follow the path of discrimination, using their intellect.

There is a popular saying:

स्वदेशे पूज्यते राजा विद्वान् सवृत्र पूज्यते ।

The king is honoured only in his kingdom whereas a learned person is honoured everywhere.[31]

(g) Helps in Sorting out Psychological Problems Born out of Tensions, Conflicts, etc.[32]

What most psychologists ask their patients to do is to yield to the demands of the unconscious. In some cases this may release the inner tensions. But this may not be permanent and may even be more harmful. The super conscious is at present unknown to us, but that does not mean that it is the same as the unconscious mind of the psychologists. It can be attained through spiritual disciplines. It is the source of supreme peace and bliss. More than all, it gives man the feeling of wholeness, the feeling of supreme fulfilment.

(h) Strengthen Will Power

Development of will power is a problem that is often faced by everyone of us. If we can exercise our body and buildup its strength gradually, there is no reason why the same cannot be done with our mind ! By denying ourselves small pleasures and temptations to begin with, we can gradually but surely build up our will power. The example given by the Holy Mother of the farmer who could lift a bull because he used to carry it daily since the time it was a small helpless calf, can give us much-needed encouragement here also.[33]

Fear is the greatest of all foes. It is a devil residing with. Fearlessness is the first rung on the ladder of freedom.

To cultivate the quality of humility is one step toward enlightenment. By being humble we gain much and lose nothing. Prayer and contemplation strengthen our willpower in cultivating this inner quality.

(i) Understanding the Purpose of Life

Swami Rama feels that "If a human being remains constantly aware of the purpose of his life and directs all his actions toward the fulfilment of that purpose, there remains nothing impossible for him. Those who are not aware of the purpose of life are easily caught by the whirlpool of miseries."

A human being is fully equipped with all necessary healing powers, but does not know their usage. The moment he comes in touch with the healing potentials within, he can heal himself. All the powers belong to only one God. A human being is only an instrument.

(j) Nutrition for Yogic Persons

Swami Vishnu Devananda in his book Meditation and Mantras has rightly said that, What is consumed by the human body correlates directly to the efficiency with which the brain functions. Recent studies show that certain red food colouring creates hyperactivity in children, and that refined sugar can cause emotional instability. These are just two examples of substances that are often heedlessly consumed without understanding their effect on the body and mind.

Several years ago vegetarianism was, in a sense, an underground practice. A person who refrained from eating meat was viewed with a certain amount of curiosity, if not suspicion. Today it is quite a different story. Health food stores and vegetarian restaurants are prevalent. There is a growing awareness that our health is directly affected by what we eat. Many diseases can be cured by a change in diet or a short period of fasting, with no medications at all. This is true not only of physical disorders, but of many mental difficulties as well. It is particularly important that pregnant mothers have this awareness; too often they do not realize the effect of their diet on the developing fetus.

There is no doubt that, "You are what you eat", a subtle part of what is consumed becomes the consciousness. Those who have changed from a meat to vegetarian diet notice a corresponding change in consciousness. There is a certain grossness that disappears, and the awareness becomes finely tuned.

In the Bhagavad-Gita three types of food have been mentioned which produce three different types of dispositions in individuals.

A person becomes healthy, moral, religious, intelligent and creative by regularly taking, sattvika food.

Sattvika spreads sattvika and the cumulative effect is purity of environment

आयु: सत्वबलारोग्यसुखप्रीतिविवर्धना: ।
रत्या: सिनगधा: स्थिरा हरद्या आहारा: सात्त्विकप्रिया: ।। xvii / 8 Bhagavad Gita.

Foods which promote longevity, intelligence, vigour, health, happiness and cheerfulness, and which are sweet, bland, substantial and naturally agreeable, are dear to the Sattvika type of men."

कटृवम्ललवणात्युश्णतीक्षणक्षविदाहिन: ।
आहारा राजसस्येश्टा दु:खशोकामयप्रदा: ।। xvii / 9 Bhagavad Gita.

Foods which are bitter, acid, salty, overhot, pungent, dry and burning, and which cause suffering, grief and sickness, are dear to the Rajasika type of men.

यातायामं गतरसं पूति पयुणितं च यत् ।
उच्छिश्टमपि चामोध्यं भोजन तामसप्रियम् ।। xvii / 10 Bhagavad Gita.

Food which is half-cooked or half-ripe, insipid, putrid, stale and polluted, and which is impure too, is dear to men of a Tamasika disposition.

RESEARCH STUDIES ABOUT IMPACT OF YOGA ON LIVES OF PEOPLE

P.K. Hassanagas *et. al.* in their article, "Yoga in the Culture of Labour" based on research have come out with the following conclusions:[34]

1. Practising yoga helps in improving the general health of the volunteers.
2. The psycho condition is reinforced and the mental capabilities are increased. The concentration and the memory are developed. Self-confidence, self-discipline and working capability are increased.
3. The capability for removing the psychophysical fatigue is increased.
4. The influence of the harmful factors from the working conditions to health is decreased because the immunity and the resistance of the body is reinforced and the participants learn how to protect themselves.

5. The number of the injuries is decreased as a result of increase of the self-consciousness, self-control of the body and the brain.
6. The number of absences due to illness is decreased.
7. The efficiency and the productivity increases leading to profits.

Nedungade V. Haridas in the article, "Physiological and Philosophical Aspects of Yoga" states that[35]—

Yoga science is a well proven treasure and it is up to us to tap the yoga power to relax and rejuvenate our mind, increase our physical strength, expand our spiritual awareness, improve our concentration, help our body use oxygen and nutrients more effectively and to prevent illness and retard old-age.

In conclusion, a quotation is taken from His Holiness Swamy Vishnudevananda, "Health is wealth—peace of mind is happiness—yoga shows the way."

Pavlos K. Hassanages *et. al.* in their article, "Yoga and Cardio-Vascular Diseases" state:[36]

Our results show remarkable influence of yoga on eliminating and alleviating of chronic psycho-stresses, increasing of self-control, self-confidence and self-discipline which help to eliminate other risk factors and to undertake responsibility for improving one's own health and the quality of living which in turn helps in preventing coronary disease.

Dr. (Mrs.) Hemalatha Murthy in his article, "Management of Respiratory Diseases by Yoga",[37] states that yoga gives us solace, confidence, redeems all our miseries, obsession, conflicts. It is suitable to all and all times. It helps the persons to change their attitude and bring a tremendous change in way of life which is simple and which is very necessary, unless, there is no true solutions to all the problems and illnesses. Right knowledge of yoga burns out the likes and dislikes, ego and ignorance and there is establishment of Pure Bliss, which is natural state of a being.

For the management of stress in order to combat the so-called stress-induced disorders all the above discussed areas should be tapped. Yoga way is more holistic, which offers the lifestyle of bliss, efficiency, emotional equipoise, mental clarity, intellectual sharpness and physical well-being.

Swami Harshananda in his article, "Attainment of Yoga" mentions that knowingly or unknowingly, all of us are struggling to get peace. As long as our mind is in pieces and the pieces are in ceaseless mutual conflict, peace eludes us. It is only when we learn to put these pieces together so as to make the mind whole and integrated that we gain the peace of Kaivalya. This is easier said than done. However, with competent guides like Patanjali who are ever eager to help out of infinite compassion, this task should not be that difficult.

Patanjali, the great master of the Yoga system, calls these pieces of the mind as vrttis, modifications, which are ever arising and never subsiding. Yoga or union of the individual self with the Supreme Self will result through Yoga or Samadhi, when these Vrttis are controlled, suppressed and eliminated, by the right kind of discipline and training. This discipline and training is also Yoga.[38]

Dr. S.C. Manchanda,[39] Professor and Head; Department of Cardiology, All India Institute of Medical Sciences, New Delhi has depicted the role of Yoga lifestyle in Coronary Artery diseases in his "Research Study of Reversal of Coronary Heart Disease through Preksha Meditation with Reference to Coronary Atherosclerotic Reversal Potential of Yoga Lifestyle Intervention." According to the study, forty-two male patients (mean age 51.0 + 9.5 range 32-72 years) with angiographically proven CAD were included. Patients in the control group (n=21) were managed on conventional medical therapy (with control of risk factors, AHA step 1 diet, moderate aerobic exertion), while those in the yoga group (n=21) were advised strict lifestyle modifications and yogic exercises as detailed below. The yogic lifestyle intervention programme consisted of:

(a) Yogic Lifestyle Methods—
   (i) Health rejuvenating exercises: a set of movements for improving the general tone of the body and to improve coordination.
   (ii) Relaxation exercise (Kayotsarg): a method of complete relaxation to prepare the body and mind for meditation.
   (iii) Breathing exercises (Pranayama).
   (iv) Yogic postres for stretch relaxation (Asanas).
   (v) Preksha meditation (preksha means seeing deeply within).
   (vi) Reflection on moral values (Anuvrat and Anupreksha).
(b) Stress Management (relaxation, breathing exercises and Preksha meditation).
(c) Dietary control.
(d) Moderate aerobic exercises.

The change in the lesion severity was classified into regression (10% absolute reduction in diameter stenosis), no significant change «10% change in diameter stenosis) or progression (>10% absolute increase in diameter stenosis). In the Yoga group, 3 (5%) lesions showed progression, 46 (75%) lesions showed no change while 12 (20%) lesions showed regression. In the control group 22 (37%) lesions showed progression, 36 (61%) showed no change while 1 (2%) showed regression.

Yoga lifestyle intervention is beneficial in improving the symptoms and exercise capacity, lowering weight and serum lipid levels. It also retards the progression of coronary atherosclerosis in patients with severe coronary artery diseases and reduces revasularisation procedures.

In ancient India the early Yogis were a group of mystics and scientists to whom the relationship between the mortal man and an immortal spirit was of great interest. They set about to find ways and means of uniting these two during the earthly life of man. They spent not decades but centuries in making their experiments with different methods of concentration, meditation and relaxation; with various breathing processes, postures and foods. When they finally succeeded in their experiments, they systematized the result of their findings and called it the science of Yoga. The aim of Yoga is to achieve reintegration of the individual consciousness with the cosmic consciousness.[40]

The aim of Yoga is to completely alter one's personality and outlook so that he is able to face all problems of life with equanimity, while pursuing to achieve the ideals which he cherishes. It is a complete break with normal waking consciousness. It is neither a condition of vain pursuits and frustrations of waking life, nor a condition of mere dreaming, nor even condition of absence of quality as in deep sleep, but a condition of calmness and tranquility of mind in daily pursuits. As Gita describes with an analogy, he is one into whom all desires enter as waters into these and is ever motionless though constantly being filled (11.70). He enjoys and suffers like all human beings; he has passions, fears and rages like all human beings; but unlike the ordinary human beings, he is able to maintain tranquility through them all.

YOGA EDUCATION

Universities and colleges can translate the potential benefits of Yoga through Yoga education. Without Yoga education, the benefits of Yoga cannot be obtained. So, it is essential for universities and colleges to start "Yoga departments to impart theory and practice of Yoga Education through morning or evening classes.

From the time you are quite young, the work of your educators is to teach you to control your impulses and obey only those which are in conformity with the laws under which you live or with the ideal you wish to follow or the customs of the environment in which you are. The value of this mental construction which will govern your impulses depends a great deal on the surroundings in which you live and the character of the parents or people who educate you. But whether it be good or bad, mediocre or excellent, it is always the result of a mental control over the impulses. When your parents tell you, "You should not do this", or when they say, "You have to do that", this is a beginning of education for the mind's control over the impulses.

Usually education, all culture, all refinement of the senses and the being is one of the best ways of curing instincts, desires, passions. To eliminate these things does not cure them; to cultivate, intellectualize, refine them, this is the surest means of curing. To give the greatest possible development for progress and growth, to acquire a certain sense of harmony and exactness of perception, this is a part of the culture of the being, of the education of the being . . .

Education is certainly one of the best means of preparing the consciousness for a higher development.

Mental culture, intellectual education changes the constitution of your brain, enlarges it considerably, and as a result the expression becomes more complete and more precise.

In yoga one can do in a very short time what takes otherwise an interminable time. But it is always in the body and always upon earth that it is done, not elsewhere. That is why when one is in a body one must take advantage of it and not waste one's time, not say, "A little later, a little later." It is much better to do it immediately. All the years you pass without making any progress are wasted years which you are sure to regret afterwards.

Thirst for knowledge is inherent in man and no one likes to be ignorant. Knowledge alone can remove ignorance. A beautiful verse in Chanakya Niti (XVII-17) says:

ज्ञानं नराणामधिको विर्षेशः ।
ज्ञानेन हीनाः पशुभिः समाना ॥

"What distinguishes a man from an animal is his capacity to acquire knowledge. Without knowledge men are equal to animals."

Spiritual knowledge comes through direct experience of Truth, but very few can reach that state. Others have to follow the path of discrimination, using their intellect.

There is a popular saying:

"The king is honoured only in his kingdom whereas a learned person is honoured everywhere."[41]

स्वदेशे पूज्यते राजा विद्वान् सर्वत्र पूज्यते ।

The universities and colleges can adopt the following strategy:

1. Starting Part-time courses for students and general public in theory and practice of yoga.
2. Starting Diploma courses.
3. B.A., M.A. and Ph.D. in Yoga philosophy and science.

Though Yoga Education, the Institutions of higher education would find the change in atomosphere, i.e. from indiscipline and restlessness to intellectual and peaceful environment where there is bliss alround. The students can enjoy not only their life in universities and colleges but the rest of life in a highly dignified way.

ROLE OF UGC

The UGC initiated a scheme in 1993 for promotion of Yoga Education and Practice in Universities. This scheme aims at assisting universities in setting up Yoga Education and practice centres in their campuses for which they may identify and involve one of the eminent Yoga Institutions in the country. Assistance is provided to universities for meeting the recurring expenditure incurred on managing the Yoga center. The recurring expenditure consists of the amount the university would be required to pay to the Yoga Institutions whose instructors would manage the Yoga center and conduct Yoga classes, or pay directly.

The university would be required to levy a fee of Rs. 50 per month per person from the participating teachers/students for meeting the needs of consumables and for maintenance of the Yoga center.

The Commission had constituted an Expert Committee to consider the proposals for financial assistance for the establishment of Yoga centres in universities during the Ninth Plan period.

On the recommendations of the Committee the Commission approved the revision in the guidelines of the scheme for providing financial assistance to Yoga centres, which is also applicable to the already existing Yoga centres during Ninth Plan, w.e.f. 0.01.2000 as shown on next page.

The Commission also approved the following guidelines for the appointment of Instructors priority-wise:

- Post-graduate degree (full time course) in Yoga/Yogic Science/ Yoga Therapy/Yoga Studies, etc. from Universities.
- Post-graduate Diploma (full time one year course) in Yoga/ Yogic Science/Yoga Therapy/Yoga Studies, etc. from Universities.
- Post-graduate Diploma (full time course) in Yoga/Yogic Science/Yoga Therapy/Yoga Studies, etc. from eminent Institutions other than the Universities.

The Commission has approved, so far, 42 universities for the establishment of Yoga centres. The commission further decided to support at least ten universities for establishing/strengthening of Departments of Human consciousness and Yogic Science with the following staff:

1. Professor	One
2. Reader	One
3. Lecturer	Two
4. Lab. Assistant	One
5. Lab. Attendant	One
6. Computer Operator	One

The financial assistance to run the Department of Human consciousness and Yogic Science would be available as under:

Sl. No.	Item(s)	Existing	Proposed
(a)	Initial Furnishing, equipment and contingency (one time grant)	Rs. 50,000	Rs. 1,00,000
(b)	Honorarium to Instructors for A and B class cities	Rs. 6,000 p.m.	Rs. 7,500 p.m.
(c)	Honorarium to instructors for remaining places	Rs. 5,000	Rs. 6,500 p.m.

(a) Non-Recurring	
(i) Lab. (Human Performance)	Rs. 5,00,00
(ii) Computer Lab.	Rs. 4,00,000
(b) Recurring	
(i) Salary	Actual
(ii) Book and Journals	Rs. 1,00,000

The Expert Committee identified ten universities out of the proposals received from 50 universities for creating an independent Department of Human Consciousness and Yogic Science.

These are:

1. Andhra University, Visakhapatnam (A.P.).
2. Bharathidasan University, Tiruchirapalli (T.N.).
3. Dr. H.S. Gour University, Sagar (M.P.).
4. Gurukula Kangri Vishwavidyalaya, Haridwar (Uttaranchal).
5. Jawahar Lal Nehru University, New Delhi.
6. Karnataka University, Dharwad (Karnataka).
7. Mahatma Gandhi Gramodaya Vishwavidyalaya, Chitrakoot (M.P.).
8. Mangalore University, Mangalore (Karnataka).
9. Mumbai University, Mumbai (M.S.).
10. University of Allahabad, Allahabad (U.P.).

A grant of Rs. 1,000 lakhs each to all the above universities was also released during the financial year 2000-2001 for starting the Department of Human consciousness and Yogic Science. The courses and the syllabi for the Department of Human Consciousness and Yogic Science as approved by the Expert Committee/Commission have been sent to all the concerned universities for implementation.[42]

CONCLUSION

Systematic and regular practice of Yogic techniques viz. Postures, Pranayama, Mudras, Bandas, Shat-Kriyas, Concentration, Meditation and diet regulations under experts guidance and certainly not from books alone, will go for to build up the lost muscle tone of various organs, glands, nerves, etc. mental clarity, positive attitude towards life, and in removing physical and mental restlessness and physiochemical process as the stress creates nerves disorders due to modern hectic, pressurized, frustrated living.

It has been reported in the ancient literature that Yogic practice brings change in various hormonal and physiochemical process in the human body by operating at the higher levels in the nervous system.[43]

"Yoga helps in maintaining good health
and gives resistance, stamina, vitality and vigour to the body.
Yoga is the best curative and preventive medicine.
Yoga leads to chittanasa which is moksha.
Yoga practitioners should not become Bhogi.
If no Yoga—no health, no peace, no life."

Notes and References

1. Xth Plan of University Grants Commission, New Delhi, 2002, p. 51.
2. Dr. H.R. Nagendra and Dr. R. Najarathna, News Perspectives on Stress Management, Swami Vivekananda Yoga Prakashana, Bangalore, 2003, Preface.
3. *Ibid.*, pp. 2-3, 27.
4. YB ; ii (2).
5. YS I (2).
6. YS (i) 12.
7. R.H. Singh, "Yoga and Health, Science and Philosophy of Indian Medicine, Baidyanath Bhawan, Nagpur, 1978.
8. Dr. C.H. Sudarshan, Yoga for Better Health, in NIS Argopcar Varta, National Institute of Naturopathy, Pune, May 2001.
9. Y.S. H. 30.
10. Y.B. R.M. ii 30.
11. Swami Srikantananda, The Intelligent Way to Yoga, Sri Ramakrishna Math, Chennai, 2001, pp. 30-31.
12. Swami Srikantananda, *op. cit.*, p. 66.
13. Manual of Ethics, 1935, p. 341.
14. Y.S. R.M. Y.B. (i) 46.
15. Y.S. ii 49, 50.
16. Y.S. ii 53, U.B. R.M. ii 52.
17. Swami Sivananada, Practice of Yoga Quoted in Swami Devananda, *op. cit.*, p. 60.
18. Swami Vishnu Devananda, *op. cit.*, p. 161.
19. Y.S. Y.B. M.P. ii 54.
20. YB iii, Y.S. Y.B. iii 7.
21. R.M. iii 2.

22. Y.S. Y.B. iii, 4, 7, 8.
23. Swami Siddhinathananda, Yoga in Srimod Bhagavata, *Yoga and Its various Aspects,* Sri Ramakrishna Math, Madras, pp. 160-61.
24. Swami Srikantananda, *op. cit.,* pp. 7-11.
25. Swami Siddhinathananda, Yoga in Srimad Bhagavata, *Yoga and Its various Aspects,* Sri Rama Krishna Math, Madras, pp. 160-61.
26. Swami Vishnu Devananda, *op. cit.,* p. 177.
27. Bata K. Day, Ethics: Maladies and Remedies, in *IJPA,* July-Sept, 1995, p. 46.
28. Swami Srikantananda, *op. cit.,* pp. 56-57.
29. *Ibid.,* pp. 40-41.
30. *Ibid.,* p. 17.
31. *Ibid.,* 65-66.
32. Swami Yatishwarananda, Meditation and Spiritual Life, Ramakrishna Ashram, Bangalore, 1983, pp. 17-18.
33. *Ibid.*
34. P.K. Hassanagas, "Yoga in the Culture of Labour based on Research", Arya Vidya Sala Kottakhal and University of Calicut, Holistic Life and Medicine, Sixth World Congress on Holistic Life and Medicine held at Calicut, Kerala, 5-7 July 1996, pp. 127-28.
35. Nedungade, V. Hardias, Physiological and Philosophical Aspects of Yoga.
36. *Ibid.,* p. 150.
37. Dr. (Mrs.) Hemlatha Murly, "Management of Respiratory Disesase by Yoga", National Institute of Naturopathy, Pune, *op. cit.,* p. 12.
38. Swami Harshanand, "Attainment of Yoga Maladies and Remediese", in *Yoga: Its various Aspects,* Sri Ramakrishana Math, Madras, pp. 203-04.
39. Manchanda, S.C. *et. al.,* "Research Study of Reversal of Coronary Heart Disease through Preksha Meditation with reference to coronary atherosclerotic reversal potential of yoga lifestyle intervention", A Research Study conducted by AIIMS, Deptt. of Cardiology, New Delhi, pp. 1-8.
40. Swami Prabuddhananda, Yoga in Daily Life, In *Yoga: Its various Aspects,* Shri Ramakrishna Math, Madras, pp. 70-71 and 121-22.
41. Swami Srikantananda, *op. cit.,* p. 66.
42. UGC Annual Report 2001-02, New Delhi, p. 89.
43. Dr. C.H. Sudarshan, *op. cit.,* p. 20.

APPENDIX 7.1

THE UGC SCHEME FOR PROMOTION OF YOGA EDUCATION AND PRACTICE AND POSITIVE HEALTH IN UNIVERSITIES

1. Introduction

Yoga promotes physical and mental health. It disciplines the mind and improves the power of concentration. Therefore, it is ideally suited for those who are involved in intellectual pursuits. The concepts of positive health and lifelong learning are relatively new and need to be strengthened. Yoga is a discipline, based on meticulous practice and requires very modest infrastructure and money. The Commission has formulated a scheme for promotion of yoga education and practice in the Xth Plan and a new component of positive health is being added to this scheme.

2. Objective

To impart special education in various areas like yoga, positive health, career, personality development, etc. for the overall development of students, teachers and non-teaching staff of universities.

3. Eligibility/Target Groups

All eligible universities which are included under Section 2 (f) and have been declared fit to receive central assistance under Section 12(b) of the UGC Act of 1956, are covered under the scheme. The target group is students, teachers and non-teaching staff of universities.

4. Nature of Assistance

The UGC will provide grants to the selected universities upto the end of Xth Plan period only, i.e. 31st March, 2007. Thereafter the scheme is required to be taken over by the concerned universities under its maintenance budget. The UGC will provide financial assistance as under:

Yoga

Sl. No.	*Items*	*Financial Assistance under the scheme*
1.	Equipment/Furnishing	Rs. 1,00,000 (one time grant)
2.	Honorarium to instructors – maximum two (2)	Rs. 1,80,000 p.a. @ Rs. 7500 p.m. (Rs. 7500 x 12 x 2 = 1,80,000

The Universities may charge Rs. 50 p.m. per head as a token fee from the students/teachers non-teaching staff interested to participate in its yoga center activities for meeting the recurring expenditure.

The minimum qualifications for yoga instructors shall be as under:

1. Post-graduate degree (full time course) in Yoga/Yogic Science/

Yoga Therapy/Yoga Studies, etc. from a recognized university.

Or

2. Post-graduate diploma (full time of at least one year course) in Yoga/Yogic Science/Yoga Therapy/Yoga Studies, etc. from a recognized university or an eminent institution with a well established reputation in the field of yoga, with a minimum experience of two years in yoga teaching and practice.

Positive Health

Assistance will be provided for organizing 3-5 days awareness programme by inviting guest speakers/experts, etc. These programmes could be from amongst the following:

1. General counselling,
2. AIDS,
3. Drug Abuse,
4. Sex education and reproductive health,
5. Art of healthy living,
6. Stress management, and
7. Sound Body and mental health.

Any other programme on similar subject/nature can also be covered.

Sl. No.	*Activity*	*Financial Assistance*
1.	For organizing 3-5 days awareness programme	Rs. 25,000 per programme

CHAPTER 8

HUMAN EXCELLENCE EDUCATION: VITAL FOR HEALTH EDUCATION

God, Give us Men!
God, give us men! A time like this demands,
Strong minds, great hearts, true faith and ready hands;
Men whom the lust of office does not kill
Men whom the spoils of office cannot buy;
Men who possess opinions and a will;
Men who have honour; men who will not lie.

—*Josiah Gilbert Holland*

Our power of life lies in thoughts. Thought is the secret key in our mental software.
Lead us from negative thoughts (darkness) to positive thought (light), from Untruth to Truth from Immortality to Mortality

तमसो मा ज्योतिर्गमय
असतो मा सद् गमय
मृत्योर्माऽमृतं गमय

From Negative Thought
To Positive Thoughts
From Untruth
To Truth
From Immortality
To Mortality

Human Excellence Education: Vital for Health Education

> Transformation of individuality into personality, thus, is an essentially for spiritual growth—for the manifestation of all potentialities lying latent in the man. When this happens excellence naturally come in its trail. . . . Spiritual intelligence is always to be regarded as the supreme guide in all human exercises, because it is this spiritual intelligence that leads to fulfilment of human march, it is this spiritual growth, which enables the man to discharge his obligations to the community in an excellent manner
>
> —*Prof. Ramaranjan Mukherji*
> "Sanskrit and Human Excellence" In *Souvenir*,
> World Sanskrit Conference,
> New Delhi, 5-9 April, 2001.

We mention below the following essentials which can be developed through right education which can ensure holistic development of people and keep them from modern influence of materialistic tendencies . . . responsible for stresses and strains and other mental problems.

Dr. M. Lakshmi Kumari in her forward to "Yoga in Education", Vol. I by Dr. H.R. Nagendra and Sri T. Mohan Swami Vivekananda Yoga Prakashan state that the aim of all education, undoubtedly, is the attainment of human excellence and perfection, not just in any field of knowledge or activity but life in totality. Education should be the means to fashion excellent characters out of the very ordinary human raw material. This means culturing of the qualities of head and heart in a way congenial to the growth and development of oneself and other around him. In practical life, this has to be translated as qualities of truthfulness, righteous living, purity in personal life, self-confidence, integration of body, mind and intellect, love and compassion towards all living beings and surrender to Almighty. These are steps leading to the unfoldment of perfection already in man. Such a truly education and cultured man alone can meet the challenges, internal and external, in a positive way, converting them into opportunities, helping in his ultimate evolution. Pursued further, one's entire thought, behaviour and life itself would come to express the spiritual oneness of the creation and this would be the manifestation also of the divinity inherent in man. A truly educated man, like a true scientist, satisfied with nothing but the one truth, has to be necessarily spiritual as well.

Swami Vivekanand stressed on man-making, character-building education. To quote him, "Education is not the amount of information that is put into your brain and runs riot there undigested all your life. We must have life-building, man-making, character-making assignmilation of ideals. We want education by which character is formed, strength of mind is increased, the intellect is expanded, by which one can stand on one's feet. What we want is Western science coupled with Vedanta, Brahmacharya as the guilding motto and also Shraddha and faith in one's own life." Education is the panacea for all the ills affecting us individually, socially, nationally.

The education as is obtained today is not at all aimed at character-building with the result that we find even highly educated men who have so much of power and service machinery at their command fail miserably when tackling problems in the right way, in the human way, in the interest of our nation. Highly talented individuals are there in every field, second to none, but devoid of patriotic fervour and personal integrity, the impact they produce is minimal. Today, we are urgently in need to men and women of character, integrity and dedication and of tremendous capacities happily blending dignity of man with dignity of labour.

Concentration of mind, its purity and chastity alone can bring out the amazing qualities and capacities that lie hidden in the human mind. Lack of these has created a student community who are debilitated, inhuman, selfish and indifferent to human values. Swami Vivekananda stresses the value of Shraddha, faith, as one of the most potent factors capable of elevating human life. He wanted this, "Life saving, great, ennobling, grand doctrine" to be taught to our children from their very birth. Where the different streams of consciousness in man, namely concentration of mind, purity of life, faith in oneself, strength of body and fearlessness of mind are combined together in a single personality, the force of that character becomes invincible. Men of such stature alone can rebuild a shattered society. It is such men that our educational system should create to safely carry over our country to the 21st century.

Excellence in Sanskrit Literature differs a lot from the ordinary definition given in general description. Excellence in general discussion is generally associated with outward manifestation and temporary achievement e.g. a person solving an issue on a temporary basis. However, the real definition of excellence is in Ancient Sanskrit Literature which is permanent and based on spiritually. Though the reality is every where, we can only make contact with it in our own hearts. Swami Prabhavananda in his Patanjali Yogasutras quotes the poem of Saint Kabir which emphasizes that God is within us.

I laugh when I hear that the fish,
in the water is thirsty.
You wander restlessly from forest to forest
while the reality is within your own dwelling
the truth is here! Go where you will.
To Benarus or to Mathura until you have found
God in your own Soul,
the whole world will seem meaningless to you.

Excellent character is the first and foremost an essential quality of a man of excellence. It is very difficult to remain firm in character. We generally find unsteadfast people in day-to-day life. They are not steadfast. Let us quote an example.

We find the wonderful character of Nachiketa in the Katha Upanishad; a boy of eleven years, but what maturity! At such a tender age he wanted to know the Truth about man. He asked Yama and Lord of death (1.1.20):

येयं प्रेते विचिकित्सा मनुष्येऽस्तीत्येके नायमस्तीति चैके ।
एतद्विद्यामनुशिष्टस्त्वयाऽहं वराणामेष वरस्तृतीयः ॥

'When a man dies there arises a doubt: some say that he exists; some others say that he does not. Which is right, I should like to know, being taught by you.'

Nachiketa's question regarding this profound truth was like a bombshell to Yama. How could he impart this great truth to a mere boy? Instead of answering his question he tried his best to divert the boy's mind by offering him tempting alternatives. He offered him plenty of wealth sense enjoyments, progeny, a kingdom on earth. But the boy stood firm. He said: (1.1.26)

श्वोभावा मर्त्यस्य यदन्तकैतत्
सर्वेन्द्रियाणां जरयन्ति तेजः ।
अपि सर्वं जीवितमल्पमेव
तवैव वाहास्तव नृत्यगीते ॥

'All these pleasures that you have offered, are transient. O Death, they also wear out the vigour of all the sense organs of mortal man. Moreover, all life, long or short, is only little compared to eternal life. Let your chariots, dance and song remain with you only.'[1]

The man of excellence does not follow blindly. He exercises his mental faculty to discriminate between real and unreal. He gets guidance from authoritative sources like our Ancient Sanskrit literature.

Sri Krishna clearly says that even to perform work in the right spirit one must exercise his intellectual faculty. Even a little work, done with the spirit of self-sacrifice and dedication, gives a sense of fulfilment. Therefore, intelligent people always choose the path of selfless work using their discriminative faculty. To work and yet to be free from the effects of work requires subtle understanding of the secret of work and such understanding comes from Buddhi. Sri Krishna says in the Bhagvad Gita (2.39).

बुद्ध्या युक्तो यथा पार्था कर्मबन्धं प्रहास्यसि ।

'Being endowed with such intellect you will get rid of the bondage of actions, O partha.'.

Discrimination between the real and the unreal is called Viveka. Buddhi alone has the capacity to determine the real nature of an object. In the path of knowledge, the aspirant has to realize the Truth by constant reasoning and through Buddhi alone this can be done. Shankaracharya emphasizes this view in the Vivekachudamani (verse: 16):

मेधावी पुरुषो विद्वानूहपोहविचक्षण: ।
अधिकार्यात्मविद्यायामुक्तलक्षणलक्षित: ।।

An intelligent and learned man skilled in arguing in favour of the Scriptures . . . is the recipient of the knowledge of the Atman.[2]

The person of excellence should develop positive attitude and firm faith in himself and the scriptures. This will create respect towards scriptures and such a person would welcome challenges and solve them intelligently.

A man with a positive attitude does not like an easy going life. He welcomes challenges, obstacles, difficulties, problems and faces them with great courage. He always likes an adventure in life. Such heroic spirit is a quality needed to become a successful leader. He alone can lead the society who has developed a positive intellect.

Shankaracharya defined this attitude in the Vivekachudamani (Verse: 25):

शास्त्रस्य गुरुवाक्यस्य सत्यबुद्ध्यवधारणम् ।
सा श्रद्धा कथिता सभ्दिर्यया वस्तू2पलभ्यते ।।

'The firm conviction that the words of the scriptures and the Guru are true is called sraddha, by which the Real is attained.[3]

A man of excellence does not believe in his own welfare and development. He is keen to promote the welfare of all as in their welfare lies his own welfare. In Mahabharata, the Victory of Pandvas was because, the persons on their side were highly skilled, spiritual and desireless while on the other side, that is Kaurvas were desirous of usurping the territory of legal heirs. Ram Rajya in Ramayana was based on the Character of Ram and his brothers.

When we pray for the welfare of others, all our petty and selfish feelings will go away and our intellect will expand. There are many such prayers in the Vedas and the Puranas, such as:

सर्वे भवन्तु सुखिनः सर्वे सन्तु निरायाः ।
सर्वे भद्राणि पश्यन्तु मा कश्चिद् दुःखभाग् भवेत् ।।

'May all be happy, may all be free from disease, may all realize what is good, may none be subject to misery.'[4]

A man of excellence is keen to pursue knowledge as knowledge is power. A person is great not because of money but because of knowledge.

Knowledge alone can remove ignorance. A beautiful verse in Chanakya Niti (XVII-17) says:

ज्ञानं नराणामधिको विशेषः ।
ज्ञानेन हीनाः पशुभिः समानाः ।।

'What distinguishes a man from an animal is his capacity to acquire knowledge. Without knowledge men are equal to animals.'

There is a popular saying:

स्वदेशे पूज्यते राजा विद्वान सर्वत्र पूज्यते ।

"The king is honoured only in his kingdom whereas a learned person is honoured everywhere."[5]

A man of excellence should understand that all life is a continuous struggle with temptation and evil which can be avoided by a disciplined life.

Neither by work, nor through progeny nor through wealth but by renunciation alone is life eternal reached (Mahanarayana Upanisad VIII. 14.) Sacrifice of self is the best sacrifice.

By speculative knowledge, we come nearer to the gates of reality but we cannot approach Truth by means of thought alone. It can be reached only through the perfection of the whole human nature, we must practice the tortures of body, mind and spirit. The control of passions means transmutation into spiritual energy and bliss. This state of poise can be attained only by vigorous practice.

Patanjali Yoga Sutras, Chapter 2, Sloka 4 says that Ignorance creates all other obstacles. They may exist either in potential or a Vestical form or they may have been temporarily overcome or fully developed. Patanjali

CHART 8.1

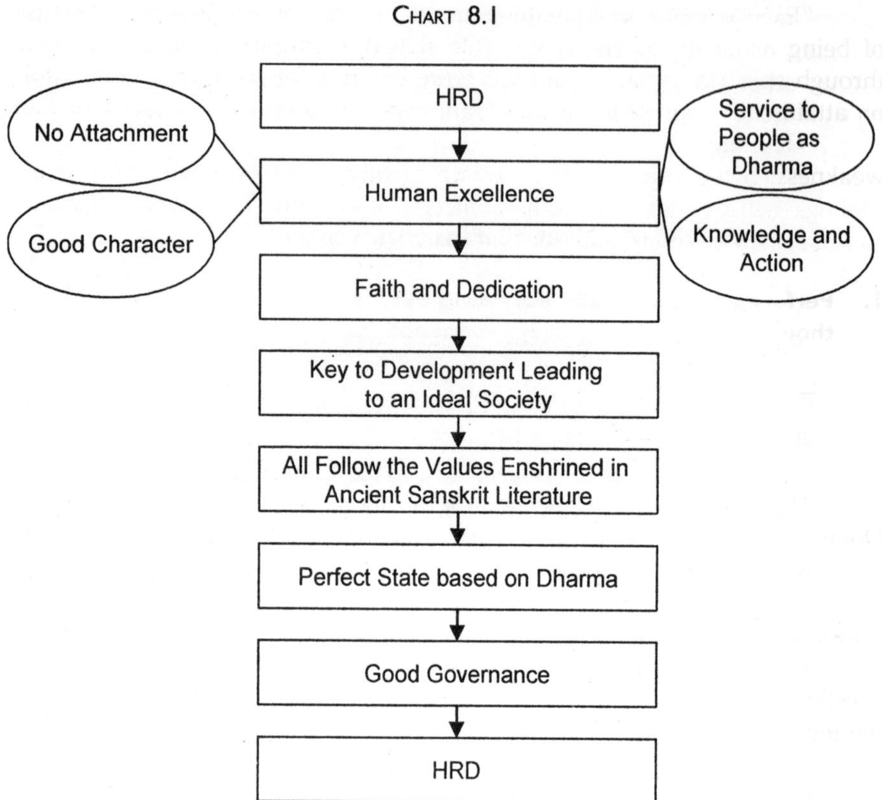

Yoga Sutras, Chapter 1, Sloka 30 says that sickness, mental laziness, doubt, lack of enthusiasm, sloth, craving for sense pleasure, false perception, despair caused by failure to concentrate and unsteady in concentration, these distractions are the obstacles to knowledge.

Mahayana Buddhism makes out that the Buddha's appear on earth for the redemption of mankind, "The exalted one appears in the world for salvation to many people, for joy to many people, out of compassion for the world, as a blessing, as a salvation, as the joy of Gods and men."

The excellence, therefore is not purely for brightening one's life but it is to help other people in this world to achieve salvation.

(Sadharma Pundarika, XV)

In advanced countries, people are following what is written in our scriptures and that is why they are developed materially while people in developing countries are not following their own ideas enshrined in Ancient Sanskrit Literature resulting in backwardness. However, the people in advanced countries concentrate only on material advancement which is causing imbalance in development. What is needed is to imbibe qualities of service to humanity along with material advancement to make this world a real place of enjoyment and bliss.

"Excellence", consequently, is not a figment of imagination, incapable of being achieved at any stage; it is a reality capable of being obtained through spiritual growth. And the prescription given by Sanskrit Literature on attainment of Excellence in all spheres is unique and is itself excellent.

Human excellence is based on human strength and not human weakness. Swami Vivekananda was a great exponent of this view.

ESSENTIAL VALUES FOR HUMAN EXCELLENCE

1. Performance of ones duty without attachment, i.e. without the thought of personal benefit or nepotism

तस्मादसक्तः सततं कार्यं कर्म समाचर ।
असक्तो ह्याचरन् कर्म परमाप्नोति पूरुषः ॥ 3/19 Bhagavad Gita

Therefore, go on efficiently doing your duty without attachment. Doing work without attachment man attains the Supreme, i.e. excellence.

Renunciation of attachment implies renunciation of desire as well; for it is from attachment that desire springs up (II.62). It is, therefore, that renunciation of the desire for fruit has not been separately mentioned.

People who become attached to senses, they cannot achieve excellence. They become slaves of their senses. They should work without having any personal interest.

ध्यायतो विषयान् पुंसः सङ्गस्तेषूपजायते ।
सङ्गात्संजायते कामः कामात्क्रोधोऽभिजायते ॥ 2/62 Bhagavad Gita

The man dwelling on sense objects develops attachment for them; from attachment springs up desire, and from desire (unfulfiled) ensues anger.

Sri Krishna explains Yoga as 'balance of mind' (Chap. II, 48). When an action is motivated by desire, anxiety as to whether the desired result is going to be obtained or not will surely disturb the peace of mind of the doer. Again, when an action is inspired by self-interest, the doer is likely to lose sight of what is right or what is wrong. Even when he has chosen to do the right thing, undue eagerness for obtaining the result is likely to make him swerve from the path of rectitude; whereas a doer, if he is detached towards the result, is saved from all anxiety. There is nothing to divert him from the righteous path. This teaching that we ought to discharge our obligations, social or otherwise, with a sense of responsibility, at the same time banishing from our minds all thought of obtaining personal benefit therefrom and in a spirit dedication to the Lord is what is meant by Karma-Yoga.[6]

By constantly dwelling on objects of enjoyment man develops an intensive form of attachment for them. This awakens in his mind a keen desire to obtain various forms of enjoyment. This is what is meant by attachment giving rise to desire. And when some hindrance appears in the fulfilment of this desire, he develops hatred for the cause of this hindrance, and the hatred is transformed into anger. This is what is meant by desire producing anger. Anger causes stress and poor mental status.

मा वाऽकर्ता भव प्राज्ञ किमकर्तृतयेहिते ।
साध्यं साध्यमुपादेयं तस्मात्स्वस्थो भवानघ ॥7॥

Neither think yourself as actor, because no actor can attempt to do anything. Discharge whatever is your duty, and remain at your ease with having done your part. Yoga Vasistha-Utpatti-Prakarana, Book 3). If you want to secure real happiness, then renounce all. By so renouncing you will secure happiness infinitely greater than what you could have had through your property. You can enjoy more as you will remain stress free.

The essential nature of true penance is not to possess anything. Nothing. Even a single thing will bring back the delusion of property.

Only those who have completely renounced will reach the highest goal of life, Moksha; the others still with the delusion get entangled in the net of Samsara with all the mental problems associated with it.

The object of Gita is to discover a golden mean between the two ideals of action and of contemplation, preserving the merits of both. Karma-yoga is that golden mean in which the merits of both the ideals are happily integrated. It advocates a life of activity with detachment as the guiding spirit and one's spiritual unfoldment as the goal of one's activities. Thus, it discards neither ideal but integrating the spirit of renunciation of the one and the activism of the other, it purifies and elevates man. This fusion of the two ideals in Karma-yoga gives due regard to social welfare on the one hand and the other leads an individual to the fulfilment of his spiritual aspirations. Thus, the Gita ignores neither the society nor the individual. It does not advocate a life of inaction but instead recommends a life of intense action in which self is effaced in all its aspects.[7] (*Ibid.*, pp. 25-26)

The first verse of the Isa Upanishad says:

All the changing things and events of this world have to be covered with Isa (God—the Supreme Reality). Live your life in a spirit of non-attachment. Don't crave for possessions which are not yours.[8]

The Chandogya Upanishad, for example, prescribes:

All this is Brahman. Mediate calmly on Him as the One from whom everything is born, by whom everything is maintained and annihilated.[9] Such feelings would develop integrated personalities free from all modern ailments—anxiety, fear, tension, stress, etc.

2. Dedication towards one's work and doing it honestly

मयि सर्वाणि कर्माणि संन्यस्याध्यात्मचेतसा ।
निराशीर्निर्ममो भूत्वा युध्यस्व विगतज्वरः ॥ 3/30 Bhagavad Gita

Therefore, so long as while performing actions or enjoying their fruit a participant is found to have the feeling of possession and desire with regard to those actions and their fruit, or so long as his mind is subject to morbid feelings such as attraction and repulsion, joy and grief, etc., it should be clearly understood that all his actions have not been dedicated to god.

Pt. Jawaharlal Nehru, while addressing the Fourth Annual General Body Meeting of the Indian Institute of Public Administration, appropriately remarked that:

"In a period of dynamic growth, however, we want as civil servants—persons who are not, if I may use the word without any disrespect, merely head clerks but people with minds, people with vision, people with desire to achieve, who have some initiative for doing a job and who can think how to do it. But, the person who is to be completely neutral is a head clerk and no more. He would do his work efficiently as a head clerk, no doubt but nothing more. Can a person be neutral, I ask you, about basic things which we stand for, our state stands for, our plan stands for e.g. a socialist pattern of society."[10]

N. Rajagopalan in his article, "Political Neutrality of the Public Service: A Perspective Study", in the *Indian Journal of Public Administration* (January-March, 1977) has rightly said:

"As a human being no public servant can be psychologically neutral on issues and problems which confront him. No public servant can possibly take neutral position between action and inaction. A commitment to the goals and objectives of the state is inescapable, neutrality cannot be allowed to degenerate into unconcern, political sterilization, ought not become political desensitization. There is a crying need, more than ever before, for developing sense of responsiveness and positive concern in the public administrators to the goals and programmes of the state in democratic governments, if public administration is to deliver the goods and take its rightful place in the international polity."

Swami Jagadatmananda in his book, "Learn to Live", Vol. 2, talks about honesty which is the most essential ingredient of excellence. He says that: Honesty is another essential quality like patience. Honesty is a great force. Honesty means integration of the three aspects of personality, thought, speech and deed. For instance, when you give a promise to the workers, honesty demands that you act accordingly or at least make a sincere attempt to act according to the promise. Otherwise, it is dishonesty or deceit. A victim of deception does not easily forget the humiliation or shock that he has left. It explodes one day or the other, in some form or the other. It doesn't explode, it remains simmering within. Honesty can win the hearts of men. Though one may not be able to fulfil one's promise or keep one's word, if the effort is sincere, it has its value, it will earn respect, it will have a good effect.

The public officials should dedicate their whole energy upon the task on which they are engaged to optimise the results. This would be beneficial as both public officials and citizens can lead a life of harmony and not conflict.

3. Acquire complete knowledge about the work in which one is engaged

तद्विद्धि प्रणिपातेन परिप्रश्नेन सेवया ।
उपदेक्ष्यन्ति ते ज्ञानं ज्ञानिनस्तत्त्वदर्शिनः ॥ 4/34 Bhagavad Gita

Understand the true nature of that Knowledge by approaching illumined soul. If you prostrate at their feet, render them service, and question them with an open and guileless heart, those wise seers of Truth will instruct you in that Knowledge.

For the attainment of Knowledge, faith, reverence and guilelessness of heart are of primary importance. The intention is to make it clear that spiritual instruction given to a man devoid of faith and reverence cannot be properly received and retained by him. Illumined souls need no prostrations, personal services, respect and homage for themselves. But they do not feel inclined to discuss the higher truths when someone asks them impertinent questions with a heart full of pride and mischief and with a view to testing their knowledge. Therefore, he who desires to attain Knowledge should in the first instance approach the preceptor with faith and reverence in his heart, and surrendering himself to serve him to the best of his ability.

The object of true knowledge is the integral Brahma or God, who is Truth, Consciousness and Bliss solidified for it is He who is realized through such knowledge. Constantly visualizing that transcendent. Reality as equally present everywhere is what is meant by "seeing that object of true knowledge."

The opposites of virtues, viz., lust for honour and glory, hypocrisy, violence, anger, duplicity, crookedness, malice, impurity, fickleness, covetousness, attachment, egotism, the sense of mineness, differentiation, impiety, association with civil man and other such evil propensities are conducive to the growth of ignorance, which is the cause of birth and death and degrade the soul. Hence they are the same as ignorance and as such should be totally abandoned.

True, that spiritual illumination shines of itself in a pure heart, and, as such, it is not something acquired from without; but to attain this purity of heart means long struggle and constant practice. It has also been found, on careful enquiry in the sphere of material knowledge, that those higher truths which have now and then been discovered by great scientific men, have flashed like sudden floods of light in their mental atmosphere, which they had only to catch and formulate. But such truths never appear in the mind of an uncultured and wild savage. All these go to prove that hard Tapasya, or practice of austerities, in the shape of devout contemplation and constant study of a subject, is at the root of all illumination, in its respective spheres.[11]

Knowledge is powerful and without this public official cannot discharge their duties. In this context, it may be of interest to note that without the expert trainers and desirous trainees, there can be no knowledge. Knowledge depends both on the teacher and taught.

Men should act according to buddhi or understanding. If we are victims of our impulses, our life is as aimless and devoid of intelligence as that of the animals. If we do not interfere, attachments and aversions will determine our acts. So long as we act in certain ways because we like them and abstain from others because we dislike them, we will be bound by our actions. But if we overcome these impulses and act from a sense of duty, we are not victims of the play of prakrti. The exercise of human freedom is conditioned and not cancelled by the necessities of nature.[12]

न हि ज्ञानेन सदृशं पवित्रमिह विद्यते ।
तत्स्यवं योगसंसिद्धः कालेनात्मनि विन्दति ।। 4/38 Bhagavad Gita

There is no purifier as great as Knowledge, he who has attained purity of heart through a prolonged practice of Karmayoga automatically sees the light to Truth in the self in course of time.

There is nothing that can replace the special intelligence that a worker has about the workplace. No matter how smart a boss is or how great a leader, he/she will fail miserably in tapping the potential of employees by working against employees instead of with them

—*Ronald Cantino*, former Deputy Commissioner, New York City Sanitation Department

Swami Jagadatmananda in his book, "Learn to Live", Vol. 2 talks about honesty which is the most essential ingradient of excellence. He says that:

Honesty is another essential quality like patience. Honesty is a great force. Honesty means integration of the three aspects of personality, thought, speech and deed. For instance, when you give a promise to the workers, honesty demands that you act accordingly or at least make a sincere attempt to act according to the promise. Otherwise, it is dishonesty or deceit. A victim of deception does not easily forget the humiliation or shock that he has felt. It explodes one day or the other, in some form or the other. If it doesn't explode it remains simmering within. Honesty can win the hearts of men. Though one may not be able to fulfil one's promise or keep one's word, if the effort is sincere, it has its value, it will earn respect, it will have a good effect.[12]

4. Action Oriented

Mere accumulation of knowledge would be of no use unless put to action. Words written or spoken are of no use unless put to action.

सन्यासः कर्मयोगश्च निःश्रेयसकरावुभौ ।
तयोस्तु कर्मसंन्यासात्कर्मयोगो विशिष्यते ।। 5/2 Bhagavad Gita

The Yoga of Knowledge and the Yoga of Action both lead to supreme Bliss. Of the two, however, the Yoga of Action (being easier of practice) is superior to the Yoga of Knowledge.

What I've noticed about bureaucratic programmes is that for all their rules and red tape, they keep very little track of what actually happens to the people they're serving. If that's built in from the beginning—if you keep track of the results—you can dispense with a lot of red tape.

—*Tom Fulton*, President of the Minneapolis/
St. Paul Family Housing Fund

We may follow Gandhiji's ideals, the key to making Gandhi's vision a reality and practicing his values is to persistently subvert selfish worldly pursuits with ethical livelihood. This is the immediate struggle every Indian on an individual and collective basis, has to non-violently and passionately wage. Will the political leadership, policy-makers and administrators listen to this call and put things back on the right track? If they realize and do, it is good. The sooner the better.

A person who possesses all other powers but is wanting in the power of action will not be appreciated as a desirable person by the world at large.

Shri Radha Krishnan says that there is more happiness in doing one's own work even without excellence than in doing another's duty well. Each one must try to understand his psycho physical make-up and function in accordance with it. It may not be given to all of us to lay the foundations of systems of metaphysics or clothe lofty thoughts in enduring words. We have not all the same gifts, but what is vital is not whether we are endowed with five talents or only one but how faithfully we have employed the trust committed to us. We must play our part, manfully, be it great or small. Goodness denotes perfection of quality. However distasteful one's duty may be, one must be faithful to it even unto death.[13]

Whatever result a persons intends to achieve he may succeed in realising it according to his idea provided he pursues his end with a steadfastness of will.

In executing an action that is clearly discerned to be the right one, the adequate course must be pursued with the steadfast will without hesitation or procrastination.

Swami Jagadatmananda in his book, "Learn to Live", Vol. I rightly says:

Instability and indecision mark the state of mind which is not subject to any discipline. The energies of an undisciplined mind are scattered in many directions and are wasted. A person with an unsteady mind can not achieve any thing worth while. By doing all work, big or small, with concentration and methodically, one gathers the ability to work with efficiency and ease.[14]

5. Control over senses to avoid any temptation to do wrong actions

योगयुक्तो विशुद्धात्मा विजितात्मा जितेन्द्रियः ।
सर्वभूतात्मभूतात्मा कुर्वन्नपि न लिप्यते ॥ 5/7 Bhagavad Gita

The Karmayogi, who has fully conquered his mind and mastered his senses, whose heart is pure, and who has identified himself with the Self of all beings, remains untainted, even though performing action.

So long as one's mind and senses are not controlled, they naturally run after sense enjoyments; and so long as impurities in the form of likes and dislikes exist in the mind it is difficult to remain equipoised in success and failure. Hence, until the mind and senses are fully controlled and perfect purity of heart is attained a practicant, cannot be called a real Karmayogi.

प्राज्ञे यथार्थभूतेयं वस्तुदृष्टिः प्रसीदति ।
दृगिवेन्दौ निरम्भोदे सकलामलमण्डले ॥

Yoga Vasistha Mumuksu Prakarana, Book 2, Sloka 71.

The true light of things dawns only in the minds of the wise, as the gentle moon appears to sight only in the clear and cloudless sky.

पूर्वापरविचारार्थचारुचातुर्यशालिनी ।
सविकासा मतिर्यस्य स पुमानिह कथ्यते ॥

Yoga Vasistha Mumuksu Prakarama, Book 2, Sloka 72.

He is truly called a man who can judge (the truth) by the major and minor proposition, whose mind is expanded and fraught with brilliant ingenuity.

"Some say knowledge is power,
others say, the above is not true.
Character is power and wealth." —*Satya Sai Baba*

6. Loyalty and Integrity

Loyal devotion, knowledge of the things necessary for the State, clear decision to promote them and absence of greed, he who has these four gifts must be implicitly trusted by the king.

When a man's special aptitude for a particular work is known then let him be entrusted with the execution of this work on his own personal responsibility.

Thomas Donaldson (Ethics in Business: A New Look) observes that "There is a growing realization all over the world that ethics is vitally important for any business and for the progress of any society. Ethics makes for an efficient economy; ethics alone, not government or laws, can protect society; ethics is good in itself; ethics and profits go together in the long-run. An ethically responsible company is one which has developed a culture of caring for people and for the environment; a culture which flows downwards from the top managers and leaders."

7. No temptation to take credit for action/results

Public officials should not be tempted to personify them for results to come into lime-light. This would add to the impurities in mind to make him proud.

युक्तः कर्मफलं त्यक्त्वा शान्तिमाप्नोति नैष्ठिकीम् ।
अयुक्तः कामकारेण फले सक्तो निबध्यते ॥ 5/12 Bhagavad Gita

Offering the fruit of action to God, the Karmayogi attains everlasting peace in the shape of God-Realization; whereas he who works with a selfish motive, being attached to the fruit of actions through desire, gets tied down.

सन्तुष्टिपरतृप्तस्थ महतः पूर्णचेतसः ।
क्षीराब्धेरिव शुद्धस्य मुखे लक्ष्मीर्विराजते ॥
Yoga Vasistha Mumuksu Prakarana, Book 2, Saloka 13.

There is a beauty shining in the face of one, whose mind has the satisfaction of contentment, the fullness of magnanimity and the purity of thoughts likes that of the milky ocean in it.

8. Avoidance of lust and anger

Everybody in the world seeks happiness. But very few know what is real happiness and how to attain it. Due to this ignorance they run away with the wrong idea that happiness consists only in enjoying the objects of senses. That is why they hanker after them and strive to attain them. And when they find themselves balked in their efforts, they are seized with anger. But as a rule one who is habitually under the sway of lust and anger can never be happy. One who is under the sway of anger, both be take themselves to all sorts of mischief's and vice—the former for the sake of a wife, progeny, wealth and honour, etc. and the latter with a view to harming others. They thereby expose themselves to illness, grief, ignominy, infamy, perturbation, unrest, anxiety and various kinds of agonies in this world.

He alone is a real 'Nara' or man, who having thus subdued his evil propensities like lust and anger and developed dispassion and quietism attains God, the embodiment of Truth, Knowledge and Bliss. The word 'Narah' signifies such a person, no matter to which sex he belongs.

शक्नोतीहैव यः सोढुं प्राक् शरीरविमोक्षणात् ।
कामक्रोधोद्भवं वेगं स युक्तः स सुखी नरः ॥ 5/23 Bhagavad Gita

He alone who is able to stand in this very life the urges of lust and anger is a yogi and he alone is a happy man.

He who lives a holy life with his gentle and peaceful conduct, is said to be truly living in this world and no other.

समयाशमशालिन्या वृत्या यः साधु वर्तते ।
अभिनन्दितया लोके जीवतीह स नेतरः ।।

Yoga Vasistha Mumuksu Prakarana, Sloka 70.

We have to remember one thing today. The maladies, difficulties and distress which mankind is facing throughout the world, are spiritual in nature. That is why medical science has almost failed; that is why psychology has almost failed; that is why technological wealth and prosperity have almost failed. That is why most civilized, organized disciplines and political orders have almost failed, because the malady that man is suffering from today is spiritual. It is related to the quality of his mind; it is related to the quality of his soul; it is related to the quality of his philosophy.

9. Love and affection for people to achieve peace

Administration is manned by and meant for people. We must attend their problems with love and affection which would in return give strength and bliss.

Happiness on earth and bliss above are certainly the fruits of living the life of love. The changeless abode of the soul is reached by the path of love. Those that are devoid of love are just the skeleton covered with skin.

The journey of this world is delightful to one, who after the removal of his errors and dispersion of the cloud of his ignorance, has come to the knowledge of truth.

परिक्षीणे मोहे विगलतिधने ज्ञानजलदे परिज्ञाते तत्वे समधिगतात्मन्यतितते ।
विचारर्यायैः सार्द्ध चलितवपुषै वै सदृशतो घिया दृष्टे तत्त्वे रमणमटनं जागतमिदम् ।।

Yoga Vasistha, Mumuksu Prakarana, Book 2, Sloka, 20.

In Isavasya Upanishad, Sloka 6 it has been advised that the wise man who perceives all beings as not distinct from his own self at all and his own self as the self of everything he does not by virtue of that perception hate anyone love and emotions are a great strength and source of tremendous power. Swami Vivekananda has beautifully put: "If there is a conflict between the intellect and the heart, always follow heart" the above mentioned teaching has to be perfected through constant use to achieve excellence. To quote Swamiji again, "the various feelings in the human heart are not wrong in themselves; only they have to be carefully controlled and given a higher direction, until they attain the very highest condition of excellence.[15]

Swami Harshananda in his Article, "Attainment of Yoga: Maladies and Remedies" suggest the method of attainment of peace based on Patanjali: To quote him:[16]

Knowingly or unknowingly, all of us are struggling to get peace. As long as our mind is in pieces and the pieces are in ceaseless mutual conflict, peace eludes us. It is only when we learn to put these pieces together so as to make the mind whole and integrated that we gain the peace of Kaivalya.

This is easier said than done. However, with competent guides like Patanjali who are ever eager to help out of infinite compassion, this task should not be that difficult.

Patanjali, the great master of the Yoga system, calls these pieces of the mind as vrttis, modifications, which are ever arising and never subsiding. Yoga or union (yuj=to yoke) of the individual self with the Supreme Self will result through Yoga or Samadhi (yuj=to get samadhi or perfect concentration) when these Vrttis are controlled, suppressed and eliminated, by the right kind of discipline and training. This discipline and training is also Yoga.

10. Selfless Service

The great secret of true success, of true happiness, then, is this; the man who asks for no return, the perfectly unselfish man, is the most successful. It seems to be a paradox. Do we not know that every man who is unselfish in life gets cheated, gets hurt? Apparently, Yes, "Christ was unselfish, and yet he was crucified." True, but we know that his unselfishness is the reason, the cause of a great victory—the crowning of millions upon millions of lives with the blessings of true success.

Swami Harshanand says that Ask nothing; want nothing in return. Give what you have to give; it will come back to you—but do not think of that now. It will come back multiplied a thousand fold—but the attention must not be on that. Yet have the power to give; give, and there it ends.[16]

"Man is born to give not to grab" grabber pays the penalty in the form of misery"; the giver reaps the reward in the form of joy.

The resources, the bodily effort and the mental disposition becomes multiplied in the man of yajna. Such a man is never in want, always in affluence. His bounteous mind is the real Kamdehnu. Becaue of his frame of mind he is ever in prosperity. This is the plan and purpose of cosmos.

इष्टान् भोगान् हि वो देवा दास्यन्ते यज्ञभाविता: ।
तैर्दत्तानप्रदायैभ्यो यो भुङ्क्ते स्तेन एव स: ।। 3/12 Bhagavad Gita

When the Creator said that fostered by sacrifice, the gods would surely bestow on man all the desired enjoyments unasked, he meant that, for his own part; man should go on scrupulously performing his duty. If man did not fail in the performance of his duty, there could be no doubt that fostered and nourished by his sacrifice, the gods could ever continue to supply him with all the means of leading a happy and contented life; for the gods were bound to perform their part of duty.

The essence of the spirit of service is contained in the following words of Vivekananda: "This is the gist of all worship—to be pure and to do good to others. He who sees Shiva in the poor, in the weak, and in the diseased, really worships Shiva; and if he sees Shiva only in the image, his worship is but preliminary. He who has served and helped one poor man seeing Shiva in him, without thinking of his caste, or creed, or race, or anything, with him Shiva is more pleased than with the man who sees Him only in the temples. He who wants to serve the father must serve the children first. He who wants to serve Shiva must serve His children must serve all creatures in the world first."[17]

11. Self-introspection and self-understanding to make ourselves perfect

We are to take care of ourselves—that much we can do—and give up attending to others; for a time. Let us perfect the means; the end will take care of itself. For the world can be good and pure, only if our lives are good and pure. It is an effect, and we are the means. Therefore, let us purify ourselves. Let us make ourselves perfect.

Besides we should always remember that we have no separate identity. We are made of the same elements as others are.

In sixth chapter of Chandogya Upanishad, a father tells his son Svetaketu with example like the rivers coming from different directions, merge with ocean loosing their identity, i.e. "the individuality has merged into sat" (Chandogya Upanishad, 6.8.1)

The father further advises his son Svetaketu thus:

"Crave to know that from which all these beings take birth by which they live after being born and towards which they move and into which they merge. That is Brahman." (Chandogya Upanishad 3.1.1.)

The same view has been propounded by the Mundaka Upanishad:

"The fifteen constituencies (of the body) go back to their causes and all the senses to their respective deities, the actions and the limited intelligent self (jivatma) become one with the highest imperishable Brahman which is the self of all" (Mundaka Upanishad 3.2.7.)

Man, therefore, according to Vedanta philosophy, is the greatest being that is in the universe, and this world of work the best place in it, because only herein is the greatest and the best chance for him to become perfect. Angles or gods, whatever you may call them, have all to become men, if they want to become perfect. This is the great center, the wonderful poise, and the wonderful opportunity—this human life.

न विचारं विना कश्चिदुपायऽस्ति विपश्चिताम् ।
विचारादशुभं त्यक्त्वा शुभमायाति धीः सताम् ॥

Yoga Vasistha Mumuksu Prakarana, Book 2, Sloka 5.

There is no expedient for the learned and wise except reason; it is by means of reason that the minds of good people can avoid evil and secure their good.

युक्तायुक्त महादीपमभिवांछितसाधकम् ।
स्फारं विचारमाश्रित्य संसारजलधिं तरेत् ।।

Yoga Vasistha Mumuksu Prakarna, Book 2, Sloka 7.

Reason is the lamp to show us the right and wrong, and the instrument for accomplishment of our desires: by reliance on right reason, one crosses over easily the wide ocean of the world.

सन्तुष्टिपरतृप्तस्थ महतः पूर्णचेतसः ।
क्षीराब्धेरिव शुद्धस्य मुखे लक्ष्मीर्विराजते ।।

Yoga Vasistha Mumuksu Prakarana, Book 2, Sloka 13.

There is a beauty shinning in the face of one whose mind has the satisfaction of contentment, the fulness of magnanimity and the purity of thoughts like that of the milky ocean in it.

विचारवता पुरुषेण सकलमिदमाधिपञ्जरं सर्पेण त्वचमिव परिपक्वं संत्यज्य विगतज्वरेणं शीतलान्तःकरणेन । विनोदादिन्द्रजालमिव जगदखिलमालोक्यते सम्यग्दर्शनवता असम्यग्दर्शनवतो हि परं दुःखमिदम् ।। 13 ।।

The reasoning man gets released from his worldly sickness, and quits his frame which is full of diseases, as a snake castes off his time worn slough; and looks with a placid mind and clam composure upon the magic scenes of the world. Hence the fully wise man is not subject to the misery of the imperfectly wise.

विषमो ह्यतितरां संसाररागो भोगीव दशति असिरिव च्छिछिनति कुन्त इव वेधयति रज्जुरिवावेष्टयति पावक इव दहति रात्रिरिवान्धयति अशंकितपरिपतितपुरुषान्पषाण इव विवशीकरोति हरति प्रज्ञां नाशयति स्थिति पातयति मोहान्धकूपे तृष्णा जर्जरीकरोति न तदस्ति किंचिदुःखं संसारि यत्र प्राप्नोति ।। 14 ।।

The rough and uneven pleasure of the world is but a disease to men, and stings them like a snake. It cuts them as a sword, and pierces them as a spear. It binds them fast as by a rope, and burns them as with the fire, and blindfolds, their understanding as in the darkness of the night. It makes them as prostrate and dull as a slab of stone. It destroys one's prudence and lowers his position. It casts them into the pit of error, and torments them with avarice. Thus, there is almost no kind of trouble which does not betide worldly minded men.

दुरन्तेय किल विषयविषूचिका यदि न चिकित्स्यते ।
तन्नितरां नरकनगरनिकरफलानुबन्धिनी तत्तत्करोति ॥ 15 ॥

Worldliness is as dangerous a diseases as cholera, which unless it is healed in time, is sure to trouble its patient with the torments to hell.

The journey of this world is delightful to one, who after the removal of his errors and dispersion of the cloud of his ignorance has come to the knowledge of truth.

12. Independent Thinking

Human beings should develop the quality of independent thinking: God is seemingly indifferent, for he leaves the decision to Arjuna's choice. His apparent indifference is due to His anxiety that each one of us should get to Him of his own free choice. He constrains no one since free spontaneity is valuable. Man is to be wooed and not coerced into co-operation. He is to be drawn, not driven, persuaded, not compelled. The Supreme does not impose His command. We are free at any moment to reject or accept the Divine call. The integral surrender should be made with the fullest consent of the seeker. God does not do the climbing for us, though He is ever ready to help us when we stumble, comfort us when we fall. God is prepared to wait in patience till we turn to Him.

13. Objectivity

Human beings should think objectively and avoid any bias: God is equally present in all beings from Brahma down to the smallest clump of grass as their inner witness. Therefore, He looks upon all with an equal eye, has no partiality for or prejudice against anyone. This is what is meant by the first half of this verse.

14. Speaking as befits the occasion and the context

An excellent person should not speak irrelevant things but should also not resist to put forth his views based on Dharma forcefully, Kautilya has explained this in the following verse.

प्रस्तावसदृशं वाक्यं
स्वभावसदृशं मनः
आत्मशक्तिसमं कोपं
यो जानाति स पण्डितः

15. Good Character

All good character traits have a common denominator of social courage, usefulness, common sense besides self-acceptance and self-confidence. Men of character may not be popular, but they are respected and followed. They are true leaders of men and times. They will fight but not quarrel, differ but will not oppose or criticise, will be firm but not rigid, dogmatic, appreciate without flattery, cooperate without surrendering, self-confident but not self-important, cooperate, compromise and reconcile on non-essentials but put up a valiant, relentless fight for basic principles, act and never react.

Will power and patience are basic to personality development. Both provide fibre and tone to it. Will is the motive power, driving force and patience is the period over which this force works to develop character.

All human endeavors achievements require minimum necessary time to mature and fulfil. Impatience only wastes vital energy, tires, confuses, sickens and impairs our will power. Our personality does not register on others if we are impatient with them who can benefit or be friend you without your giving him time.[18]

CONCLUSION

Human Excellence can do wonders. Swami Vivekananda says that India is no more to be a mere geographical expression. Our ancestors conceived of India as a cultural entity, the Punyabhumi. But Swami Vivekananda advances a step further and breathes life into it by making India, the symbol of the great 'Virat'. The reformers and workers bent on serving India socially, politically, or otherwise, are to be imbued with this grand idealism of the Virat, concretized in India. It is this transformation of vision with regard to our holy land which the Swami teaches as one of the potent means for spiritualizing our national activities.

"For the next fifty years, this alone shall be our keynote—this, our great Mother India. Let all other vain Gods disappear for a time from our minds. This is the only God that is awake, our own race, everywhere His hands, everywhere His feet everywhere His ears, He covers everything. All other Gods are sleeping. What vain Gods we shall go after and yet cannot worship the God that we see all round us, the Virat? When we have worshipped this, we shall be able to worship other Gods."

May we have firm faith in Mother India and in her spiritual culture as well as in the Swami's vision of a future India more glorious than her past !—a vision which inspired him to utter:

"I do not see into the future, nor do I care to see. But one vision I see clear as light before me. That the ancient Mother has awakened once more seating on her throne, rejuvenated, more vigorous than ever. Proclaim her to all the world, with the voice of peace and benediction."

May the appeal to unity as made by the Vedic Rishi find a response in the hearts of all !

"Common be your desires, united be your hearts, united be your intention, so that there be a thorough union among you."

Awake, arise, and stop not till the goal is reached.

'Nowadays, everybody blames those who constantly look back to their past. It is said that so much looking back to the past, is the cause of all India's woe. To me, on the contrary, it seems that the opposite is true.

So long as they forget the past, the Hindu nation remained in a state of stupor; and as soon as they have begun to look into their past, there is on every side a fresh manifestation of life'.[19]

Life is a rugged Journey, over hills and plains and dreary deserts. But say not 'die' in struggle of life. Be Brave and cheerful all through the battle. Husband your strength and resources. Be Vibrant in the battle of life. Keep calm in the hour of adversely yogic (M.K. Spencer, How I found God?), p. 324.

Prem Saran in his article, "Right Brain Management: Need of the Hour" in *MIG*, July-September, 2000 defines HRD.

"Human Resource Development has become the key functional area in Public Administration, and in Management generally, since technology *per se* no longer grants sufficient competitive advantages in today's global world of accelerated dissemination of information and knowledge. People as resources are, therefore, to be optimally tapped for organizational excellence, and here again the over emphasized left brain skills of analysis and logical manipulation are being found to be insufficient to meet the transformational needs generated by quickening change."

Excellence is a state of mind which prepares the employees to perform duties with dedication. It also creates self-reliance and helps him/her to have a vision and an urge to do better and better.

HRD approach focuses on the optimum utilization of valuable human resources through tapping their potential energy to vitalize, activate and renew an organization to generate dynamism and development.

The final, ultimate, complete and eternal methodology of rising to the challenges of the future is to take on the form of divine trinity for effective HRD.

Preserve the relevant,
Destroy the irrelevant,
Create what is needed.

This is the eternal magic formula valid for all times to come.

For ordinary men, ethical principles are formulated on the basis of these truths, as Swami Vivekananda has done in formulating his 'Practical Vedanta':

This is the gist of all worship—to be pure and to do good to others. He who sees Siva in the poor, in the weak, and in the diseased, really worships Siva; and if he sees Siva only in the image, his worship is but preliminary. He who has served and helped one poor man seeing Siva in him, without thinking of his caste, or creed, or race, or anything, with him Siva is more pleased than with the man who sees Him only in temples.

The emergence of a Renascent India was as clear as daylight to Swami Vivekananda who has left the following universal religion for posterity:

"Each soul is potentially divine.

"The goal is to manifest the divine within, by controlling nature, external and internal.

"Do this either by work, or worship, or psychic control, or philosophy, by one, or more, or all of these, and be free.

"This is the whole of religion. Doctrines, or dogmas, or rituals, or books, or temples, or forms, are but secondary details."

Human excellence is the only need of the 21st century as all other programmes depend upon him. We should devise ways and means to rejuvenate human excellence which can change the world culture and make this earth worth living a life of quality and excellence.

Dr. S.S. Gupta, has rightly said that our Rishis were social scientists par excellence and their social science included all the disciplines. Dr. Gupta suggests the following to improve human excellence.[20]

(i) The individual is the central point of the society and also the nation. So there should not be any scope of a conflict between interests of individuals, the society and the nation. There should be complete homogeneity and uniformity among the three. In the western thought this uniformity and homogeneity is missing. In socialist literature conflict is an essential ingredient.

(ii) That life is one whole. It should not be divided into watertight independent segments like social, political, economic, etc. By doing so, an invitation is given to tensions and split of life which will become competitive instead of complimentary.

(iii) That the perfect coherence between individuals, between different segments of life and between individuals and these segments is possible when the guiding principles (or fundamentals of all are same and not different. Today we find different guiding principles of all these segments of life and no competition and conflicts among them. This is leading to growing tensions in individuals and their split personalities.

(iv) That the guiding principles of the entire life, which can promote simultaneously, the happiness of individuals, the whole society and the world, should be natural, scientific and achievable. The Rishis-*cum*-Social Scientists of India gradually developed them and called them human-values of social values such as truth simplicity, self-control, purity, non-stealing, non-anger, The number of these basic principles was not static. It went on changing as per the needs of time and new researches.

(v) That the sum total of these guiding principles will be called Dharma, which is distinct from the rituals of religion. It is unfortunate that today people, specially the politicians and even so called scholars do not understand the meaning of Dharma and confuse it with religion. The ancient Rishis-*cum*-Social Scientists explained the meaning of Dharma. They gave it multi-dimensional meaning. One important meaning was that every thing has a nature, i.e. Dharma. For example, fire has a Dharma (Nature) to burn and air has a Dharma to blow. Similarly, the Dharma of the people of the world should be these basic Human-values. So, by Dharma, they meant a code of conduct. Certainly, this is not Religion.

S. Radhakrishnan in "the Bhagavad Gita" has beautifully explained the path to achieve excellence:[21]

How is the goal of perfection to be attained? Samsara is historical becoming. It is the temporal (Katha Upanisjad, Vol. II, p. 10) procession of changes from one state into the next. What keeps the world going is action of karma. If the world is nothing but ebb and flow, continual becoming, it is due to action. At the human level action is caused by desire or attachment, kama the root cause of desire is avidya or ignorance of the nature of things. The roots of desire lie in the ignorant belief in the individual's self-sufficiency, in the attribution of reality and possible to escape from the vicious circle of becoming. We cannot cure desires by fresh desires; we cannot cure action by more action. The eternal cannot be gained by that which is temporal. Whether we are bound by good desires or bad desires, it is still a question of bondage, it makes a little difference whether the chains which bind us are made of gold or of iron. To escape from bondage we must get rid of ignorance, which is the parent of ignorant desires and so of ignorant actions. Vidya or wisdom is the means of liberation from chain of avidya kama karma.

Wisdom is not to be confused with theoretical learning or correct beliefs, for ignorance is not intellectual error. It is spiritual blindness. To remove it, we must cleanse the soul of its defilement and kindle the spiritual vision. The fire of passion and the tumult of desire must be suppressed (Katha Upanishad, IV.39). The mind, inconstant and unstable, must be steadied so as to reflect the wisdom from above. We must control the senses, possess the faith which no intellectual doubts, disturb and train the understanding (buddhi). (Katha Upnishad, Vol. II, p. 94)

Wisdom is direct experience which occurs as soon as obstacles to its realization are removed. The effort of the seeker is directed to the elimination of the hindrances, to the removal of the obscuring tendencies of a vidya. According to advaita vedanta, this wisdom is always present. It is not a thing to be acquired; it has only to be revealed. Our casual apprehensions, backed by our wishes and prejudices, do not reveal reality. Utter silence of the mind and the will, an emptying of the ego produces illumination, wisdom, the light by which we grow into our true being. This is life eternal, the complete fulfilment of our capacity of love and knowledge, the completely simultaneous and perfect possession of unlimited life at a single moment, to use the words of Boethius.

Jnana and Ajnana, wisdom and ignorance are opposed as light and darkness. When wisdom dawns, ignorance dies and the evil is cut-off at the root. The liberated soul overcomes the world. There is nothing to conquer or create. Action no more binds. When we grow into this wisdom, we live in the Supreme. This consciousness is not an abstract one. It is that by which thou shall see all existences without exception in the self, then in me, the true human individual pursues this ideal of perfection with a devotion similar to that which he offers to an adored woman. (Muktikanta)

Perfection at the human level is a task to be accomplished by conscious endeavor. The image of God operating in us produces a sense of insufficiency. Man has a haunting sense of the vanity, the transience and the precariousness of all human happiness. Those who live on the surface of life may not feel the distress, the laceration of spirit, and may not feel any urge to seek their true good. They are human animals (purusapasu), and like animals they are born, they grow, they mate and leave offspring and pass away. But those who realize their dignity as men are acutely aware of the discord and seek a principle of harmony and peace.

To quote S. Radhakrishnan again:[22] Human nature has immeasurable potentialities and the world process has no predestined goal. The power of free choice gives us hope for the future. We can remake the world. Whatever flaws of character or deficiencies of mind we have we can remove them. If we strive to do so, the forces of the universe will assist us. We can consciously direct the process of human evolution. Nature comes to its fulfilment in the human individual, who is the bearer of the creative process. He is the unique representative of the universe in whom the unconscious creativity of nature becomes conscious creativity. The inner discord means that he can contend with the disruptive forces, conquer them and attain peace.

Indian thought asks us to liberate ourselves from bondage. We must pass from samasara, life in time subjects to discords to moksa or enlightenment or eternal life.

To a person
Who is thoughtless, and
Negligent of Duties,
His enormous wealth
And Property
Will be of no value
THE THIRUKKURAL
O man
Do not be afraid of performing
Your marital duties
With courage and conviction
Fellow the path of Dharma
Endowed with strength,
Honour and Valour
May you obey
Your god assigned duties
And be happy
Yajurveda.

Notes and Reference

1. Walter R. Sharp, Field Administration in the United Nations System, London, 1961, p. 19.
2. Prof. Ramarajan Mukherji, Sanskrit and Human Excellence, in *Souvenir*, ed. (Prof. Vachaspati Upadhyaya, World Sanskrit Confernece, 5-9 April 2001, New Delhi, Shri Lal Bahadur Shastri Rashtriya Sanskrit Vidyapeeth, pp. 14-16.
3. Complete Works of Swami Vivekananda, Vol. III, p. 237.
4. *Ibid.*, Vol. II, p. 3.
5. *Ibid.*, p. 225
6. Swami Vijnananda, Gita on Karma Yoga, in *Yoga: Its Various Aspects*, Sri Ramakrishna Math, Madras; pp. 24-25.
7. *Ibid.*, pp. 25-26.
8. Isha Upanishad 1.1.
9. Chondogya Upanishad, 3.4.1.
10. V. Jaganadham, Jawaharlal Nehru and Public Administration, *IJPA*, New Delhi, 1975.
11. Verinder Grover, Swami Vivekananda, A Biography of his Vision and Ideas, Deep & Deep, New Delhi, 1998, p. 114.
12. Radhakrishnan, The Bhagavad Gita, Harper Collins, New Delhi, 1996, p. 146.
13. *Ibid.*, p. 147.
14. Swami Jagadatmananda, Learn to Live, Vol. I, Chennai, Shri Ramakrishna Math, pp. 106-07.
15. Complete Works of Swami Vivekananda, 1965 (ed.) Vol. II, p. 78.
16. Swami Harshananda, Attainment of Yoga: Maladies and Remedies" in *Yoga: Its Various Aspects*", Shri Ramakrishna Math, Madras, pp. 203-04.
17. Swami Jagadatmananda, Learn to Live, Vol. I, Chennai, Shri Ramakrishna Math, p. 256.
18. Ram Parshad Gupta, Food for Thought, New Delhi, 1996, pp. 18-23.
19. The Complete Works of Swami Vivekananda, Vol. IV, p. 324.
20. S.S. Gupta, *op. cit.*, pp. 159-60.
21. S. Radhakrishnan, Bhagavad Gita, New Delhi, Harper & Collins, 1996, pp. 51-53.
22. S. Radhakrishnan, Recovery of Faith, An Orient Paperback, 1967, pp. 95-96.

APPENDIX 8.1

PROTECTING AND PROMOTING HUMAN HEALTH

Introduction

Health and development are intimately interconnected. Both insufficient development leading to poverty and inappropriate development resulting in over-consumption, coupled with an expanding world population, can result in severe environmental health problems in both developing and developed nations. Action items under Agenda 21 must address the primary health needs of the world's population since they are integral to the achievement of the goals of sustainable development and primary environmental care. The linkage of health, environmental and socio-economic improvements requires inter-sectoral efforts. Such efforts, involving education, housing, public works and community groups, including business, schools and universities and religious, civic and cultural organization, are aid at enabling people in their communities to ensure sustainable development. Particularly relevant is the inclusion of prevention programmes rather than relying solely on remediation and treatment. Countries ought 10 develop plans for priority actions, drawing on the programme areas in this chapter, which are based on cooperative planning by the various levels of government, non-governmental organizations and local communities. An appropriate international organisational organization, such as WHO, should coordinate these activities.

The following programme areas are contained in this chapter:

(a) Meeting primary healthcare needs, particularly in rural areas;
(b) Control of communicable diseases;
(c) Protecting vulnerable groups;
(d) Meeting the urban health challenge; and
(e) Reducing health risks from environmental pollution and hazards.

PROGRAMME AREAS

A. MEETING PRIMARY HEALTHCARE NEEDS, PARTICULARLY IN RURAL AREAS

Health ultimately depends on the ability to manage successfully the interaction between the physical, spiritual, biological and economic/social environment. Sound development is not possible without in healthy population; yet most developmental activities affect the environment to some degree which in turn causes or exacerbates many health problems. Conversely, it is the very lack of development that adversely affects the health conditions of any people, which can be alleviated only through health sector cannot meet basic needs and objective on its own; it is dependent and sustainable water policies to ensure safe drinking water and sanitation to preclude both microbial and chemical contamination; and promotion of health education, immunization and provision of essential drugs. Education and appropriate services regarding resource planning of family size, with respect for cultural, religious and social aspects, in keeping with freedom, dignity and personally held values and talking into account ethical and cultural considerations, also contribute to these intersectoral activities.

Objectives

Within the overdue strategy to achieve health for all by the year 2000, the objectives are to meet the basic health needs of rural peri-urban and urban populations; to provide the necessary specialized environmental health services; and to coordinate the involvement of citizens, the health sector, the health-related sectors and relevant non-health sectors (business, social, educational and religious institutions) in solutions to health problems. As a matter of priority, health service coverage should be achieved for population groups in greatest need, particularly those living in rural areas.

Activities

National government and local authorities, with the support of relevant non-governmental organizations and international organizations, in the light of countries specific conditions and needs, should strengthen their health sector programmes, with special attention to rural needs to:

(a) Build basic health infra-structures, monitoring and planning systems

(i) Develop and strengthen primary healthcare systems that are practical, community-based, scientifically sound, socially acceptable and appropriate to their needs and that meet basic health need for clean water, safe food and sanitation;

(ii) Support the use and strengthening of mechanisms that improve coordination between health and related sectors at all appropriate levels of government, and in communities and relevant organizations;

(iii) Develop and implement rational affordable approaches to the establishment and maintenance of health facilities;

(iv) Ensure and, where appropriate, increase provision of social services support;

(v) Develop strategies, including reliable health indicators, to monitor the progress and evaluate the effectiveness of health programmes;

(vi) Explore ways to finance the health system based on the assessment of the resources needed and identify the various financing alternatives;

(vii) Promote health education in schools, information exchange, technical support and training;

(viii) Support initiatives for self-management of services by vulnerable groups;

(ix) Integrate traditional knowledge and experience into national health systems, as appropriate;

(x) Promote the provisions for necessary logistics for outreach activities, particularly in rural areas; and

(xi) Promote and strengthen community-based rehabilitation activities for the rural handicapped.

(b) Support research and methodology development

(i) Establish mechanisms for sustained community involvement in environmental health activities, including optimization of the appropriate use of community financial and human resources;

(ii) Conduct environmental health research, including behaviour research and research on ways to increase coverage and ensure greater utilization of services by peripheral, underserved and vulnerable populations, as appropriate to good prevention services and healthcare; and

(iii) Conduct research into traditional knowledge of prevention and curative health practices.

Means of implementation

(a) Financing and cost evaluation

The Conference secretariat has estimated the average total annual cost (1993-2000) of implementing the activities of this programme to be about $40 billion, including about $5 billion from the international community on grunt or concessional terms. These are indicative and order of magnitude estimates only and have not been reviewed by Governments. Actual costs and financial terms, including any that are non-concessional, will depend upon, *inter alia,* the specific strategies and programmes Governments decide upon for implementation.

(b) Scientific and technological means

New approaches to planning and managing healthcare systems and facilities should be tested, and research on ways of integrating appropriate technologies into health infrastructures supported. The development of scientifically sound health technology resources, including the maintenance and repair of equipment used in healthcare. Programmes to facilitate the transfer and sharing of information and expense should be developed, including communication methods and educational materials.

(c) Human resources development

Intersectoral approaches to the reform of health personnel development should be strengthened ensure its relevance to the "Health for All" strategies. Efforts to enhance managerial skills at the district level should be supported, with the aim of ensuring the systematic development and efficient operation of the basic health system. Intensive, short, practical training programmes with emphasis on skills in effective communication, community organization and facilitation of behaviour change should be developed in order to prepare the local personnel of all sectors involved in social development for carrying out their respective roles. In cooperation with the education sector, special health education programmes should be developed focusing on the role of women in the health-care system,

(d) Capacity-building

Government should consider adopting enabling and facilitating strategies to promote the participation of communities in meeting their own needs, in addition to providing direct support to the provision of healthcare services. A major focus should be the preparation of community-based health and health-related workers to assume an active role in community health education, with emphasis on team work. Social mobilization and the support of other development workers, National programmes should cover disctrict health systems in urban, peri-urban and rural areas, the delivery of health programmes at the district level, and development and support of referral services.

B. CONTROL OF COMMUNICABLE DISEASES

Basic for Action

Advances in the development of vaccines and chemotherapeutic agents have brought many communicable diseases under control. However, there remain many important communicable diseases for which environmental control measures are indispensable, especially in the field of water supply and sanitation. Such diseases include cholera, diarrhoeal diseases, leishmaniasis, malaria and schistosomiasis. In all such instances, the environmental measures, either as an integral part of primary healthcare or undertaken outside the health sector, form an indispensable component of overall disease control strategies, together with health and hygiene education, and in some cases, are the only component.

With HIV infection levels estimated to increase to 30-40 million by the year 2000, the socio-economic impact of the pandemic is expected to be devastating for all countries, and increasingly for women and children. While direct health costs will be substantial, they will be dwarfed by the indirect costs of the pandemic—mainly costs associated with the loss of income and decreased productivity of the workforce. The pandemic will inhibit growth of the service and industrial sectors and significantly increase the costs of human capacity-building and retraining. The agricultural sector is particularly affected where production is labour-intensive.

Objective

A number of goals have been formulated through extensive consultations in various international forums attended by virtually all Governments, relevant United Nations, organizations including WHO, UNICEF, UNFPA, UNESCO, UNDP and the World Bank and a number of non-governmental organizations. Goals (including but not limited to those listed below) are recommended for implementation by all countries where they are applicable, with appropriate adaptation to the specific situation of each country in terms of phasing, standards, priorities and availability of resources, with respect for cultural, religious and social aspects, in keeping with freedom, dignity and personally held values and taking into account ethical considerations. Additional goals that are particularly relevant to a country's specific situation should be added in the country's national plan of action (Plan of Action for Implementing the World Declaration on the Survival, Protection and Development of Children in the 1990s). Such national level action plans should be coordinated and monitored from within the public health sector. Some major goals are:

(a) By the year 2000 to eliminate guinea worm disease (dracunculiasis);
(b) By the year 2000 to eradicate polio;
(c) By the year 2000 to effectively control onchocerciasis (river blindness) and leprosy;
(d) By 1995 to reduce measles deaths by 95 per cent and reduce measles cases by 90 per cent compared with pre-immunization levels;
(e) By continued efforts, to provide health and hygiene education and to ensure universal access to safe drinking water and universal access to sanitary measures of excreta disposal, thereby markedly reducing waterborne diseases such as cholera and schistosomiasis and reducing:
    (i) By the year 2000, the number of deaths from childhood diarrhoea developing countries by 50 to 70 per cent; and
    (ii) By the year 2000, the incidence of childhood diarrhoea in developing countries by at least 25 to 50 per cent;
(f) By the year 2000, to initiate comprehensive programmes to reduce mortality from acute respiratory infections in children under five years by at least one-third, particularly in countries with high infant morality;
(g) By the year 2000, to provide 95 per cent of the world's child population with access to appropriate care for acute respiratory infections within the community and at first referral level;
(h) By the year 2000, to institute anti-malaria programmes in all

countries where malaria presents significant health problem and maintain the transmission-free status of areas freed from endemic malaria;

(i) By the year 2000, to implement control programmes in countries where major human parasitic infections are endemic and achieve an overall reduction in the prevalence of schistosomiasis and of other trematode infections by 40 per cent and 25 per cent, respectively, from a 1984 baseline as well as a marked reduction in incidence, prevalence and intensity of filarial infections;

(j) To mobilize and unify national and international efforts against AIDS to prevent infection and to reduce the personal and social impact of HIV infection;

(k) To contain the resurgence of tuberculosis, with particular emphasis on multiple antibiotic resistant forms; and

(1) To accelerate research on improved vaccines and implement to the fullest extent possible the use of vaccines in the prevention of disease.

Each national Government in accordance with national plans for public health. Priorities and Objectives, should consider developing a national health action plan with appropriate international assistance and support including at a minimum, the following components:

(a) National public health systems

(i) Programmes to identify environmental hazards in the causation of communicable diseases;

(ii) Monitoring systems of epidemiological data to ensure adequate forecasting of the introduction, spread or aggravation of communicable diseases;

(iii) Intervention programmes, including measures consistent with the principles of the global AIDS strategy; and

(iv) Vaccines for the prevention of communicable diseases.

(b) Public information and health education

Provide education and disseminate information on the risks of endemic communicable diseases and build awareness on environmental methods for control of communicable diseases to enable communities to playa role in the control of communicable diseases.

(c) Intersectoral cooperation and coordination

(i) Second experienced health professionals to relevant sectors, such as planning, housing and agriculture; and

(ii) Develop guidelines for effective coordination in the areas of professional training, assessment of risks and development of control technology.

(d) Control of environmental factors that influence the spread of communicable diseases

Apply methods for the prevention and control of communicable diseases, including water supply and sanitation control, water pollution control, food quality control. integrated vector control, garbage collection and disposal and environmentally sound irrigation practices.

(e) Primary healthcare system

(i) Strengthen prevention programmes, with particular emphasis on adequate and balanced nutrition;
(ii) Strengthen early diagnostic programmes and improve capacities programme and improve capacities for early preventative/ treatment action; and
(iii) Reduce the vulnerability to HIV infection of women and their offspring.

(f) Support for research and methodology development

(i) Intensify and expand multidisciplinary research, including focused efforts on the mitigation and environment control of tropical diseases;
(ii) Carry out intervention studies to provide a solid epidemiological basis for control policies and to evaluate the efficiency of alternative approaches; and
(iii) Undertake studies in the population and among health workers to determine the influence of cultural, behavioural and social factors on control policies.

(g) Development and dissemination of technology

(i) Develop new technologies for the effective control of communicable diseases;
(ii) Promote studies to determine how to optimally disseminate results from research; and
(iii) Ensure technical assistance, including the sharing of knowledge and know-how.

Means of Implementation

(a) Financing and cost evaluation

The Conference secretariat has estimated the average total annual cost (1993-2(8) of implementing the activities of this programme to be about

$4 billion, including about $900 million from the international community on grant or concessional terms. These are indicative and order of magnitude estimates only and have not been reviewed by Governments. Actual costs and financial terms, including any that are non-concessional, will depend upon, *inter alia,* the specific strategies and programmes Governments decide upon for implementation.

(b) Scientific and technological means

Efforts to prevent control diseases should include investigations of the epidemiological, social and economic bases for the development of more effective national strategies for the integrated control of communicable diseases. Cost effective methods of environmental control should be adapted to local development conditions.

(c) Human resources development

National and regional training institutions should promote broad intersectoral approaches to prevention and control of communicable diseases including training in epidemiology and community prevention and control, immunology, molecular biology and the application of new vaccines. Health education materials should be developed for use by community workers and for the education of mothers for the prevention and treatment of diarrhoeal diseases in the home.

(d) Capacity-building

The health sector should develop adequate data on the distribution of communicable diseases, as well as the institutional capacity to respond and collaborate with other sectors for prevention, mitigation and correction of communicable disease hazards through environmental protection. The advocacy at policy and decision-making levels should be gained, professional and social support mobilized, and communities organized in developing self-reliance.

C. PROTECTING VULNERABLE GROUPS

Basis for Action

In addition to meeting health needs, specific emphasis has to be given to protecting and educating vulnerable groups, particularly infants, youth, women, indigenous people and the very poor as a prerequisite for sustainable development. Special attention should also be paid to the health needs of the elderly and disabled population.

Infants and children

Approximately one-third of the world's population are children under 15 years old. At least 15 million of these children die annually from such preventable causes as birth trauma, birth asphyxia, acute respiratory infections, malnutrition, communicable diseases and diarrhoea. The health of children is affected more severely than other population groups by malnutrition and adverse environmental factors, and many children risk exploitation as cheap labour or in prostitution.

Youth

As has been the historical experience of all countries, youth are particularly vulnerable to the problems associated with economic development, which often weakens traditional forms of social support essential for the healthy development of young people. Urbanization and changes in social mores have increased substance abuse, unwanted pregnancy and sexually transmitted diseases, including AIDS. Currently more than half of all people alive are under the age of 25 and 4 of every 5 live in developing countries. Therefore, it is important to ensure that historical experience is not replicated.

Women

In developing countries, the health status of women remains relatively low, and during the 1990s poverty, malnutrition and general ill-health in women were even rising. Most women in developing countries still do not have adequate basic educational opportunities and they lack the means of promoting their health, responsibly controlling their reproductive life and improving their socio-economic status. Particular attention should be given to the provision of pre-natal care to ensure healthy babies.

Indigenous people and their communities

Indigenous people had their communities make up a significant percentage of global population. The outcomes of their experience have tended to be very similar in that the basis of their relationship with traditional lands has been fundamentally changed. They tend to feature disproportionately in unemployment, lack of housing, poverty and poor health. In many countries the number of indigenous people is growing faster than the general population. Therefore, it is important to target health initiatives for indigenous people.

Objectives

The general objectives of protecting vulnerable groups are to ensure that all such individuals should be allowed to develop to their full potential (including healthy physical, mental and spiritual development); to ensure that young people can develop, establish and maintain healthy lives; to allow women to perform their key role in society; and to support indigenous people through educational, economic and technical opportunities.

Specific major goals for child survival, development and protection were agreed upon at. The World Summit for children and remain valid also for Agenda 21. Supporting and sectoral goals cover women's health and education, nutrition, child health, water and sanitation, basic education and children in difficult circumstances.

Government should take active steps to implement, as a matter of urgency, in accordance with country specific conditions and legal systems, measures to ensure that women and men have the same right to decide freely and responsibly on the number and spacing of their children, to have, access to the information, education and means, as appropriate, to enable them to exercise this right in keeping with their freedom, dignity and personally held values, taking into account ethical and cultural considerations.

Governments should take active steps to implement programmes to establish and strengthen preventive and curative health facilities which include women-centred, women managed, safe and effective reproductive healthcare and affordable, accessible services, as appropriate, for the responsible planning of family size, in keeping with freedom, dignity and personally held values and taking into account ethical and cultural considerations. Programmes should focus on providing comprehensive healthcare, including pre-natal care, education and information on health and responsible parenthood and should provide the opportunity for all women to breast-feed fully, at least during the first four months post-panum. Programmes should fully support women's productive and reproductive roles and well-being, with special attention to the need for providing equal and improved healthcare for all children and the need to reduce the risk of maternal and child morality and sickness.

Activities

National Government, in cooperation with local and non-governmental organizations, should initiate or enhance programmes in the following areas:

(a) Infants and children

(i) Strengthen basic healthcare-services for children in the context of primary healthcare delivery, including prenatal care, breast-feeding, immunization and nutrition programmes;

(ii) Undertake widespread adult education on the use of oral rehydration therapy for diarrhoea, treatment of respiratory infections and prevention of communicable diseases;

(iii) Promote the creation, amendment and enforcement of a legal framework protecting children from sexual and workplace exploitation; and

(iv) Protect children from the effects of environmental and occupational toxic compounds.

(b) Youth

Strengthen services for youth in health, education and social sectors in order to provide better information, education, counselling and treatment for specific health problems, including drug abuse.

(c) Women

(i) Involve women's groups in decision-making at the national and community levels to identify health risks and incorporate health issues in national action programmes on women and development;
(ii) Provide concrete incentives to encourage and maintain attendance of women of all ages at school and adult education courses, including health education and training in primary, home and maternal healthcare; and
(iii) Carry out baseline surveys and knowledge, attitude and practice studies on the health and nutrition of women throughout their life cycle, especially as related to the impact of environmental degradation and adequate resources;

(d) Indigenous people and their communities

(i) Strengthen, through resources and self-management, preventative and curative health services; and
(ii) Integrate traditional knowledge and experience into health systems.

Means of Implementation

(a) Financial and cost evaluation

The Conference Secetariate has estimated the average total annual cost (1993-2000) of implementing the activities of this programmes to be about $3.7 billion, including about $400 million from the international community on grant or concessional terms. These are indicative and order of magnitude estimates only and have not been reviewed by Governments. Actual costs and financial terms, including any that are non-concessional, will depend upon, *inter alia,* specific strategies and programmes Government decide upon for implementation.

(b) Scientific and technological means

Educational, health and research institution should be strengthened to provide support to improve the health of vulnerable groups. Social research on the specific problems of these groups should be expanded and methods for implementing flexible pragmatic solutions explored, with emphasis on preventive measures. Technical support should be provided to Governments' institutions and non-governmental organizations for youth, women, indigenous people in the health sector.

(c) Human resources development

The development of human resources for the health of children, youth and women should include reinforcement of educational institutions, promotion of interactive methods of education for health and increased use of mass media in disseminating information to the target groups. This require the training of more community health workers, nurses, midwives, physicians, social scientists and educators, the education of mothers, families and communities and the strengthening of ministries of education, health, population, etc.

(d) Capacity-building

Governments should promote, where necessary: (i) the organization of national, inter-country and inter-regional symposia and other meetings for the exchange of information among agencies and groups concerned with the health of children, youth, women and indigenous people's organizations to facilitate health and consult them on the creation, amendment and enforcement of legal frameworks to ensure a healthy environment for children, youth, women and indigenous peoples.

D. MEETING THE URBAN HEALTH CHALLENGE

Basis for Action

For hunderds of millions of people, the poor living conditions in urban and peri-urban areas are destroying lives, health, and social and moral values. Urban growth has outstripped society's capacity to meet human needs, leaving hundreds of millions of people with inadequate incomes, diets, housing and services. Urban growth exposes populations to serious environmental hazards and has outstripped the capacity of municipal and local governments to provide the environmental health services that the people need. All too often, urban development is associated with destructive effects on the physical environment and the resource base needed for sustainable development. Environmental pollution in urban areas is associated with excess morbidity and mortality. Overcrowding and inadequate housing contribute to respiratory diseases, turberculosis, meningitis and other diseases. In urban environments, many factors that affect human health are outside the health sector. Improvements in urban health therefore will depend on coordinated action by all levels of government, healthcare providers, business, religious groups, social and educational institutions and citizens.

Objectives

The health and well-being of all urban dwellers must be improved so that they can contribute to economic and social development. The global objective is to achieve a 10 to 40 per cent improvement in health indicators by the year 2000. The same rate of improvement should be achieved for environmental, housing and health service indicators. These include the development of quantitative objectives for infant morality, maternal morality, percentage of low birth weight newborns and specific indicators (e.g. tuberculosis as an indicator of crowded housing, diarrhoeal diseases as indication of inadequate water and sanitation, rates of industrial and transportation accidents that indicate possible opportunities for prevention of injury, and social problems such as drug abuse, violence and crime that indicate underlying social disorders).

Activities

Local authorities, with the appropriate support of national Governments and international organizations should be encouraged to take effective measures to initiate or strengthen the following activities:

(a) Develop and implement municipal and local health plans
- (i) Establish or strengthen intersectoral committees at both the political and technical level, including active collaboration on linkage with scientific, cultural, religious, medical, business, social and other city institutions, using networking arrangements;
- (ii) Adopt or strengthen municipal or local "enabling strategies" that emphasize "doing with" rather than "doing for" and create supportive environments for health;
- (iii) Ensure that public health education in schools, workplace, mass media, etc. is provided or strengthened;
- (iv) Encourage communities to develop personal skills and awareness of primary healthcare; and
- (v) Promote and strengthen community-based rehabilitation activities for the urban and peri-urban disabled and the elderly.

(b) Survey, where necessary, the existing health, social and environmental conditions in cities, including documentation of intra-urban differences.

(c) Strengthen environmental health services:
- (i) Adopt health impact and environmental impact assessment procedures; and
- (ii) Provide basic and in-service training for new and existing personnel.

(d) Establish and maintain city networks for collaboration and exchange of models of good practice.

Means of Implementation

(a) Financing and cost evaluation

The Conference Secretariat has estimated the average total annual cost (1993-2000) of implementing the activities of this programme to be about $222 million including about $22 million from the international community on grant or concessional terms. These are indicative and order of magnitude estimate; only and have not been reviewed by Governments. Actual costs and financial terms including any than are non-concessional will depend upon, *inter alia,* the specific strategies and programmes Governments decide upon for implementation.

(b) Scientific and technological means

Decision-making models should be further developed and more widely used to assess the costs and the health and environment impacts of alternative technologies and strategies. Improvement in urban development and management requires better national and municipal statistics based on practical standardized indicators. Development of methods is a priority for the measurement of intra-urban and Intra-district variations in health status and environmental conditions and for the application of this information in planning and management.

(c) Human resources development

Programmes must supply the orientation and basic training of municipal staff required for the healthy city processes. Basic and in-service training of environmental health personnel will also be needed.

(d) Capacity-building

The programme is aimed towards improved planning and management capabilities in the municipal and local government and its partners in Central Government the private sector and universities. Capacity development should be focused on obtaining sufficient information improving coordination mechanisms thinking all the key actors, and making better use of available instruments and resources for implementation.

E. REDUCING HEALTH RISKS FROM ENVIRONMENTAL POLLUTION AND HAZARDS

Basis for Action

In many locations around the world the general environment (air, water and land). Workplaces and even individual dwellings are so badly polluted that the health of hundreds of millions of people is adversely affected. This is *inter alia,* due to past and present developments in consumption and production patterns and lifestyles. in energy production and use, in industry in transportation, etc. with little or no regard for environmental protection. There have been notable improvements in some countries but deterioration of the environment continues. The ability of countries to tackle pollution and health problems is greatly restrained because of lack of resources. Pollution control and health protection measures have often not kept pace with economic development. Considerable development-related environmental health hazards exist in the newly industrializing countries. Furthermore, the recent analysis of WHO has clearly established the interdependence among the factors of health environmental and development and has revealed that most countries are lacking such integration as would lead to an effective pollution control mechanism. Without prejudice to such criteria may be agreed upon by the international community, or to standards which will have to be determined nationally it will be essential in all cases to consider the systems of values prevailing in each country and the extent of the applicability of standards that are valid for the most advanced countries but may be inappropriate and of unwarranted social cost for the developing countries.

Objectives

The overall objective is to minimize hazards and maintain the environment to a degree that human health and safety is not impaired or endangered and yet encourage development to proceed. Specific programme objectives are:

(a) By the year 2000, to incorporate appropriate environmental and health safeguards as part of national development programmes in all countries;
(b) By the year 2000, to establish, as appropriate, adequate national infrastructure and programmes for providing environmental injury, hazard surveillance and the basis for abatement in all countries;
(c) By the year 2000, to establish, as appropriate, integrated programme for tackling pollution at the source and at the disposal site, with a focus on abatement actions in all countries; and
(d) To identify and compile, as appropriate, the necessary statistical information on health effects to support cost/benefit analysis, including environmental health impact assessment for pollution control prevention and abatement measures.

Activities

Nationally determined action programmes with international assistance, support and coordination, where necessary in this area should include:

(a) Urban air pollution

(i) Develop appropriate pollution control technology on the basis of risk assessment and epidemiological research for the introduction of environmentality sound production processes and suitable safe mass transport; and
(ii) Develop air pollution control capacities in large cities, emphasizing enforcement programmes and using monitoring networks, as appropriate.

(b) Indoor air pollution

(i) Support research and develop programmes for applying prevention and control methods to reducing indoor air pollution, including the provision of economic incentives for the installation of appropriate technology; and

(ii) Develop and implement health education campaigns, particularly in developing countries, to reduce. the health impact of domestic use of biomass and coal.

(c) Water pollution

(i) Develop appropriate water pollution control technologies on the basis of health risk assessment; and

(ii) Develop water pollution control capacities in large cities.

(d) Pesticides

Develop mechanisms to control the distribution and use of pesticides in order to minimize the risks to human health by transportation, storage, application and residual effects of pesticides used agriculture and preservation of wood.

(e) Solid waste

(i) Develop appropriate solid waste disposal technologies on the basis of health risk assessment; and

(ii) Develop appropriate solid waste disposal capacities in large cities.

(f) Human settlements

Develop programmes for improving health conditions in human settlements, in particular within slums and non-tenured settlements, on the basis of health risk assessment.

(g) Noise

Develop programme for maximum permitted safe noise exposure levels and promote noise assessment and control as part of environmental health programmes.

(h) Ionizing and non-ionizing radiation

Develop and implement appropriate national legislation, standards and enforcement procedures the basis of existing international guidelines.

(i) Effects of ultraviolet radiation

(i) Undertake, as a matter of urgency, research on the effects on human health of the increasing ultraviolet radiation reaching the earth's surface as a consequence of depletion of the stratospheric layer; and

(ii) On the basis of the outcome of this research, consider taking appropriate remedial measures to mitigate the above-mentioned effects on human beings.

(j) Industry and energy production

(i) Establish environmental health impact assessment procedures for the planning and development of new industries and energy facilities;
(ii) Incorporate appropriate health risk analysis in all major industries for ,the surveillance of workers' exposure to health hazards;
(iii) Establish industrial hygiene programme in all major industries for the surveillance of workers' exposure to health hazards; and
(iv) Promote the introduction of environmentally sound technologies within the industries and energy sectors.

(k) Monitoring and assessment

Establish as appropriate, adequate environmental monitoring capacities for the surveillance of environmental quality and the health status of populations.

(l) Injury monitoring and reduction

(i) Support, at appropriate, the development of systems to monitor the incidence and cause of injury to allow well-targeted intervention/prevention strategies;
(ii) Develop, in accordance with national plans strategies in all sectors (industry, traffic and others) consistent with the WHO safe cities and safe communities programmes, to reduce the frequency and severity of injury; and
(iii) Emphasize preventive strategies to reduce occupationally derived diseases and diseases caused by environmental and occupational toxins to enhance worker safety.

(m) Research promotion and methodology development

(i) Support the development of new methods for the quantitative assessment of health benefits and cost associated with different pollution control strategies; and
(ii) Develop and carry out interdisciplinary research on the combined health effects of exposure to multiple environmental hazards including epidemiological investigations of long-term exposures to low levels of pollutants and the use of biological markers capable of estimating human exposures adverse effects and susceptibility to environmental agents.

Means of Implementation

(a) Financial and cost evaluation

The Conference Secretariat has estimated the average total annual cost (1993-2000) of implementing the activities of this programme to be about $3 billion, including about $115 million from the international community on grant or concessional terms. These are indicative and order of magnitude estimates only and have not been reviewed by Government. Actual costs and financial terms, including any that are non-concessional, will depend upon, *inter alia*, the specific strategies and programmes Governments decide upon for implementation.

(b) Scientific and technological means

Although technology to prevent or abate pollution is readily availably for a large number of problems, for programme and policy development countries should undertake research within an intersectoral framework. Such efforts should include collaboration with the business sector. Cost effect analysis and environmental impact assessment methods should be developed through cooperative international programmes and applied to the setting of priorities and strategies in relation to health and development.

(c) Human resource development

Comprehensive national strategies should be designed to overcome the lack of qualified human resources, which is a major impediment to progress in dealing with environmental health hazards. Training should include environmental and health officials at all levels from managers to inspectors. More emphasis needs to be placed on including the subject of environmental health in the curricular of secondary schools and universities and on educating the public.

(d) Capacity-building

Each country should develop the knowledge and practical skills to foresee and identify environmental health hazards, and the capacity to reduce the risks. Basic capacity requirements must include knowledge about environmental health problems and awareness on the part of leaders, citizens and specialists; operation mechanisms for inter-sectoral and inter-governmental cooperation in development planning and management and in combating pollution; arrangements for involving private and community interests in dealing with social issues; delegation of authority and distribution of resources to intermediate and local levels of governments to provide front-line capabilities to meet environmental health needs.

Source: Agenda 21: United Nations Conference on Environment and Development, Rio de Janeiro, Brazil, June 3-14, 2002, pp. 37-53.

CHAPTER 9

HEALTH EDUCATION FOR SELF-CONFIDENCE AND POSITIVE ATTITUDE

> Vedanta uncompromisingly insists that man is essentially perfect, and therefore infinite are the possibilities that lie lurking in him. The Rishis cry, we must realize that we have within ourselves all the resources, ability, energy and power for building-up a supremely successful life for ourselves and for others in the world. There is one great and covertable gift which is distinctly ours at all times, and this is our profound capacity to discover, develop and usefully employ the Infinite Essence in us.
>
> —*Swami Chinmayananda*

Health Education for Self-Confidence and Positive Attitude

"Stand up, be bold, be strong. Take the whole responsibility on your shoulders and know that you are the creator of your own destiny. All the strength and succour you want is within you. Therefore, make your own future."

—*Swami Vivekananda*

"There is one corner of the Universe you can be certain of improving and that is your own self."

—*Aldous Huxley*

"Begin to change your attitude, and your vision of the world will change. Everything will be peaceful and good. This is the non-dualism of the Vedantic vision. This is the highest knowledge."

—*Swami Tejanandynanda*

Let people say whatever they like, stick to your own convictions, and rest assured, the world will be at your feet. They say, "Have faith in this fellow or that fellow", but I say, "Have faith in yourself—all power is in you—be conscious and bring it out. Say, "I can do everything." "Even the poison of a snake is powerless, if you can firmly deny it." (VI.274)

We are responsible for what we are, and whatever we wish ourselves to be, we have the power to make ourselves. If what we are now has been the result of our own past actions, it certainly follows that whatever we wish to be in future can be produced by our present actions; so we have to know how to act. (I.31).

Swami Chinmayananda states,

A man or woman becomes what he or she thinks about him or her.

CHART 9.1

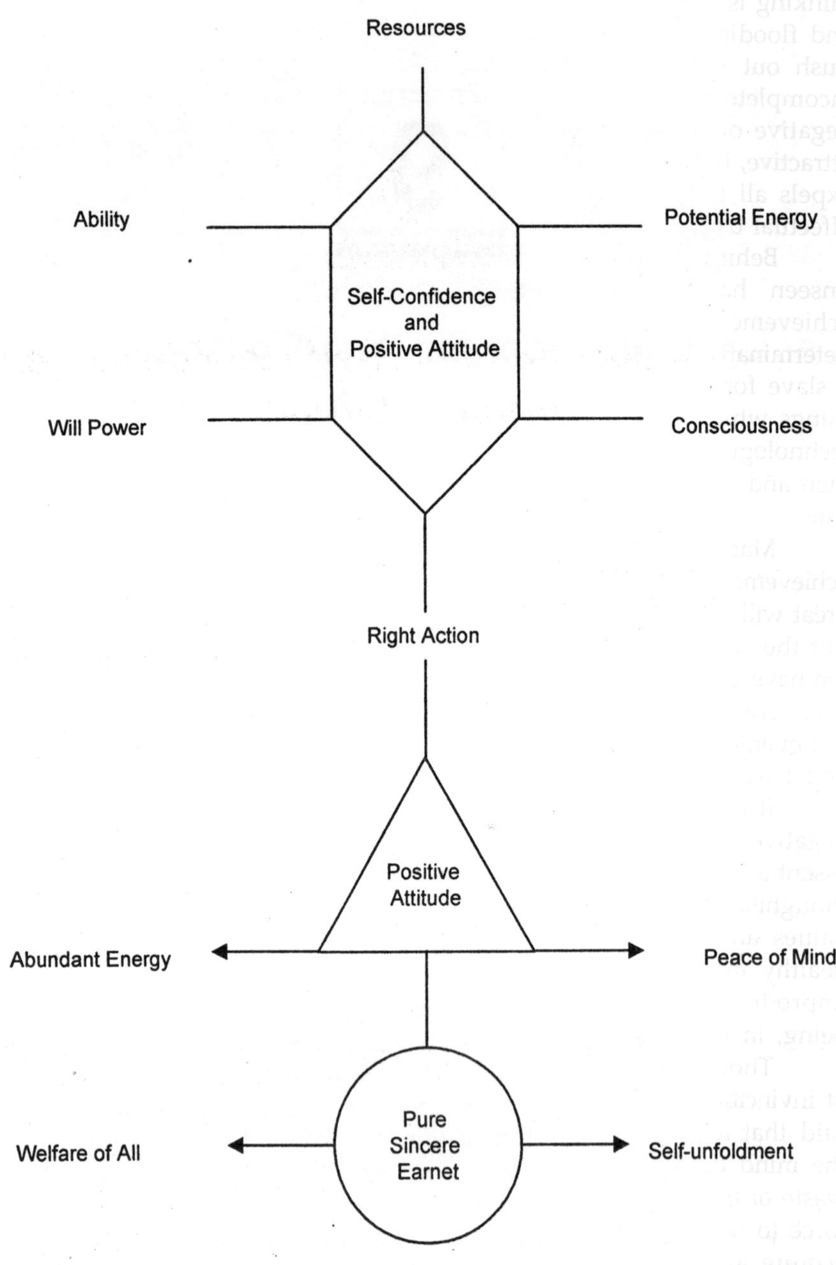
Resources
Ability
Potential Energy
Self-Confidence
and
Positive Attitude
Will Power
Consciousness
Right Action
Positive
Attitude
Abundant Energy
Peace of Mind
Pure
Sincere
Earnet
Welfare of All
Self-unfoldment

Thinking is very powerful. Positive thinking can do miracles and one can achieve whatever one wants. Systematically, therefore, we must train and discipline the mind for right thinking and correct diligent activity. Right thinking is a habit that can be cultivated. Substitution of positive thoughts and flooding the mind with creative ideas are methods by which we can flush out the floor of the mind, littered as it is now with the filth of incomplete thoughts and decaying ideas. Having recognized a thought as negative or wrong, do not waste time in upholstering it to look neat and attractive, but reject it immediately and totally—the owner of right thinking expels all false thoughts and induces healthy conceptions, adding to the effectual dynamism in the seeker.[1]

Behind every achievement that we see in this world today, is the unseen hand of the human will. The material comforts scientific achievements are all the products crystallized out of the human will and determination. The human will-power has conquered Nature, and made her a slave for the welfare of mankind, and in the process, has even created things which were not even available in the world before. Behind all the technological progress are the determined efforts of hundreds of dedicated men and women, who faced all the challenges to make their dreams come true.

Many of what we see today as solid facts of life and proof of man's achievements were only mere ideas yesterday in the minds of a few men of great will power. Those ideas would not have become realities, had they not put the will and determination to their ideas into practice. Our scriptures too have given us examples of men of great will, like Viswamitra who could even create a new world outfit sheer out of will power. All men of achievement had the blessing of tremendous will-power in their makeup, and History is full of names of such men of achievement.[2]

It is everywhere seen that in this remaking of one's destiny, there is negative and there is a positive approach. The negative approach essentially is the careful observance of the quality and texture of our thoughts, detecting the dissipations within, and eradicating those false values and wrong tendencies in our thought-patterns. To have, thus, a healthy mind within—one that has learned to negate and weed out its unproductive jungles of thought—is the secret of living in physical well-being, in harmony and happiness.

Thought is a force, and when properly harnessed it can be a power of invincible strength. Thoughts propel us to action. That is why it has been said that advance thinking can lead to positive action. Thoughts arise in the mind constantly and trickle out into the world around. This is tragic waste of the personality vitality. By conscious effort we can trains the mind-force to flow into chosen channels where it can be an irresistible power to acquire and to achieve. It has been rightly said in a poem that as lack beholds in cloud and fire, the shape that answers his own desire.

As in life, so at the moment of death and also after death. When you think of your club and go out of the house, you move towards the club, and not towards the market or theatre or office ! the powerful intentions in us are expressed in our actions. Our external movements are vivid amplifications of our deeper desires and intentions.[3]

STEPS OF POSITIVE THINKING (Chart 9.2)

(I) Set a Positive Goal of Life—Decision-making

To activate the latent abilities, we have to fix a goal for our life. The goal need not be just the desire for salvation. There should be a specific and clear goal in everybody's life. Of course, a momentary desire is not a goal. And it is not enough to have a desire to succeed in the task we have set for ourself. It is necessary to act in the proper manner so that it is carried out within the prescribed time. Unless we have a working plan, our valuable mental energy and time will be wasted.

To be able to overcome uncertainty and vacillation, we have to ask ourself what it is that we most desire for ourself. Then it becomes clear to us what main goal we should have for ourself in our life. Then our mind devotes its energy to the fulfilment of the desire.[4]

Deciding clearly, on what and how to achieve success and how to go about it is the first step to victory. One who selects a particular field and tries to reach to the top in that will receive greater respect and recognition. The target should be realistic. The field should be one in which you have interest, reasonable knowledge and enthusiasm, and you have confidence that you can achieve something. Keeping these considerations while selecting the goal, will enable one to work easily and whole heartedly and move forward.

Webster's dictionary defines decision-making as "the art of determining in one's own mind upon an opinion or course of action." Shull and his associates define the decision-making process as " . . . a conscious and human process, involving both individual and social phenomena, based upon factual and value premises, and which includes a choice of one behavioural activity from among one or more alternatives with the intention of moving toward some desired state of affairs." According to Ishwar Dayal, "decision is the commitment of the decision-maker to act, thereby committing the personnel, material and financial resources of the organization towards the action objectives." *Emory and Niland view a decision as only one step in an intellectual process of differentiating among relevant alternatives*. It is . . . "the point of selection and commitment the decision-maker chooses the preferred purpose the most reasonable task statement, of the best course of action." According to Hodge and Johnson, "Decision-making is to solve any obstacle (problem) that stands between decision-maker and the accomplishment of the organization." According to Donald J. Clough, "the decision-making process involves a problem to be solved, a number of conflicting objective to be reconciled, a number of possible alternative courses of action from which the 'best' has to be chosen and some way of measuring the value or pay off of alternative courses of action."

CHART 9.2

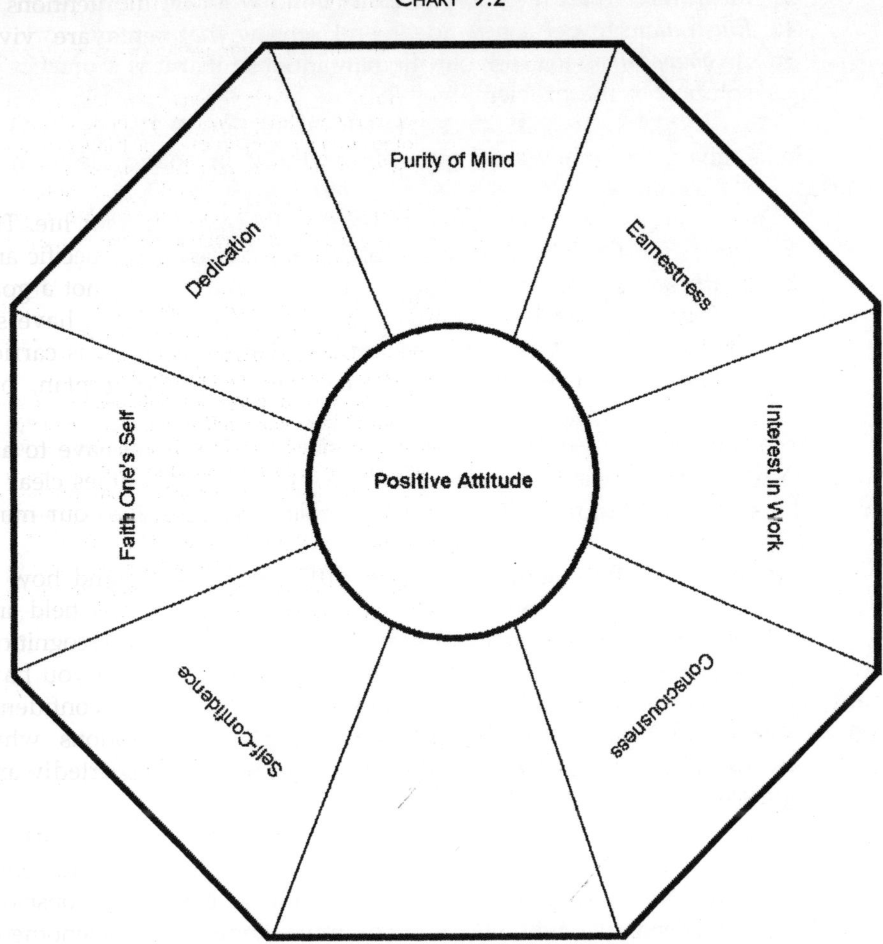

According to Kreitner; 'Decision-making is a process of identifying and choosing alternative course of action in a manner appropriate to the demand of the situation. The act of choosing implies that alternative courses of action must be weighed and weeded out'.

According to Manley H. Jones: "Broadly, decision-making involves making organization committed to adoption of a specific course of action and use of resources in a particular manner."

New problems demand new solutions and the Chief Executives who can come out from the routine are highly prized. This requires creativity in the sphere of decision-making. Newmann has indicated five distinct stages which can help the Chief Executive in this process:

1. *Saturation*: to be familiar with the problem.
2. *Deliberation*: to consider alternative solutions and to rearrange them.

3. *Incubation*: to let the sub-conscious mind work on the problem.
4. *Illustration*: to get a new ideas and sensing that it may work.
5. *Accommodation*: to work out the new ideas so that it is a practical solution to the problem.

Hicks gives the following types of creativity in sound decision-making:

1. *Innovative*: Creativity to think totally new ideas.
2. *Synthesis*: Creativity to absorb, combine and use ideas from different sources and making it new.
3. *Extension*: Creativity to use old or new ideas.
4. *Duplication*: Creativity to use the other's successful ideas.

According to W. Brooke Groves, "Decision-making is the selection from two or more reasonable possibilities of a course that will, at the time and under circumstances, provide the most suitable solution of the problem at hand."

Nepoleon says that nothing is more difficult and therefore more precious than to be able to decide.

Keen desire and ardent aspiration are the forces that take US to an environment that is conducive to the fulfilment of our goal. Even in the spiritual world, if we have very keen desire and very ardent longing we will be able to attain God. If we have intense yearning, it means there is the dawn; the sun is not far behind said Bhagawan Sri Ramakrishna. Just see the miracle of intense yearning !

If a man doesn't feel in his heart an ardent desire to know something, if he doesn't develop a keen aspiration to achieve something, he will see only darkness before his eyes. The thing doesn't appear before him at all.[5]

What we need, we will get. But we must know what we need. Otherwise there will be no result. From a goalless life we earn nothing but dejection, humiliation, inferiority complex and sorrow. In shot, this is a life of utter debility, of utter tragedy.[6]

A life barren in aspirations to work out good plans, to fulfil great schemes, to realize nobly visions, is indeed tragic, empty and insufferably blistering. The deeper enthusiasm of our inner soul is invoked only when our towering vision thrusts our eyes, our hands and our hearts upward to heavenly heights of thought and action.

Our life must grow entirely into dedicated, cheerful work and selfless, undemanding service. When these two are ignored by members of a community, in that community poverty and discord, sin and sickness, fear and anxiety, war and insecurity are inevitable. These are all self-invited sorrows, made-to-order by a society infested with idlers and selfish men.[7]

To have a great ideal, a high motive, a gracious goal, is to bring a rhythem and purpose to life. Even in the world we find that a man of ambition, of a definite political goal, of a great scientific, literacy or artistic vision has neither the time nor the urge for the idle life of dissipation. One who is fired by his deep devotion to the Self can have no fascination for sensuous pleasures and worldly preoccupations. He pursues the Self alone (मामेव ये प्रमद्यन्ते) and does, transcend the mind (मायामेतां तरन्ति ते).[8]

Thus, our first step should be spelt out in clear terms so that we can reach the goal. Ritu Bhatia in her article, "The Power of the Self" in *Life Plus*, Jan.-March, 2004 observes:

Self-esteem soars when you discover what you love to do and find a way to offer it to others. Talk show host Oprah Winfrey believes that what gives a person worth is what they can give back, "knowing who you are and what you are about, where you fit into the universe and feeling good about it," is how she puts it.

One of the preconditions to making a dream happen is to befriend, protect and nurture your spirit. This means paying attention to your real needs, treating yourself kindly and standing up for yourself even if that displeases the people around you. An intact soul is needed to support the healthy development of the life you were meant to have. Success comes from taking that first small step. Then another, and another, till they all combine to make one giant leap. Everything big comes from pushing the boundaries of the possible, and then allowing the energy of the universe to lead you.

Victor Franki, feels that "Man needs to struggle for a goal worthy of him, and find meaning waiting to be fulfilled."

(2) Faith in one self

Faith is a quality of the self. It is a great power of the mind. It can be used beneficially by everyone, at all times. Faith is certain to have a positive effect on our life, health, profession and our mind. Faith is the key with which we can open the secret treasures of this universe. It is the path that leads to the Supreme Being who is the repository of all power and glory that manifests in this world. It is also the means of acquiring tremendous energy. It is faith that gives us the steadiness to hold on, with optimism in the midst of gloom and destruction. "With true faith, one can attain enlightenment, says the Gita.

Those who tend to believe that they are culturally, socially and intellectually inferior should, first of all, shake-off their inferiority complex. Though it might be deep-rooted, it should be possible to weed it out. Of course, it is not so easy as throwing away an unwanted article. Our first and foremost need—nay, duty, is to develop confidence in our own immense power, which is latent. In the past, seers and men of spiritual insights tried to impress upon us that behind the apparently limited powers of man are hidden unlimited mysterious powers, if only we had the skill to discover them. Today, psychologists are reaffirming the same fact with the help of their experimental observations. To arouse the powers, nothing more than self-confidence is required. We should strive to rise from the state in which we are right now. We should gradually attain success, scaling each step through efforts.[9]

Swami Vivekananda repeatedly stressed the need for cultivating the faith in one self: "the ideal of faith in ourselves is of the greatest help to us. If faith in ourselves had been more extensively taught and practiced, I am sure a very large portion of the evils and miseries that we have would have vanished. Throughout the history of mankind if any motive power has been more potent than another in the lives of all great men and women, it is that of faith in themselves. Born with the consciousness that they were to be great, they became great. Let a man go down as low as possible; there must come a time when out of sheer desperation he will take an upward curve and will learn to have faith in himself. But it is better for us that we should know from the very first. Why should we have all bitter experiences in order to gain faith in ourselves? We can see that all the difference between man and man is due to the existence or non-existence of faith in himself. Faith in ourselves will do everything."

Unlimited energy is latent in each one of us. But because of our restricted imagination we act as if we have hypnotized ourselves into inaction. Self-confidence will activate the spirit of enthusiasm and lead us along the path of achieving great things in life.[10]

Self-confidence and the conviction that virtuous acts lead to one's highest good and success have their source in the power of faith, faith in God. A scientist and a religious person both pay their tribute to faith. Faith is life, William James, remarked: "Faith is one of the forces by which men live and the total absence of it means collapse." Faith is the foundation of spiritual life. It is the means to acquire the grace of the Lord. Everything is possible through faith. Is it possible in one day to have such unflinching, unshakeable trust? Faith begets faith.

To possess such trust or faith in God one has to struggle day and night giving up luxuries and comforts, ignoring one's failure and success on the path, ever holding on to learning and humility, and remembering god all the time. One has to step into the water in order to learn swimming. So also to gain faith one has to jump into the sea of efforts. One who tries to swim is scared and may fail initially. But can one swim if he gives up after initial setbacks? similarly, sincere and persistent efforts are necessary in spiritual life. What if we meet with failures? We must not stop marching ahead. Let us use all the available relaxation techniques to release the mental tension but at the same time not forget that lasting peace is possible only through spiritual practice.

Barbara Briggs in an article, "Source of the Courage" mentioned that in the *Life Plus*, January-March, 2004: Courage and inner strength in the individual spring from that which is the unified source of power, wisdom and energy in the universe. Those with a devotional temperament call it God; those with a scientific bent of mind call it the unified field of natural law, but both are referring to the same unlimited source of life-giving energy in the universe. This omnipresent, beneficent power instills in us the courage to move forward into the vast unknown. Although invisible, it is none-the-less the invincible power deep within our hearts that we always call upon in our hour of need. This omnipresent being, this nameless wholeness of life, is a source of inner strength that will never fill us as long as we trust in it.

There is a saying, faith, even the size of a mustard seed, can move mountains. Courage is born of faith in oneself and in God. Faith springs from our awareness of the Oneness that underlies, supports and governs the diverse field of life. The faith we have in ourselves enriches our faith in God and *vice-versa,* for atman and Brahman are essentially one. Yatha pinde, tatha brahmande—as in the individual, so in the cosmos; as in the microcosm, so in the macrocosm. Faith stems from an intuitive awareness of a benevolent power that nourishes and protects all living beings in the universe. Faith is an inner anchor that bestows mental equilibrium in the face of danger. It enables us to meet the crises in our lives without losing our balance. The more we want to achieve, the more courage and faith are needed. The higher the building we wish to erect, the deeper we must dig the foundation.

The invincible power that infuses life with energy, intelligence and creativity, is always involved consciously or unconsciously in any act of courage. This power alone guides all actions towards achievement and fulfilment. Without faith, courage will be lacking and without courage, we cannot accomplish anything of significance in life.

In the Bhagavad Gita (4:39-40), Sri Krishna says to Arjuna: "He gains knowledge who is possessed of faith, is active of purpose and has subdued the senses. Having gained knowledge, swiftly he comes to the supreme peace. But the man who is without knowledge, without faith and of a doubting nature, perishes. For the doubting mind there is neither this world nor another nor any happiness."

The qualities that are necessary for an individual to be assured of the Knowledge-Divine are being enumerated here as vividly as from the leaf of a Science text-book. Three great qualities have been indicated and to understand them is to understand why the so-called seekers, in spite of their claims to sincere self-applications, do not actually reach anywhere near the ladder of development. Faith, devotion, and self-control are the three imperative necessities to be acquired before we can hope to evolve to the diviner stature from our present mortal encumbrances.

The Lord says that such men who "Doubt the Self" will not find any joy or happiness ANYWHERE—NEITHER HERE NOR IN THE HEREAFTER." In explaining Thus, the Geeta seems to express that there may be a small chance perhaps, for one who is devoid of knowledge and faith to discover some kind of a happiness in this world, here and now, but that those who are constant doubters can enjoy neither here nor there. Such men are psychologically incapable of enjoying any situation, because the doubting tendency in them will poison all their experiences. He whose teeth have become septic must constantly poison the food that he is taking; so too, those who have this tendency of doubting everything.

Lack of awareness of the underlying oneness wholeness and unity in the midst of life's diverse expressions is born of lack of faith, which in turn gives rise to doubt and despair. Doubts emerge when one focuses on the field of differences to such an extent that one forgets or ignores the field of oneness. When he unified wholeness of life is forgotten, one is unable to feel the interconnectedness between the whole and its parts.

One ignores the eternal, immortal, imperishable aspect of life and instead identifies with the perishable, ever-changing aspect and so becomes increasingly vulnerable. One reacts to changing circumstances like a leaf tossed about by the blowing wind. The mind is caught between conflicting emotions and desires. One is forced to choose between 'this' and 'that'. The weak mind is always caught in the conflict born of the duality between mind and heart.

It is said in the Upanishads: Dvitiyad vai bhayam bhavati—certainly fear is born of duality. Whenever there is a sense of two, fear can arise. In the Vivek Chudamani, Adi Shankara says: "whenever the wise man sees the least difference in the infinite Brahman, at once that which he sees as different through mistake, becomes a source of terror to him."

When Arjuna, the greatest archer of his time, was caught in a state of suspension in the battlefield, Sri Krishna taught him the knowledge of sankhya, pertaining to the indestructibility of the spiritual content of life. In the Bhagavad Gita (2:17-24), Krishna says: "Know that to be indeed in destruction by which all this is pervaded. None can work the destruction of this immutable being. He is uncleavable; he cannot be burned; he cannot be wetted, nor yet can he be dried. He is eternal, all-pervading, stable, immovable, ever the same."

Armed with this knowledge and after directly experiencing the transcendence of the field of duality, Arjuna was able to rise to the occasion and fulfil his dharma. By the end of three hours, Arjuna succeeds in becoming established in the immovable wholeness of life and in conquering not only his inner enemies, in the form of ears and doubts, but his external enemies as well and in re-establishing dharma, the rule of righteousness for the good of all beings. As Krishna says in the Bhagavad Gita (5:19): "Even here, in this life, the universe is conquered by those whose mind is established in equanimity."

Courage is the quality of a conqueror. He who would conquer the world must conquer the mind and become established in the being, the omnipresent wholeness of life. Only then can one truly work towards nourishing, supporting and uplifting the world.

3. Control over Mind

The mind is the instrument which translates into action the ideas and convictions which are already in the intellect. In our home we learn from the teachers and books. From these we get the bulk of our intellectual ideas. We understand and analyse them with our head. Still whatever mass of knowledge we may acquire, we can be an utter failure in our life, unless we can produce that knowledge in the outside world. In order to send it out into the world, we will have to direct the knowledge through our mind. Therefore, mental control, mental development as the modern educationists say, is important. The student who develops a certain amount of mind control is marked as one who will have the greatest success in life. This idea, developed throughout the ages of Hinduism, is called yoga. Disciplining the mind is called yoga; not that which is popularly called as yoga: sitting with folded legs, the nose held between two fingers.

The mind can cause or cure a disease! Patience, love, sympathy, generosity, selflessness—such positive attitude leads to a smooth, healthy, cheerful functioning of all parts of this machine called the human body. But from negative thoughts arise fear, anxiety, hatred, jealousy, frustration and selfishness, which affect the whole body and lead to disease. Let me repeat it, so that this truth is firmly imprinted on your mind. The mind can cause or cure disease. Cheerfulness, transquility, courage, self-confidence, determination—such positive states of mind are more efficacious than any tonic in keeping the body healthy.[11]

Mind is a mere thought-flow. Just as "water flowing continuously in a given direction" is a river, so too thought-flow is the mind. Just as continuous flow of gallons of water give us the magnitude of the river, though flowing continuously from an individual toward the world of objects is the "mind." Naturally as the character of the river is the character determined by the nature of its waters, so too, the mind is also conditioned by its own thoughts. If the waters are clean, the river is clean. If the waters flow fast, the river is fast. The similarity is so complete that the same can be applied to the mind. The nature and behaviour of thought in an individual bosom at a given moment, must condition and define the type of mind the individual possesses at that time. Thus, if the thoughts are good, the mind is good. If the thoughts are agitated, the mind is agitated.[12]

Ramana Maharsi says that the mind causes all thoughts to arise. Apart from thoughts, there is no such thing as mind. Therefore, thought is the nature of mind. Apart from thoughts, there is no independent entity called the world... Just as the spider emits the thread (of the web) out of itself and again withdraws it into itself, likewise the mind projects the world out of itself and again resolves it into itself.

The human body and mind act as an antenna which transmits thought waves, propagates and interacts with other human beings and influences them accordingly. So ones good thought spreads globally and influences others to become good and do good and similarly the *vice versa*. In the same way the human body and mind act as receiving antenna and receives all thought waves of others and are being influenced by them. So one is not fully responsible for his activity, as he is governed and influenced by so many such radiations but human brain with its intellect structural arrangements can plan, act and lead a harmonious life on understanding the nature of these radiations.

4. Love

Love is the elixir of life. It has been found to have power even to cure physical and mental disorders. One who has hatred in his mind not only loses his mind, but also undermines his health and life. On the other hand, love, sympathy, and friendship not only contribute towards building one's peace of mind, but also create a balanced outlook. A man who develops these qualities will acquire serenity, joy and peace in spite of all external circumstances.

Concentrating is very important to achieve victory. If the issue is of interest to you, concentration comes automatically. But even otherwise, once you have chosen a goal, keeping in view the demand *vis-a-vis* your interest, you should try to have concentration with auto-suggestions and by developing interest.

5. Need of Enthusiasm and Dynamism

To make life worthwhile and fruitful, we must generate enthusiasm within ourselves. Generation of enthusiasm will take place when we discover for ourselves a goal and attach ourselves to the Altar with a spirit of dedication, reverence and love. Once we have surrendered ourselves to it, the ideal itself will provide us with the inspiration and strength. Then nothing can hinder the progress of our march towards that Goal and the ideal. The love for the ideal will overcome and vanquish all the hurdles from the ideal, and if it comes to that, life itself will be cast-off with a smile in dedication at that Altar. That was how Bhagat Singh could walk to the gallows with a smile on his face. What is important is that one should choose the right ideal . . . an ideal worthwhile even if it comes to sacrificing one's own life in the endeavour. The ideal should be inspiring, it should arouse the spring of activity in us. Thus, the discovering of the ideal is the secret of generating in ourselves Dynamism and Vitality in its fullness.[13]

6. Right Actions and Implementation

Right actions strengthen and enrich our vitality. The inspiration derived from the ideal has to be conserved, enriched and strengthened by cultivating and living right values of life. Living the right values of life is like building a dam on a river. Just as the dam raises the water—level, the right values raise the stock and wealth of our inner vitality.[14]

The path of Action called karma yoga—, is a highly scientific way-of-life which all of us can easily adopt, when once we have understood its entire implications. The world of objects and beings remaining the same, everyone of us, in whatever condition we may be at present, can learn to slowly grow to unbelievable heights—gathering to ourselves a new stature, undreamt by anyone around us at any time.

Life is ever active and positive. Life is never passive and negative. Dynamic expressions in action are "life." When all actions have ended, the organism is "dead", while living, no organism can ever remain, even for a moment, without activity; work expresses the life within, in every living organism. All work outside and activities of thoughts within one, are stopped only when the organism is dead. To escape work is to escape "life" and run into "death", it is suicidal.

Worlds, written or spoken, are of no use unless put into action. The emphasis should be more on performance rather than paper planning. Khalil Gibran has rightly said that, "Believing is a fine thing, but placing those beliefs into execution is a test of strength. Many are those who talk like the roar of the sea, but their lives are shallow and stagnant, like the rotting marshes. Many are those who lift their heads above the mountain tops, but their spirit remain dormant to the obscurity of the caverns."

The Tribune Editorial has rightly commented that "Man's future was in his own hands and assisted by science he could be trusted to shape it to his own liking. The disappearance of this belief has left our minds a waste land, empty of hope, lacking in ideals, devoid of aspirations. In a world, skepticism, apathy and disillusion go wider and cut deeper than they have ever done before.

Swami Vivekananda has also mentioned that we must act decisively to regenerate the potentialities of our country:

"What our country now wants, are muscles of iron and nerves of steel, gigantic wills which nothing can resist, which can penetrate into the mysteries and the secrets of the universe, and will accomplish their purpose in any fashion, even if it meant going down to the bottom of the ocean and meeting death face to face, that is what we want, and that can only be created, established and strengthened, by understanding and realizing the ideal of the Advaita, that ideal of the oneness of all. None can regenerate this land of ours without the practical application and effective operation of this ideal of the oneness of things. The truths of the Upanishads are before you. Take them up, live upto thee and the salvation of India will be at hand."

He further adds:

"Let us all work hard, my brethren; this is no time for sleep. One our work depends the coming of the India of the future. She is there ready, waiting. She is only sleeping. Arise and awake, and see her seated here, on her eternal throne, rejuvenated, more glorious than she ever was, this Motherland of ours."

Thus, the future of this budding developing democracy depends upon the attitudes of its political and administrative elite. There is no substitute for hard work which would be reflected in better life of the people. Nevertheless, without a concerted attempt to make the administration much more action-oriented than at present, these may not yield enough results.

Kaibara Ekken, the Japanese sage has nicely put it as: if by study, enquiry or thought, we have learned the truth, we should then put it into practice in both our speech and action. Let what we say be true and what we do discreet. Regulate the emotions, and suppress anger and selfish desires. Shake of evil and cling to good. Discovering our faults, let us not hesitate to correct them. Towards others let us be considerate. All this is the way of true action. Without putting what we have learned into practice, it bears no fruit.

Robert M. Hutchines states (quoted in M.R. Pinto, Value's in Public Services, *IJPA*, January-March, 1989), "Thus, all organizations can function and achieve excellence provided all its members strive to pursue the goals of the organization earnestly, sincerely, whole-heartedly and with dedication."

Our thought is the seed which determines the fruit of our action. If the seed is good, then the flowers and fruit which come from the seed must be good and must prove beneficial to ourselves and others. But if we plan in our hearts a poisonous seed, it will harm not only ourselves but all who come in contact with us. Human life is a great responsibility. Only a thoughtless man will say: I cannot help what happens, I am responsible. We are constantly influencing ourselves and our fellow-beings by what we think, because our thought shapes our inner nature and we radiate consciously or unconsciously what we are. Let us be wakeful then. Let us be thoughtful in whatever we do. Let us be faithful to our true self; for all blessings must come to us, if we prove ourselves true to our higher nature.

Face life and its upheavals around you. Be active and tirelessly dynamic. Each exertion undertaken is a shooting spark of "life" from the well of Existence in you. Fearlessly work with a clear vision plan and selflessly execute it. Fear not sweat!, hesitate not to face disappointments. Live life, so long as you are alive. Grow through work. Evolve in work. Expand while striving. Make your own life. Thus, rich and sweet. You can. You must.[15]

The highest and noblest type of an individual working in the world is known as the "man of achievement" (Yogi). Such men work, neither for the sake of wages, nor for success; they are not after mere sensual pleasures, nor do they aspire to reform the world; they delicately perform their obligatory duties finding peace and fulfilment in their very activity. Their fulfilment consists in doing their duties to the best of their ability without claiming any rights and they are totally unmindful of whether the society commends or condemns their actions.

The Path of Action called karma-yoga is a highly scientific way of life which all of us can easily adopt, when once we have understood its total implications. The world of objects and beings remaining the same, everyone of us, in whatever condition we may be at present. Can learn and slowly grow to unbelievable heights, gathering to ourselves a new stature, undreamt of us by any one around at anytime.

Action is the answer, not inaction. Running away from problems is cowardice and the result of cowardice is sorrow, shame and defeat. Facing the situation is courage and the blessings of courage are sublimity, splendor and success. Swami Visharadananda in his book, "Human Values" observes that:

Human life is not to be wasted. Time is not to be squandered. It has to be used properly. It is interesting to examine and see our life, how many things we start and how much we are able to retain.

We can start an event. But commitment does not come, because commitment comes from the emotional self not from intellectual self. Intellectual self decides and emotional self-executes. Intellectual self is the father and emotional self is the mother in us. Since emotional self-implements actions, it is good if emotional self decides also. Emotional self will not implement unless it feels fully convinced. For that we have to do analysis. The conviction that, 'This alone I have to do, I cannot waste my time anymore has to come in life. Then sthirata comes. When sthirata comes, motivation is no longer needed. External support is also no more needed. Clarity only brings sthirata. If I know very clearly what I want in my life, commitment is bound to come. People who want to earn money, power, popularity have to have so much of commitment. They cannot sleep. They have to work day and night. Similarly, a person who wants moksha will have to work harder. We should be able to apply our mind consistently wherever it has to be foucused. We should be able to contain our pursuit regardless of external situations.

Ratnaih maharghaih na tutusuh devah
Na bhejire bhima vishena bhitim;
Sudham vina na prayayuh viramam,
Na niscitarthat viramanti dhiraha.

When samudra manthanam (churning of ocean) was done, along with many attractive objects, dreadful poison also came out. Poison could not frighten gods nor could ratnas (gems) dissuade them. They continued to churn the ocean till amrta (nectar) came.

This is how we have to behave. Once we are committed, we have to work irrespective of the difficulties, till we attain the objective. If we stop before that, we have to start all over again. As stated already, persistence and consistency are very important and no result is achieved without them.

7. Achieving Consciousness

The core of the human personality is the consciousness which is the life centre around which all the activities of the body, mind and the intellect revolve. It remains even changeless and immovable, like an axle for the wheel, yet causes all changes and movements to occur. When man succeeds in identifying with this changeless, immovable. Conscious principle within himself, he is no longer victimized by the changing phenomena of perceptions, emotions and thoughts; he becomes the supreme Lord of them all. The intellectual pursuits, emotional attachments and physical cravings of such a man naturally wither and fall away like petals when the fruit emerges.

8. Firmness at Mental and Intellectual Level

In our experience in life, we find that we are what we are because of the caliber of the mental and intellectual equipment in us. If we are full of feelings of love, tenderness and kindness, we are naturally loving and kind and if the power of our discrimination is sharp and brilliant, we are bound to be brilliant. The environment and circumstances may be disagreeable and disturbing, but as long as our inner equipment is healthy and strong, none of these can influence or disturb our peace, stability and tranquility. Such a man stands erect and firm like a towering lighthouse which is unaffected by the surging waves strike against it and die away. But when this subtle equipment is neglected or kept in disuse, the individual, like a neglected boat in the ocean of life, is tossed hither and thither by the calamitous waves of challenges.

A nation is built by the individuals comprising it. When each individual in a society or nation puts forth his effort in the direction indicated in the scriptures and reconstitutes his personality, then that society or nation grows dynamically, distributing peace and glory to one and all. Let us therefore, awake, arise and rebuild ourselves and our nation.

He is an active and dynamic man of goodness, living every moment in inspired job, meeting all challenges with a smile, accepting life and death equally, unaffected by the world of turmoil around, unattached to anything, free and ever liberated from the weaknesses of the flesh. He reigns indeed he reigns as a sovereign wielding his power with infinite love and wisdom.[16]

9. Interest in Work

The first factor necessary for success is work. An individual has to work even though he or she would like to have success without work. There is only one place where success comes before work, and that is in the dictionary. So work is a must for success. We see many people working laboriously. Still, they do not seem to accomplish anything. This is because there is no efficiency in their work. Efficiency is the second factor required for success. The skill or knack of working or performing an action in such a way that it will bear the desired fruit is called efficiency. The third factor required is knowledge, for to perform work knowledge is a must. Knowledge means: (1) knowledge of our desired goal; (2) knowledge of the means to attain the goal; and (3) knowledge of the performer who is going to adopt the means and strive for the goal. This knowledge is called proficiency.

A person who has knowledge but no efficiency cannot be successful. The difference can be seen in the material progress of India as compared to other countries such as the United State or Japan. In India, more emphasis is given to theoretical knowledge. Indian universities impart a lot of information, but practical knowledge is overlooked, while in America more emphasis is given to the practical aspect and work is done efficiently. Therefore, even though so many students are graduating from universities in India with outstanding degrees, what is the condition of India materially? We are speaking only from the material point of view at the moment. India's prosperity cannot be compared to the prosperity of the United State, Canada or Japan because India has neglected the practical aspect.[17]

When a person works with inspiration, he never gets tired or exhausted. When man works only for himself, there is perspiration; but when he works for a noble goal there is inspiration. In cases where a man cannot dedicate his actions to the Lord, even if he works for some ideal or goal he will derive tremendous strength from his chosen altar of dedication. The nobler the goal, the greater will be the strength he gains. This is the beauty of love and dedication, which brings efficiency in life.[18]

Work ethic embraces work responsibility, work conscience, ethical work conduct. If one has the satisfaction that he is contributing his very best to his organisation and is not just earning the bread, then this would be the true feeling of work ethics. Work ethic demands that one works for attaining organisational objectives in its fullest measure.[19]

Today belongs to us. Success is like oxygen to a person. Every time you achieve success, enthusiasm in you increases. Your respect gets doubled. When you succeed, world gives you recognition. All will be with you or following you. Everyone will compete to say that they are acquainted with you. Your relatives will be proud of you. Failure pulls down a person. Success gives new strength. No one will hand over to you success in a golden plate. You have to make all efforts to succeed. You can forget about the efforts made and difficulties undergone after you have achieved victory. But it is not so easy to achieve success. Merely thinking that I want to become a winner is not sufficient. For that: deciding the goal, drawing up a wise plan, effort, determination, reputation, constant pursuit, concentration, strength to face defeat, desire to achieve something, personal development, time management, keen observation/examination, patience and expertise to detect a mistake and rectify it, etc., are required. Firm resolve to travel in that direction is most important.

Today belongs us, yesterday was; tomorrow will be; but today is with us. Everyday is bursting with opportunities for us to do and to serve, to act and to express, to love and to live.

We must make use of these lush chances and diligently make our life rich, fruitful and useful for others at all times. When we have such a team of even a few courageous and honest servants of God, the nation is made, the world is saved.[20]

10. Need of the Study and Practice of True Religion

There is a need of infusing the ideology of Positive Religion among people through encouraging the study and propagation of the true ideals of religion, i.e. ideals of truth, service and sacrifice. This can be supplemented through circulation of the extracts from the lives of great men who practiced the principles of true religion in their lives and are the living embodiment of true religion. This will cement the different sections of the people into cohesive unity and remove all differences based on caste, colour, creed, sex and lead to emotional integration. Mahatma Gandhi has rightly said, "No man can live without religion" and he further says, "There are some who in the egoism of their reason declare that they have nothing to do with religion. But that is like a man saying that he breathes, but that he has no nose." Again he says, "My devotion to truth has drawn me into the field of politics; and I can say without the slightest hesitation, and yet in humility; that those who say that religion, has nothing to do with politics do not know what religion means." It is obvious that he is using it in a sense—probably moral and ethical more than any other—different from that of the critics of religion. According to Prof. John Dewey "any activity pursued on behalf of an ideal end against obstacles, and inspite of threats of personal loss, because of conviction of its general and enduring value, is religious in quality." Nehru admits that true religion means inner craving and spiritual growth of human beings. A truly religious man seeks for truth at all costs with single-minded sincerity and is prepared to make any sacrifice for it. Thus, there is a need to encourage the study and practice of true religion. We can say that mechanical efficiency is not enough. What we need to develop is the human approach. As Graham Wallas says: "In the case of government officers, most of those who have had dealings with them would say that they need to be humanized. The official should be a man, should be known as a man and should be expected to behave as a man."

The people inhabiting the developing world expect their government to pull them out of the morass of distressing under-development. This would be possible only provided the efforts of the governments are comprehensive, selective, co-ordinated and sustained. Besides, timely action backed by a strong will and determination at all decision-making and operational levels can change the complexion of our socio-economic scene.

Public Administration in the developing countries has the potential and can be optimized. The need is to enforce its reputation, prestige, credibility and viability. Public services properly recruited, rightly trained, properly motivated and given the congenial environment, can help in fulfilment of the ideals of the country. Thus, the public service would have to work hard with dedication to achieve the results. (Chart 9.3)

Let us have a great ideal, an ideal that will startle us with its greatness. That is the only kind of an ideal to hold before our minds eye and to work for. Little by little our imperfections and difficulties will vanish and instead of regarding life as a drudgery, instead of shrinking from it, we shall bless this life which offers so many opportunities. We shall find joy even in the little daily tasks and wherever we are placed we shall know happiness

Pure, we Must be,
Sincere, We Must Become.

CHART 9.3

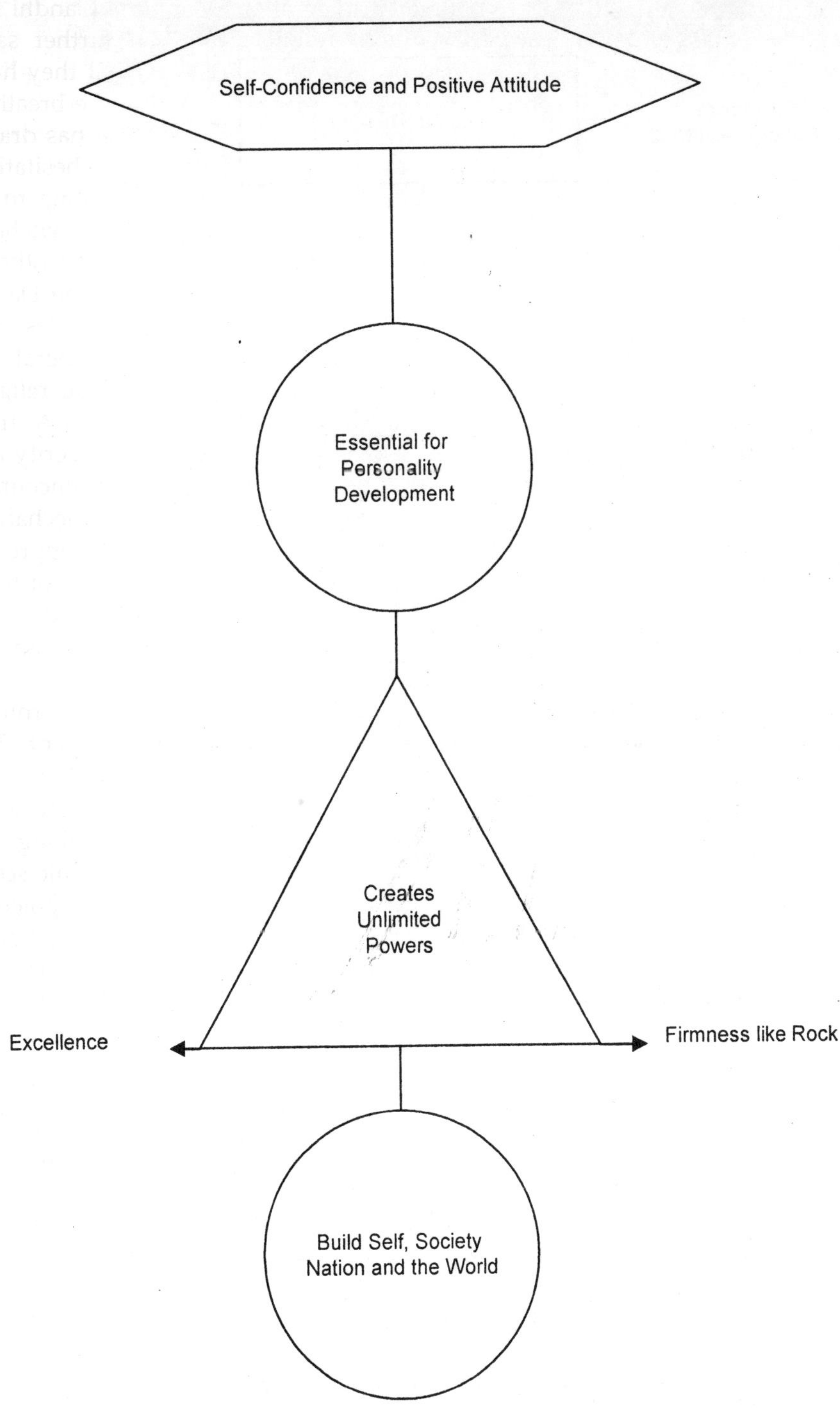
Self-Confidence and Positive Attitude
Essential for Personality Development
Creates Unlimited Powers
Excellence
Firmness like Rock
Build Self, Society Nation and the World

Chart 9.4

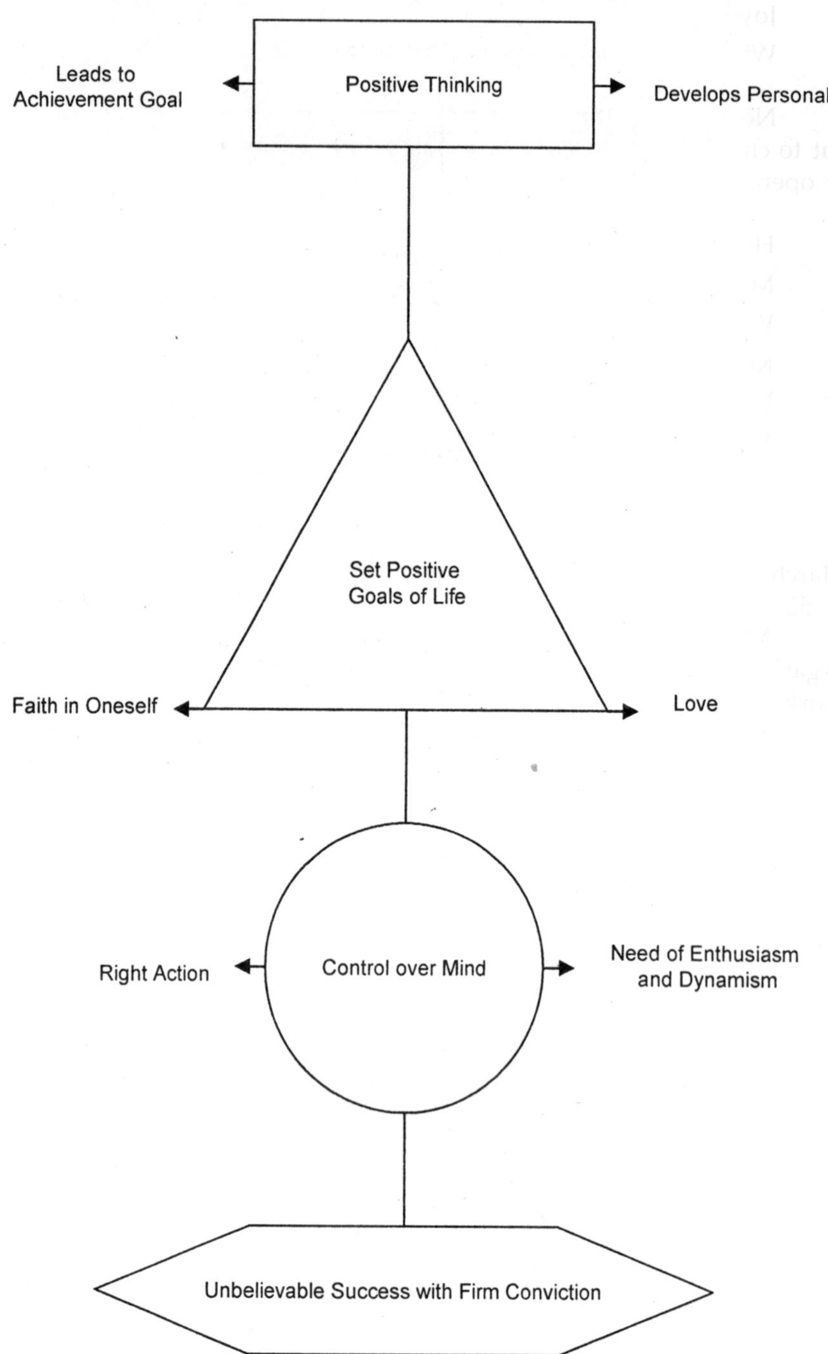
Leads to
Achievement Goal
Positive Thinking
Develops Personality
Set Positive
Goals of Life
Faith in Oneself
Love
Right Action
Control over Mind
Need of Enthusiasm
and Dynamism
Unbelievable Success with Firm Conviction

Earnestness, We Must Befriend,
Dedicated Living, We Must Bequeath.
Joyous Living, We must Behold,
When We Live in And For the beloved Alone.[21]

Not all revolutionaries set out to change the world *per se*—they set out to change their worlds. And in so doing, change how the world thinks or operates in some way.

Honour your own self
Mediate on your own self
Worship your own self
Kneel to your own self
Understand your own self
You god dwells within you as you.

—*Swami Muktananda*

Mishra Shukla in her article, "Fine Balance in Life Plus", January-March, 2004, Feels about women which are valid for men also a to a, p. 52.

Many women have achieved new heights despite all the barriers organizations and unfair bosses put to them. They did this with their hard work, perseverence, intellect and intuition. Here are some ways in which they did this:

- Understand the environment in which you work. It is better to test the waters before you take a dip.
- Adatptability and flexibility can take you a long way.
- Maintain focus on your priorities in terms of work and the goals you want to achieve.
- Work on the business priorities in terms of work and the goals you want to achieve.
- Work on the business priorities. It is too easy to get caught up in everyday emergencies and other people's requests.
- Learn to delegate and trust that your people will do their job.
- You may be phenomenal at some specific skill, but that talent will do you no good, if it's not a key element to the job you are performing.
- Be more than good at whatever job you accept—be exceptional.
- Learn to be effective with people because, believe it or not, your peers play a big role in your promotion.

Notes and References

1. Swami Chinmayanada, A Manual of Self-Unfoldment, Central Chinmaya Mission Trust, Mumbai, 2001, p. 15.
2. *Ibid.*, p. 24.
3. Swami Chinmayananda, We Must Control, Chinmaya Mission Trust, Mumbai, 2001, p. 3.
4. Swami Jagadatmananda, Learn to Live, Vol. I, Sri Ramakrishna Math, Chennai, 2000, p. 52.
5. *Ibid.*, pp. 53-54.
6. *Ibid.*, p. 55.
7. Swami Chinmayananda, We Must, Central Chinmaya Mission Trust, Mumbai, 2001, p. 84.
8. Swami Chinmayananda, The Art of Man Making, Chinmaya Mission Trust, Mumbai, 2002, p. 314.
9. Swami Jagadatmananda, Learn to Live, Vol. I, *op. cit.*, p. 243.
10. *Ibid.*, p. 251.
11. Swami Jagadatmananda, Learn to Live, Vol. II, p. 44.
12. Swami Chinmayananda, A Manual of Self-Unfoldment, *op. cit.*, p. 119.
13. Swami Chinmayananda, A Manual of Self-Unfoldment, *op. cit.*, p. 42.
14. *Ibid.*, p. 37.
15. *Ibid.*, pp. 49-50.
16. Swami Chinmayananda, The Art. of Man Making, Central Chinmaya Mission Trust, Mumbai, 2002, p. 81.
17. CCMT, Mumbai, 2002, p. 53
18. Swami Tejomajananda, Right Thinking, CCMT, Mumbai, 2002, p. 29
19. S.K. Bhatia, Business Ethics and Management Values, New Delhi, Deep & Deep, 2002, p. 14.
20. Swami Chinmayananda, We Must, Central Chinmaya Mission, Mumbai, 2001, p. 30.
21. *Ibid.*, p. 38.

CHAPTER 10

IMPORTANT VALUES EDUCATION FOR MENTAL HEALTH

"Wisdom is knowing things in different ways (Atthasaline). Give charity out of devotion, always maintain the moral precepts, find delight in meditation, and you will attain the celestial life."

—(*Dukkhappattakigathal*)

Important Values Education for Mental Health

"Abstain from all unwholesome deeds, perform wholesome ones, purify your mind."

—(*Dhammapada*, XIV, 5, 183)

"You are your own master, you make your own future. Therefore, discipline yourself as a horse trader trains a thoroughbred."

—(*Dhammapada, XXV, 21, 380*)

I. NON-VIOLENCE

Non-violence is not mere abstinence from harming others by our thoughts and deeds. Non-violence also means pure love towards all. Love, friendship and kindness are just another aspect of non-violence. When saints practise non-violence the currents of pure love emanate from their heart. There are instances where even ordinary men who have not practised any spiritual exercise like meditation and prayer have experienced peace and contentment in the presence of such great men. There are also instances where birds and animals too have experienced great joy and fearlessness in the company of such holy men.

Swami Jagadatmananda observes that Ahimsa in its spiritual import means never having cruel intentions. Non-injury is the spirit that should dominate all our motives. Our intentions should not be polluted by even a trace of cruelty or hatred. Harmlessness consists not so much in never causing physical injury to a being as in never contemplating to do harm of any sort. Practicing non-injury physically is impossible. To continue living, some kind of physical harm is unavoidable. But even while bringing about unavoidable disturbances around ourselves, if our motives are pure and clean, the harm so brought about is not regarded as injury. If you protect yourself against robber in your own home or protest against

CHART 10.1

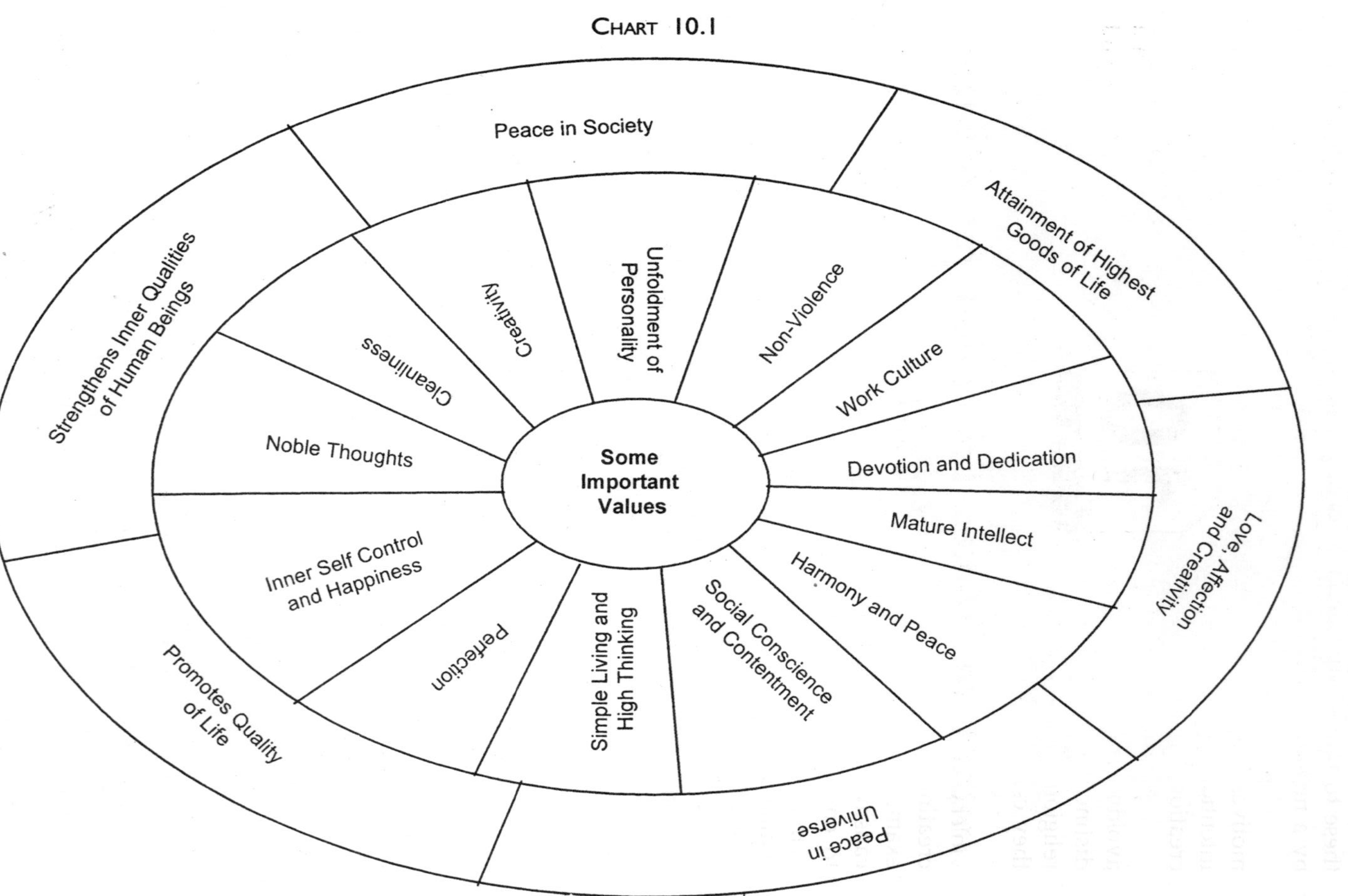
Peace in Society
Strengthens Inner Qualities of Human Beings
Attainment of Highest Goods of Life
Love, Affection and Creativity
Promotes Quality of Life
Peace in Universe
Some Important Values
Unfoldment of Personality
Creativity
Cleanliness
Noble Thoughts
Inner Self Control and Happiness
Perfection
Simple Living and High Thinking
Social Conscience and Contentment
Harmony and Peace
Mature Intellect
Devotion and Dedication
Work Culture
Non-Violence

aggressors, you are not transgressing ahimsa. To smash a serpent or a scorpion in your house is not an act of cruelty. On the contrary, to allow these to flourish in the name of non-violence is weakness sanctioned only by a misinterpreted culture.[1]

Thus, non-injury is a value of life to be applied at the level of our motives. Our motives must be non-injurious and pure. This purity of intention can arise only out of a deep sense of oneness with the Lord's creation and compassion toward all beings, good and bad alike.

Non-violence is broader in scope. Non-violence is not merely avoiding violence. It is only another name of love, love which makes no distinction between friend and foe. This is the highest ideal that any religion has preached. Certainly it cannot be meant for all and sundry as they cannot practice it.

Violence has become a greatest pollutant of this life. People do violences in the name of religion, fundamentalism and personal gains creating permanent scars on this globe. Gujarat violence is a recent example. Such incidences spoil the environment and disturb its peace causing enmity, hatred and jealousy among people causing a great danger to environment. Swami Rama has laid down some principles, based on Gandhiji's ideology which if followed can bring communal harmony, national integration and international brotherhood. All these principles are based upon the philosophy of Shrimad Bhagavad Gita, Vedas, etc. To quote:

1. Non-violence and cowardice cannot go together, because non-violence is a perfect expression of love that casts our fear. To be brave because one is armed implies an element of fear. The power of ahimsa is an extremely vital and active force which does not come from physical strength.
2. A true follower of ahimsa does not believe in disappointment. He dwells above in perennial happiness and peace. That peace and joy do not come to him who is proud of his intellect or learning; they come to him who is full of faith and has an undivided and single-pointed mind.
3. The intellect can produce many wonders, but non-violence is a matter of the heart. It does not come through intellectual exercises.
4. Hatred is not overcome by hatred, but rather by love. This is an unalterable law.
5. Devotion is not mere worship with the lips. It is self-surrender with mind, action, and speech.
6. Gandhi did not believe in the barriers created by religions, cultures, superstitions, and mistrust. He taught and lived the brotherhood of all religions.
7. Gandhi believed in the art of living without concern for the fruits of ones actions. He practiced not worrying about success or failure, but paid attention to the work at hand without feeling the slightest anxiety or fatigue.

8. In order to enjoy life one should not be selfishly attached to anything. Non-attachment means to have a pure motive and a correct means without any worry or desired result. He who gives up action falls, but he who gives up the reward rises and is liberated.
9. Yoga is the complete re-integration of all the states of mind, the intellect, senses, emotions, instincts, and every level of personality. It is a process of becoming whole.
10. One's mantra becomes one's staff of life and carries one through every ordeal. Each repetition has a new meaning and carries one nearer and nearer to God. It is capable of transforming that which is negative in the personality into that which is positive, and it can gradually integrate, divided and opposing thoughts at deeper and deeper levels of consciousness (Based on Gandhiji Ideals).[2]

If you practice non-violence out of cowardice, it is no merit at all. Real non-violence means the greatest strength and power of endurance that a man can attain to. It means the greatest courage coupled with the greatest love. It means total absence of hatred. That is what Sri Krisna tried to teach Arjuna in the Gita. He exhorted them to do his duty, which in his case happened to be fighting, without hating others.[3]

HE the Dalai Lama in his article, "Religion of the 21st Century", observes:

Just when we have entered the 21st Century, we are able to see the importancce of changing our mindset and know the potential of internal development by nurturing the ideals of non-violence and peace. Various religious heads should rather engage in a common effort to contribute to the welfare of humankind.

The goal of self-realisation (truth, which to him was god) through the practice of non-violence stamped Gandhiji every thought, word and deed. Mahatma Gandhi observed that "This ahimsa is the basis of the search for truth. I am realising every day that the search is vain unless it is founded on ahimsa as the basis . . . . "

If faith in Gandhian non-violence needs a reminder we only have to look at the examples of Martin Luther King Jr., Nelson Mandela and Anug Sen Suu Ki, all of whom have been inspired by Gandhi in fashioning their non-violent protests against tyranny, oppression and racism. Towering figures, all, they have proved once more that non-violence has a moral power that exacts our respect and reverence in a way that violence never can.

Gandhi called his overall method of non-violent action satyagraha. This translates roughly as 'truth force'. A fuller rendering would be 'the force that is generated through adherence to truth'. For Gandhi, non-violence defined a broader concept, namely a way of life based on love and compassion. Satyagraha and non-violent action do not refer to the same thing. Satyagraha is a form of non-violent action—Gandhi's own version of it.

Gandhi practised two types of satyagraha. The first was civil disobedience, which entailed breaking a law and courting arrest. When we hear this term today, our minds tend to stress the 'disobedience' part of it. But for Gandhi, 'civil' was just as important. He used 'civil' not just in its meaning of 'relating to citizenship and government' but as 'civilized' or 'polite'.[4]

The ahimsa is a high ideal. We must proceed step by step towards that ideal. The mind must be cleansed of all unclean, we get some real spiritual experience. Ahimsa as a theory and ahimsa as practised in one's own life are wide apart. In the Isavasya Upanisad you read, 'When a person sees the Self in all people and all people in the Self, then he hates no one. This is a recurring idea in the Upanisads—that self-realization is the basis of true ahimsa. When one realizes the Self, one hates none.

2. WORK CULTURE

I. Importance of Work—Work is Worship/Dharma

The first factor necessary for success is work. An individual has to work even though he or she would like to have success without work. There is only one place where success comes before work, and that is in the dictionary. So work is a must for success. We see many people working laboriously. Still, they do not seem to accomplish anything. This is because there is no efficiency in their work. Efficiency is the second factor required for success. The skill or knack of working or performing an action in such a way that it will bear the desired fruit is called efficiency. The third factor required is knowledge, for to perform work knowledge is a must. Knowledge means—

(1) knowledge of our desired goal;
(2) knowledge of the means to attain the goal; and
(3) knowledge of the performer who is going to adopt the means and strive for the goal. This knowledge is called proficiency.

A person who has knowledge but no efficiency cannot be successful. The difference can be seen in the material progress of India as compared to other countries such as the United State or Japan. In India, more emphasis is given to theoretical knowledge. Indian universities impart a lot of information, but practical knowledge is overlooked, while in America more emphasis is given to the practical aspect and work is done efficiently. Therefore even though so many students are graduating from universities in India with outstanding degrees, what is the condition of India materially? We are speaking only from the material point of view at the moment. India's prosperity cannot be compared to the prosperity of the United State, Canada or Japan because India has neglected the practical aspect.[5]

When a person works with inspiration, he never gets tired or exhausted. When man works only for himself, there is perspiration; but when he works for a noble goal there is inspiration. In cases where a man cannot dedicate his actions to the Lord, even if he works for some ideal or goal he will derive tremendous strength from his chosen altar of dedication. The nobler the goal, the greater will be the strength he gains. This is the beauty of love and dedication, which brings efficiency in life.[6]

Work ethic embraces work responsibility, work conscience, ethical work conduct. If one has the satisfaction that he is contributing his very best to his organisation and is not just earning the bread, then this would be the true feeling of work ethics. Work ethic demands that one works for attaining organisational objectives in its fullest measure.

Behind every achievement that we see in this world today, is the unseen hand of the human will. The material comforts, scientific achievements are all the products crystallised out of the human will and determination. The human will-power has conquered Nature, and made Her a slave for the welfare of mankind, and in the process has ever created things which were not even available in the world before. Behind all the technological progress are the determined efforts of hundreds of dedicated men and women, who faced all the challenges to make their dreams come true.

Many of what we see today as solid facts of life and proof of man's achievements were only mess ideas yesterday in the minds of a few men of great will-power. Those ideas would not have become realities, had they not the will and determination to put their ideas into practice. Our scriptures too have given us examples of men of great will, like Viswamithra who could even create a new world out of his sheer power of willing. All men of achievement had the blessing of tremendous will-power in their makeup, and History is full of names of such men of achievements.[7]

Bata K. Dey in his Article, 'Work Culture in India—Achievements and Failure' rightly says that culture is not something which can be imported or transplanted; it must grow from within; it grows, and it does, in fertile soil and congenial climate. Gap in capital equipment or technology can be filled by import. You can even buy management, but not dedication, commitment, culture. How to create that is a million dollar question. An inexpensive answer to such a costly question is that, work culture tends to be congruous with and is an extension of, the societal, indeed national culture. And the latter, at the moment, is the elusive commodity, despite this country ancient civilization and old culture. The search is on. And we shall succeed.[8]

Murtaza Mithani, Chairman and Managing Director of Wintech Group in his article, "The High Road", in *The Tribune,* dated June 28, 2000 expects his employees to be committed to their work. "As the head of an organization, I, expect my employees to be innovative, competitive and flexible. They should possess total commitment, be actively involved in every day work, and have no hastiness while interacting. He wants his team to be able to work in synergy with various departments. Failures and challenges should be treated as a stepping stone to success. Think big, create your own space and help yourself."

3. HARMONY AND PEACE

In the world today, we are living through an age of confusions and tensions, both within and without us. The external challenges persecute us and render our lives unhappy and sorrow ridden. The intelligent philosophy of the Rishis advises man 'to live in harmony' with the situations in life and steadily work on to meet them with discretion and constant application. When we live, thus, for a period of time, a subjective poise develops, giving us inward peace and tranquillity, which, thereafter, remains unaffected by external threats and onslaughts.[9]

Revered Shri Vethatheri, Maharishi says, "Harmony is a precious treasure of human life." Real success and satisfaction, happiness are the different facets of harmony. If one is to enjoy the benefits of life to the fullest, it is necessary to develop and maintain harmony; and for this understanding the philosophy of nature is required.

Harmony should be maintained in all spheres of life, and these are:

- Between body and life;
- Between wisdom and habits;
- Between self and society;
- Between the purpose of life and the method of living; and
- Between will and nature.

The more one understands life, the more one will achieve harmony; and success will be proportionate to that. No doubt, harmonizing life is a difficult task, but it is worth all the striving, for it is the only way to equip oneself to enjoy life to the fullest extent and to reach the goal of life, which is the perfection of consciousness. By the development of knowledge man comes to understand the cause and effect system which is the law of nature.[10]

It is clear that it is not enough for a world leader to be politically astute. It may be an additional qualification, but the essential requisite is for him to have a character that will command respect from all including those who disagree with him. People aspiring for world leadership have to have something of the moral stature that characterized Buddha and Christ. They must have the same compassion and wisdom so that the weaker nations may feel that their interests are safe in their hands. As world leaders, they must accept the responsibility of helping the weaker nations grow stronger. If there is any injustice done to them, they must see it redressed quickly. Now that technology has unified the world, they must help this unity grow stronger and more meaningful by promoting the spirit of co-operation and friendship among the nations. The world's problems are not merely political and economic. they are also moral. Life's purpose is not accumulation of wealth and pursuit of sense-pleasure, but higher development—morally and spiritually. World leaders should never tire of repeating this. But they themselves should set an example in this respect.

The Dalai Lama, while speaking on the occasion of the Theosophical Society of India's centenary celebration, put his finger on the real problem when he said that at the root of the troubles which afflicted man today lay his own pride and selfishness. He said that there could be no peace on earth so long as man continued to neglect moral values. Progress in science and technology was good, but this, he pointed out, needed to be matched by advancement in moral qualities if chances of conflicts were to be minimized.

4. DEVOTION AND DEDICATION

Of the innumerable techniques prescribed by the rishis for self-development, the most popular ones are the path of selfless dedicated service (karma yoga), the path of discriminative knowledge (jnana yoga), and the mystic path of self-development through disciplined contemplation (raja yoga).

According to Sage Narada, true devotion for the Lord is superior and nobler to all these, because devotion is the final outcome of all other methods of self-development.

This supreme devotion is indeed, as a technique, even superior to the path of action, the path of knowledge, and the path of disciplined contemplation. (Narada Bhakti Sutra, II:I:25)

All the other paths are the means that take the seekers to the final goal of spiritual experience, but in devotion there is very little difference in essence between the means and the end, between the way and the goal. Love alone is love's own end and fulfilment. Devotion is both the means and the end. As long as residual vasanas (inherent tendencies) are still lingering in the devotee's personality, so long is devotion only the path. But when, as a result of his love for the Lord, his vasanas disappear totally, a stage comes when his supreme love itself becomes the Lord of love Supreme.

Then in all other paths, devotion is the one most readily available and most easily attainable. (Narada Bhakti Sutra, VI:1:58).

Having dedicated all activities unto Him, the devotee should turn all desire, anger, pride, and so forth toward Him alone (Narada Bhakti Sutra, VI:2:65).

Having gained this supreme devotion, the devotee attains perfection and immortality and becomes extremely satisfied. (Narada Bhakti Sutra, I:1:4).

Acharya Vinoba Bhave says that knowledge, love, and constant effort are the three legs on which life stands. If one of the legs of a tripod is broken, it cannot stand, since all three legs are needed. This is also the condition of life. Even if we logically distinguish between devotion (bhakti), knowledge (jnana), and action (karma), we cannot divide them in experience. The three together make up one great entity.

Emotional intelligence can promote Devotion and Dedication.

Emotional intelligence is concerned with achieving one's goals through the ability to manage one's own feelings and emotions, to be sensitive to, and influence other key people, and to balance one's motives and drives with conscientious and ethical behaviours. The following are the characteristics of EI:

(a) Inter-personal sensitivity covering competencies like listening and sensitivity.
(b) Motivating, including impact and energy.
(c) Emotional Resilience.
(d) Influence and Adaptability covering both influencing and negotiating ability and being adaptable in various types of situations and cultures.
(e) Decisiveness and assertiveness.
(f) Integrity.
(g) Leadership including motivating other people.

5. INNER SELF-CONTROL AND HAPPINESS

Happiness that arises from consistent effort and inner self-control can yield a greater beauty and a larger sense of fulfilment. In the beginning its practice may be painful and arduous, but a person who has the necessary courage and heroism, to walk the precipitous path of self-purification, creativity, and inward balance comes to enjoy the subtlest happiness and the all-fulfilling sense of inner peace. The flimsy happiness that is gained through sense indulgence and sense gratification is a joy that is fleeting, vanishing as quickly as it comes, and after its onslaught there is a terrific undercurrent that upsets our equilibrium and drags us into ill-reputed dissipation. This happiness lasts only so long as the sense organs are actually in contact with sense objects.

Contentment with whatever has come to one as one's just share is the motto of all serious seekers. To endlessly entertain and satisfy the demands of life would be an unending game, for the mind has a knack of breeding its own demands very quickly. The policy of contentment is the only intelligent attitude to be taken up by sincere seekers or else there will be no time to seek, to strive for, and to achieve the divine goal of life. Self-integration is the reward promised for all faithful pursuits.[11]

Sense-objects are pleasure giving only because of the Self which manifests through them, and not independently, for the Self is, by its very nature, the most beloved of all. The self, therefore, is ever-blissful and can never suffer any grief or misery.

This great joy of the Self is not readily available because of mental agitations at all times. These become, as it were, a wall between the happiness which is inherent in the Self, and the world outside. The acquisition of a desired object ends the disturbances created by the desire, and the Light of Consciousness beams out from behind the mind. In our lack of discrimination we understand that the joy is in the object secured. In fact, the joy is not in the object at all. But it makes me joyful if it brings me a contact with myself. It is only because of the Atman, the Self that each one of us ekes out for himself the maximum joy.

Universally, everybody wants joy, but nobody seems to know where exactly is the source of happiness. Hence, everyone runs after sense-objects. Here the Teacher is asking us to pause for a moment, and to reflect upon the location of the fountain head of joy. Indeed, the Atman is of the nature of Bliss and Beatitude, and there is not even a trace of sorrow even to veil the face of the Atman.

Srimad Bhagawad Gita nicely points out that everybody in the world seeks happiness. But very few know what is real happiness and how to attain it. Due to this ignorance they run away with the wrong idea that happiness consists only in enjoying the objects of senses. That is why they hanker after them and strive to attain them. And when they find themselves balked in their efforts, they are seized with anger. But as a rule one who is habitually under the sway of lust and anger can never be happy. One who is under the sway of desire and the one who is under the sway of anger, both betake themselves to all sorts of mischief's and vices—the former for the sake of a wife, progeny, wealth and honour, etc. and the latter with view to harming others. They thereby expose themselves to illness, grief, ignominy, infamy, perturbation, unrest, anxiety and various kinds of agonies in this world.[12]

Bhagavad Geeta (Gita Press, Gorakhpur) in Sloka 59, Chapter 2, observes that sense objects turn away from him, who does not enjoy them with his senses; but the taste for them persists. This relish also disappears in the case of the man of stable mind when he sees the Supreme.

In the general acceptance of the term, the world 'Nirahara' is understood to mean one who gives up food and observes a complete fast. But the word has not been used in that sense in this verse, for the word 'Vaisayah' used in plural shows that abstinence not only from food but from sense-enjoyments in general is meant here. Through the renunciation of food only one object of the senses, viz. taste, is given up; the other objects, namely, sound, touch, colour and smell are not renounced. Therefore, the word 'food' (Ahara) should be understood in a wider sense; Thus, understood, every sense has its own 'food' in the shape of the object of its enjoyment. According to this interpretation the words 'Niraharasya Dehinah' should be taken to mean that human being, identifying himself with the body, who has given up the enjoyment of all the objects of senses through his senses.

The verse shows that even the unenlightened man who has given up sense-enjoyments has outwardly withdrawn his senses from sense-objects, as the tortoise draws in its limbs; but his taste for such objects will persist,—his attachment for them will not disappear. That is why his senses will continue internally to run after those objects and will Thus, keep his mind oscillating. This is what is meant by the Lord when he says that though the sense-objects turn away from that man, the taste for them persists. The following illustrations will make the point clear.

For fear of ailment, or fear of death, or due to any other cause a man who is addicted to sense-enjoyment gives up the enjoyment of one or more objects. For the time he abstains from the enjoyment of a particular object or objects, the object or objects practically cease to exist for him. Even so if he gives up the enjoyment of all objects, all objects will cease to exist for him for the time being; but such a renunciation, inspired as it is by constraint, fear or any other motive, is made notwithstanding his attachment for those objects. Such a renunciation cannot bring about real cessation of attachment or attraction for the things of the world.

When a hypocrite, in order to deceive people, gives up outwardly all activities of the five senses of perception and the five organs of action, all objects of the senses will outwardly cease to exist for him; but owing to the persistence of attachment for those objects, he will mentally continue to dwell on them (III.6). Therefore, his attachment for those objects remains as strong as ever.

In order to attain mystic powers, or with a view to obtaining any other form of worldly enjoyment, a man desiring worldly happiness may externally renounce the activities of all the ten organs, and may cease to dwell on them even mentally at the time of meditation or when absorbed in Samadhi; and yet his attraction for sense-enjoyments will continue, his attachment for them will persist.

In this way, through outward renunciation of objects, the objects no doubt will cease to exist, but the attraction for them will not cease. Herein lies the distinction between restraint of the senses as practiced by an ignorant man and that practiced by a wise man.

Construing the word 'Rasa' as mental enjoyment, the word 'Rasavarjam' may be interpreted to mean that such a person though bodily renouncing objects of enjoyment mentally goes on enjoying the same; but inasmuch as such mental enjoyment presupposes attachment for the object of enjoyment, the interpretation of 'Rasa' as attachment covers this meaning as well. Secondly, mental enjoyment of objects of senses can be avoided even before God-Realization with the help of a resolute will or discrimination or by recourse to reason; whereas the realization of God lays the axe at its very root, viz., attachment, and herein lies the fulfilment of God-Realization, not merely in suspending enjoyment with the mind of objects of the senses. Therefore, the interpretation of the Word 'Rasa' as given above is quite reasonable and proper.

The word 'Asya', in the second line of the verse, refers to the yogi of stable mind, who is the subject of discussion in these verses. This second line of the verse says that in as much as the Yogi possessed of a stable mind obtains a direct vision of God, the ocean of supreme Bliss, he ceases to have the faintest trace of any attachment for worldly objects. For attachment for worldly objects proceeds from nescience, which disappears totally when there is a direct vision of God. It is only due to their infatuation that ordinary men of the world find happiness in sense-enjoyments; that is why they feel attracted towards sense-enjoyments, whereas in reality there lies not the least happiness in sense-enjoyments. Whatever happiness is imagined to be derived from sense-enjoyments is nothing but a very faint reflection of a fraction of the Bliss which lies in God, the embodiment of supreme Bliss. Just as the light appearing in the moon that shines in a moon-lit night is nothing but a reflection of the sun's light, and with the rising of the sun the light of the moon disappears, even so the happiness which one finds in the possession and enjoyment of worldly objects is nothing but a reflection of the Bliss obtaining in the All-blissful God. Therefore, he who realizes that embodiment of supreme Bliss, viz. God, neither finds any happiness in the enjoyment of worldly objects (II.69), nor feels any the least attraction for them.

For God is such a wonderful, transcendent and supernatural object of attraction that when he is actually realized, the soul feels so enchanted; enraptured and ravished that it loses its very identity. Who can in that state think of any other object? that is why it has been said that on the realization of God all attachment for objects of enjoyment gets eradicated once for all. Thus, in the restraint of senses evinced by a man of realization it is not the sense-objects alone which turn away from him; nay, attachment itself with its root. Nescience, ceases, once for all. Herein lies the specialty of sense-restraint as practiced by the Yogi possessed of a stable mind.

6. UNFOLDMENT OF PERSONALITY

A life organised for the discovery of the potentialities already within ourselves, and the ordering of our behaviour so as to nurture and nourish them, is a life well spent. Herein our success depends upon the amount of transformation we can successfully bring about in our personality and character. The vital question is not how many talents each one of us has, but how much of our existing talents are we capable of exploring, developing and exploiting. An individual many have many talents, and yet, he can be a miserable failure in life. That person is successful who makes a practical use of at least one great talent that he possesses.

Our present and future welfare, thus, mainly depends upon ourselves. Let us never look outside ourselves for help. Let us not fall in to the delusion that the influence of others would enable us to do better or accomplish more. All our success entirely depends upon ourselves. Let us realise these fundamentals. We must.[13]

Swami Vivekanand says that follow the heart. A pure heart sees beyond the intellect; it gets inspired. It knows things that reason can never know, and whenever there is conflict between the pure heart and the intellect, always side with the pure heart, even if you think what your heart is doing is unreasonable.

When it is desirous of doing good to others, your brain may tell you that it is not expedient to do so, but follow your heart, and you will find that you make less mistakes than by following your intellect.

The pure heart is the best mirror for the reflection of truth, so all these disciplines are for the purification of the heart. And as soon as it is pure, the truth will flash upon it in a minute; all truth in the universe will manifest in your heart, if you are sufficiently pure.

There are many practices for the cultivation of dispassion, some of which are given below:

(1) One should constantly impress on one's mind by recourse to reason, the absence of any charm, love or delight in the objects of the world.

(2) One should always remember and realize that the objects of the world are transient and subject to sorrows and evils in the shape of birth and death, old-age and disease, and are the source of fear.

(3) One should study elevating scriptures reveling the real truth about God and the world.

(4) One should cultivate association with men possessed of the highest form of dispassion. In the absence of direct association, one should keep before one's mental eyes and dwell on the likenesses and lives of saints possessed of such dispassion.

(5) One should realize the ephemeral nature of the world through the sight of old, dilapidated mansions, and the ruins of deserted towns and villages.

(6) Perceiving the one and indivisible existence of Brahma, one should refuse to recognize the separate existence of anything else.

(7) One should hear again and again, from the lips of qualified souls, the indescribable virtues, glory, truth, love and mysteries of God and the glories of his divine sports as well as of his transcendental beauty and sweetness, and knowing the truth about them should have full faith in them and feel enraptured by them.

Similar to those mentioned above, there are other practices also, which may be adopted with advantage for the cultivation of dispassion.

Constant 'practice' and cultivation of dispassion, both are necessary for bringing the mind under control. 'Practice' is like a beautiful channel for the flow of thought-currents in the direction of God, and 'dispassion' is like an embankment to restrain the flow of the mind towards the objects of enjoyment. But it should be borne in mind that they are helpful to each other. Practice promotes dispassion and *vice-versa*. Therefore, the mind can be subdued and brought under control even by adopting one of these methods in the proper way.[14]

7. NOBLE THOUGHTS

The value of work is judged, not by its quantum but by the quality and texture thereof. The quality of action depends upon the ideals which guide and inspire an individual working in the world. The loftier and nobler the ideals, the greater will be the beauty of his actions and efficiency. All mighty men of superhuman achievements have been inspired by such ideals, wonderfully great and noble work in the world and the fruits of their actions are enjoyed by generations which follow them.

In the present world, man is found wanting in definite ideals for channelising his activities. He works with a selfish attitude and has no goal or vision in life to inspire him to take to better and brighter actions. He experiences monotony in any work undertaken by him, whether he be a clerk in the secretariat or a manager of an organisation. He is fatigued no sooner than he reaches his office and commerce's his work; and by evening he has hardly any energy left to reach his home. In such a state of affairs:[15]

Srimad Bhagavad Gita publised by Gita Press, Gorakhpur, Sloka 15 Chapter XVII suggests that words which cause no annoyance to others and are absolutely untainted by calumny and slander, etc., are called 'Anudvegakara'. Similarly, truthful words are those which state the bare truth in order to convey to others a correct idea of what one has actually seen, heard or experienced. Loving, sweet, artless and gentle words, which are pleasing to hear and are altogether free from acerbity, pungency, coldness, sarcasm, insolence and other faults, are known as 'Priya'. And words which are ultimately beneficial to all, which are altogether free from violence malice, jealousy and animosity, and are full of love, compassion and good wishes are called 'Hita'.

The uttering of only such words as combine in themselves all the four virtues, viz., inoffensiveness, veracity, agreeability and wholesomeness are free from all impurities of speech.

8. SOCIAL CONSCIENCE AND CONTENTMENT

Life is meant to bring us happiness. Negative actions always bring pain and sorrow, but constructive actions bring us pleasure and joy. The most important thing is transforming our minds. In our daily lives compassion is most effective. We all want to be happy and one of the most important foundations for happiness is mental peace. From my own limited experience we have found that the greatest inner tranquillity comes from the development of love and compassion. The more we care for the happiness of others, the greater our own sense of well-being. Cultivating a close, warm-hearted feeling for others automatically puts the mind at ease. This helps remove whatever fears or insecurities we may have and gives us the strength to cope with any obstacles we may encounter. It is the ultimate source of success in life.

As individuals what is particularly important is that we develop a kind heart, a sense of love, compassion and respect for others. We believe it is important that issues like working for peace in the world do not merely remain the business of politicians and diplomats; we should all be involved. The shape of the future is of great interest to all of us. I am convinced that even if only a few individuals try to create mental peace and happiness within themselves and act responsibly and kind heartedly towards others, they will have a positive influence in their community.[16]

The twentieth century was marred by conflict and war. Therefore, it is especially important that we take steps to ensure that this new century will be characterized instead by non-violence and dialogue, the preconditions of peaceful co-existence.

Contentment does not depend upon externals; it changes with our mental attitude. John Milton wrote:

> The mind is its own place, and in itself
> Can make a heaven of Hell, a hell of Heaven.

Vedanta says: We cannot change the world, we can only change ourselves. The world is like a dog's curly tail. No matter how hard we try to straighten it, it will always curl up again. We matter how hard we try to straighten it, it will always curl up again. We can only straighten ourselves.

Whatever after due consideration and analysis you find to be conducive to the good, the benefit, the welfare of all beings, that doctrine, believe in, cling to, and take as your guide.[17]

9. CREATIVITY

Creativity is defined as, "Energising connected mental communication to bring out something original, new and different." In other words, it means "creativity is the imaginatively gifted recombination of known elements into something new." We are here more concerned about the problem-solving element. It therefore suffices to say, "Creativity is keeping blocked minds open."

Creativity plays a vital role in decision-making and problem-solving. It helps individuals and the groups to arrive at better decision-making. Creative decisions are good to the extent that they depart from the routine and cut new grounds, not for its own sake, but for improving the quality of the outcomes.

Creativity is also a high risk activity. A great deal of time and efforts are required to generate new ideas. Excessive use of policies, procedures, rules and schedules impede creativity. Proper training in creativity for solving problems is very essential, so that the right type of technique is used.[18]

10. MATURE INTELLECT

Three things are necessary to develop a mature intellect:

1. Deep Thinking

Our thoughts, words and actions should arise from deep and serious thinking, and not by impulsive. Silly and controversial statements made by persons occupying responsible positions in the society are a clear sign of immature intellect.

2. Responsibility

The natural tendency of man is to avoid responsibility. However, a mature person is always ready to take the whole responsibility on his shoulder. Responsible people are honoured and respected everywhere. They fulfil their responsibilities with utmost care. Everyone should cultivate this awareness regarding his responsibility towards family, society and nation.

3. Sincerity

Every one commits mistakes but a sincere man accepts it and tries to rectify it. A sincere person never does anything wrong intentionally. Even if he makes a mistake out of ignorance it is only an error and not a mistake. If one is sincere about his purpose, he will be able to develop a mature intellect. People will have faith in his words and actions.

Subtle intellect is that capacity of the intellect which can grasp the subtle truths within a short time. There are many things in nature which we cannot perceive through our senses. Says Yama in the Katha Upanisad (I.2.20):

"This Atman is subtler than the subtle and greater than the great; it dwells in the heart of every creature."

Steady intellect is a natural and spontaneous state for a man of realization. Since he knows the truth, nothing in this world can disturb him. Even ordinary people and spiritual aspirants can derive immense benefit by cultivating a steady intellect. Intellectual, conviction about Reality may help us to develop a steady intellect to a certain extent.

He is a man of steady intellect whose mind is not disturbed by the pair of opposites, namely, happiness and misery, victory and defeat, gain and loss, praise and blame, attachment and hatred, honour and dishonour, heat and cold. Sri Krishna has given a beautiful illustration in the Bhagavad Gita (2.70), of a steady intellect.[19]

'Water enters into the sea from all directions but the sea remains full and unchanged.'

11. CLEANLINESS

Generally, only when body is clean, can the mind be clean. Cleanliness has to start from the gross level. People throw things anywhere, spit at every place. It shows a disorganized mind. One can find out the real cleanliness of a person by seeing his bathroom ! Externally the drawing room could be kept clean, since outsiders visit it. But if one enters his bathroom, his own reality will be known ! Similarly, when a table drawer is pulled open, one can see if he is organized or not. If everything is mixed up in it then person is disorganized. Having too many things gather dust and one has to work hard to maintain them. Being organized should become one's second nature. We should be clean and organized not for others but for our own sake.

After bahya souca (external cleanliness) Antahsoucham (internal cleanliness) comes. Antahsoucham is how to keep our mind clean. We must remember our behaviour itself reflects our mind. The way we speak, etc. We may carefully hide our mind from others, but it surely cannot be hidden from ourselves. Whether one lives in a hut or a palace is not important, but all of us necessarily live in our mind. Mind is our first abode. We know that we cannot get out of our physical body and that we have to live in it for whole of this life. Wherever we go, we travel with the body. Remember that the body is only for one life while mind is for every life. We are trapped in the mind first and then in the body. Taking care of the mind or tending to it is antahsoucham.

What is antahsoucham? If mind is all the time restless, makes us sad, angry, jealous, it is as if we are living with a boiler inside us. Even if one is living at a hill station, where it is always cool, it still does not make the person happy. If he stays near a boiler, he will feel only the heat. Even if the external situation is pleasant, one can have burning feelings like anger, jealousy, etc. troubling him. When jealousy or hatred enters the mind, the person burns inside. Outwardly people may not see his dvesha (hatred) but if he is angry or hates someone, he burns inside, he loses sleep. This situation needs to be corrected. This process of correction is sadhana. How do we do it? It is said in the yoga shastra:

> Maitri karuna mudita upeksanam sukha duhkha punyapunya-visayanam bhavanataha citta prasadanam.
> (Cultivate a feeling of friendliness for a happy person, compassion for miserable, cheerfulness for virtuous and indifference for evil).[20]

12. PERSEVERANCE AND CONSISTENCE

Sthairyam mean sthirata, consistency, perseverance. No work can be done in fits and starts. In order to do things consistently, a person has to be convinced about wanting to do it. To be convinced one has to do satsang and be with people who know the purpose of life. Speaking to them on how to go about with life is necessary. One has no time to lose. Before time is over, what needs to be learnt is how to reach one's destination or goal. A steady commitment in life is required to have a happy ending.

काष्ठादग्निर्जायते मथ्यमानात् ।
भूमिस्तोंय खन्यमाना ददाति ॥
सोत्साहाना नास्ति असाध्यं किञ्चित् ।
मार्गारब्धा : सर्वे यत्ना: फलन्ति ॥

When two pieces of dry twigs are rubbed, fire comes.

Bhumih toyam khanyamanat dadati;

If earth is dug it gives water

Sotasahanam nasti asadhyam kincit,

If there is enthusiasm nothing is impossible.

Margarabdhah sarve yatnaha phalanti

If you start in a proper direction and keep working, you will reach the goal.[21]

Planning and doing Work Earnestly and Sincerely

He who refuses to work with his limbs but sits brooding over the sense objects of pleasure in his mind, he the deluded fool is called a hypocrite.

But who controlling the senses by the mind, unattached, employs his organs of action in Karma Yoga service of all, he O Arjuna, indeed excels.

कर्मोन्द्रियाणि संयम्य य आसते मनसा स्मरन् ।
इन्द्रियार्थान्विमूढात्मा मिथ्याचार: स उच्यते ॥ (3-6)
यस्त्विन्द्रियाणि मनसा नियमयारभतेऽर्जुन ।
कर्मेन्द्रियै : कर्मयोगमसकत: स विशिष्यते ॥ (3-7)

The great Acharyas have said that having discovered a great goal, surrender yourself to that goal and act towards it drawing your inspiration from that goal, and thereby discover a new column of energy. Do not allow this energy to be dissipated in the futile memories of the past, regrets or failures, or in the imagined sorrows of the future, or in the excitement of the present. Thus, bring that entire energy focused into activity. That is the highest creative action in the world outside. Thereby the individual who is till now considered most inefficient finds his way to the highest achievement and success.

13. SIMPLE LIVING AND HIGH THINKING

Simplicity and high thinking leads to happiness and truthful life. The great prophets, scholars and saints believed in and practiced simple living and high thinking. The simple living and high thinking go together. Simple living while on the one hand blesses the doer, on the other hand, it helps others to ensure sustainable development Acharya's call Part 2 (H.H. Jagadguru's in his Madras Discourses) has beautifully explained the need and rationale of simple living as:

"High thinking is inconsistent with complicated material life based on high speed imposed on us by memmon worship. All the graces of life are possible only when we learn the art of living nobly."

Simplicity and high thinking promotes the following qualities in human beings:

1. Simple living protects the people practicing simplicity from evil habits like smoking, drinking, etc.
2. Simple living and high thinking help in the development of mental perfection and firmness.
3. Simple living makes the person practicing it beautiful externally and internally.
4. Simple living promotes the quality of selfless service.
5. Simple living promotes disciplined life.
6. Simple living leads to creativity and betterment of society.

A society thrives best when it is composed of men and women who are intelligent, hard-working, honest, and dutiful. A good society means a society where the average men and women are good. One or two great men do not determine its character. A great man or woman may be born in any society and under any conditions, but that is no indication that is an ideal society. An ideal society is one which gives opportunity to every individual to grow—grow physically, intellectually, and morally. It places an ideal before the individual and urges him to grow according to that ideal. Not only that, it also creates conditions conducive to such growth.

Real beauty eventually lies in simplicity. The simpler the life, the easier it is to live with.

14. PERFECTION

In the right view both of life and of yoga all life is either consciously or subconsciously a yoga. For we mean by this term a methodised effort towards self-perfection by the expression of the potentialities latent in the being and a union of the human individual with the universal and transcendent existence we see partially expressed in man and in the cosmos. When a man casts away, O Partha, all the desires of his mind, ever satisfied in himself, by himself, then he is a man of steady wisdom—

प्रजहाति यदा कामान्सर्वान्पार्थ मनोगतान् ।
आत्मन्येवात्मना तुष्टः स्थितप्रज्ञस्तदोच्यते ।। (2-55)

He is unshaken in adversity, completely unattached to pleasures, free from attachment, fear, anger. Such a one is indeed a seer of steady wisdom.

दुःखेष्वनुद्विग्नमनाः सुखेषु विगतस्पृहः ।
वीतरागभयक्रोधः स्थितधीर्मुनिरुच्यते ।। (2-56)

He who is everywhere unattached, neither rejoices at the good nor is vexed by the evil, he is a master of perfect wisdom.

यः सर्वत्रानभिस्नेहस्तत्तत्प्राप्य शुभाशुभम् ।
नाभिनन्दति न द्वेष्टि तस्या प्रज्ञा प्रतिष्ठिता ।।

Perfection is very important to impart quality To attain success in life and to reach the desired goal one must have a positive attitude. Faith in oneself and in God, courage, strength and fearlessness are the characteristics of a positive intellect. For a man of intense faith nothing is impossible in this world.

All power is within you, you can do anything and everything. Believe in that, do not believe that you are weak, stand up and express the divinity within you. Studying Swamiji will help us develop a positive attitude.

Tremendous power is hidden within each one of us, but we are not aware of that. Positive thinking helps us to release that energy. Even a little awakening of spiritual energy will make us strong. A man with a positive attitude does not like an easy going life. He welcomes challenges, obstacles, difficulties, problems and faces them with great courage. He always likes an adventure in life. Such heroic spirit is a quality needed to become a successful leader. He alone can lead the society who has developed a positive intellect.

A strong faith in the ideal, right understanding, and concentration will lead us to success and above all self-confidence. Those who struggle to cultivate these ten aspects of a pure intellect alone can succeed in this world as well as in spiritual life.

Perfection has its two aspects in man, which to some extent be separated, the perfection in being and perfection in doing. It can be imagined that through some training or compulsion, good works may possibly be extorted from a man who personally may not be good . . . where the question is not that of utility but of moral perfection, we hold it important that the individual be true to his goodness. His outer good work may continue to produce good results, but the inner perfection of his personality has its immense value, which for him is spiritual freedom and for humanity is an endless asset thought we may not know. For goodness represents the detachment of spirit from the exclusiveness of our egoism, in goodness we identify ourselves with the universal humanity. . . . In order to realise his unity with the universal, the individual man must live his perfect life which alone gives the freedom to transcend it.

Rabindranath Tagore (The Religion of Man) XIV, 120-21.

15. COMMITMENT

In Rig Veda it has been said:

एकं सत् विप्रा बहुधा वदन्ति ।

Truth is One. There are different ways to express the Truth.

In Taitryo-Upanisad, it has been rightly stated:

सह नाववतुए सह नौ भुनक्तु,
सह वीर्य करवावहै ।
तेजस्वि नावधीमस्तु,
मा विद्विषावहै ।

We should meet together, sit together, think together, and there should be no hatred amongst us.

Swami Chinmayananda beautifully sums up the Ingredients of Commitment as:

The highest and noblest type of an individual working in the world is known as the "man of achievement" (Yogi). Such men work, neither for the sake of wages, nor for success; they are not after mere sensual pleasures, nor do they aspire to reform the world; they dedicatedly perform their obligatory duties finding peace and fulfilment in their very activity. Their fulfilment consists in doing their duties to the best of their ability without claiming any rights and they are totally unmindful of whether the society commends or condemns their actions.

To one who is not ready to act in a Spirit of dedication (Yajna) there is no real gain in this world, nor does he discover his happiness and fulfilments in this life. The secret of happiness and success is to act deligently in the Yajna spirit. The responsibility of the future entirely rests on the shoulders of the day's youth. They may learn the art of hardening their mental news from the Geeta, the art of re-organising themselves to work in the Yajna Spirit.

This is the need of the hour in our country. We have irretrievably entered an era of industry and the younger generation is being geared to a life of speed and spendthrift production. At this juncture, labour can be chastened only when the workers have a philosophy of work. Without this philosophy, the best in each of us can never be brought out and poured into our productive work. The earlier we give them an uplifting philosophy of work the sooner we shall find them ready to bring into their fields of work the subtler powers of integrity, loyalty and efficiency.

अयं स्वभावः स्वतः एव यत्पर श्रमापनोदप्रवणं महात्मनाम् ।
सुधांशुरेष स्वयमर्ककर्कश प्रभभितप्तामवति क्षिति किल ।। 38 ।।

Indeed, it is the nature of the magnanimous to help remove the troubles of others, even as the moon of its own accord cools the earth scorched by the flaming rays of the sun.

This is another mellifluous verse to emphasise that the noble qualities of magnanimity, cheerfulness, etc., in a perfect Master are natural and not the products of a self-tutored habit.

Sankara compares a Seer with the moon, and directs our attention to the fact that the moon alone can, and with effortless ease does, cool the parched earth which gets baked in the burning rays of the sun. Nothing else can cool the earth so satisfactorily as moonlight. Also, there is no chance ever of the moonlight adding a single calorie of heat to the earth. The company of the wise is the surest remedy to cool down the bosom to a state of complete peace and happiness when it is in conflagration, fed by desires and hatreds, attachments and yearnings.

तदनन्तरं विश्रवामित्रेण प्रेरितः सन्
वसिष्ठ उवाच-
Tadanantaram Visvamitrena preritahsan vasistha uvaca—

सर्वदा सर्वमेवेह संयारे रघुनन्दन ।
सम्यक् प्रयुक्तात् सर्वेण पौरुषात् समवाप्यते ।। 3 ।।

(Yoga Vasistha Sangrakah)

Sarvada sarvameveha
Samsare raghunandana
Samyak prayuktat sarvena
Paurusat samavapyate (3)

Thereafter, requested by Visvamitra, Sage Vasistha said: O Raghunandana ! In this samsara (worldly existence) everything indeed is always accomplished in full by well-applied human effort.

Some people may work hard but their efforts are misdirected. Others work in fits and spurts. Yet another type of people work without thinking and some work hardly ! To bring about the desired results, our efforts should be well directed, well thought and single pointed.

As an aspiring individual, consistently maintaining his ambition in mind, walks out into his fields of activity to battle with the immediate problems, he will meet with many a tempting channel of more fascinating plans, through which he can dissipate himself and get exhausted, rendering himself incapable of conquering the highest success in his own field. To keep oneself Self-controlled, so that one may not Thus, get derailed as one shoots forward to reach the temple of success, is the third great factor that is to be kept in mind and lived fully, in order that success in life be assured.

Notes and References

1. Swami Chinmayananda, On Wings and Wheels: A dialogue on Moral Confict, CCMT, Bombay, 1995, pp. 33-34.
2. Swami Vishnu Devananda, Meditation and Mantras, Delhi, Motilal Banarsi Das, 1978, p. 179.
3. Srimad Bhagavad Gita, XVII/8, Jayadyal Goyandha, Gita Press, Gorakhpur.
4. Keshwa Setur, Ink Notes, in *Life Plus*, Oct-Dec. 2002, pp. 11, 22, 28.
5. Chinmayanand Self Discovery, CCMT, Bombay.
6. Swami Tejomayananda, Right Thinking, CCMT, Bombay, 2002, p. 29.
7. Swami Chinmayananda, A Manual of Self Unfoldment, *op. cit.*, p. 24.
8. Bata K. Dey, *IJPA*, April-June 1989, p. 175.
9. Swami Chinmayananda, We Must, CCST, Mumbai, 2002, p. 29.
10. Aliyar, 2002, p. 62.
11. Swami Chinmayananda, On Wings and Wheels, CCMT, Bombay, 1995, pp. 11, 39.
12. Bhagwad Gita (Gita Press, Gorakhpur), in Sloka 59, Chapter 2.
13. Swami Chinmayananda, We Must, *op. cit.*, p. 47.
14. Srimad Bhagavad Gita, Gita Press, Gorakhpur, p. 213.
15. Swami Chinmayananda, The Art of Living, CCMT, Mumbai, 2002, p. 13.
16. His Holiness Dalai Lama in ALIYAR, 2002.
17. Living Wisdom, *op. cit.*, p. 219.
18. P.K. Vasudeva, Training for Creativity in the 21st Century, in P.P. Arya and R.P. Gupta (ed.), pp. 150-51, 161.
19. Swami Srikantananda, The Intelligent Way to Yoga, Chennai, Sri Ramakrishna Math, 2001, pp. 26-31.
20. Swami Visharananda, Human Values, Swami Vivekananda, Yoga Prakashana, Bangalore, 2003, pp. 31-32.
21. *Ibid.*, pp. 40-42.

Bibliography

Anita, N.B. and Bhatia, Kavita, Peoples Health in People's Hand- A model for Panchayati Raj, FRCH, Mumbai. 1993.

Basch, P.E., Vaccines and World Health, New York, Oxford University Press, 1994.

Bhatnagar, S. and Goel, S.L., Development Planning and Administration. New Delhi. Deep & Deep Publications (P) Ltd., 1992.

Bhattacharjee P.J. and G.N. Shashtri, Population in India, A Study of Interstate Variation, New Delhi, Vikas, 1976.

Bosh, Ashish, From Population to People, Delhi, B.R. Publication, 1988.

Brown, Esther, Newer Dimensions of Patient Care, Russell Sage Foundation, New York, 1961.

Cartwright, A., Patients and their Doctors, A Study of General Practice, Routledge Kegan Paul, London, 1961.

Chanawongse Krasal, Rural Development Management, Research and Development Institute, Khon Kaen University, Thailand.

Chandra, R.C., A Geography of Population, Concepts, Determinants and Patterns, New Delhi, Kalyani, 1987.

Chauhan, Devraj, Anaita, N.H. and Ramdan, Sangita, Healthcare in India: A Profile, FRCH, Mumhai, 1996.

Das, K., Civil Service Reforms and Structural Adjustment, Oxford, Delhi 1998.

Duggal, R., Nandaraj, S. and Shetty, Sahana, State Sector Health Expenditure-A Database All India, FRCH, Mumbai, 1992.

P. Jurfelds, G. and Lindbergs, Pills against Poverty—A Study of Introduction of Western Medicine in a Tamil Village, Curzon Press, London, 1975.

FRCH, Panchayati Raj Information Resource Book, Mumbai, 1996.

Ghai, Sandhaya, Bursing Services Administration: A Case Study of Nehru Hospital, PGI, Chandigarh (Doctoral Thesis, Panjab University, 1998).

Ghosh, Brindra Nath, A Treatise on Hygiene and Public Health, Scientific Publishing Company, 1970, Calcutta.

Gill, Sonya, Health Status of the Indian People, FRCH, Mumbai, 1987.

Goel, S.L., Healthcare Administration Policy-making and Planning, Sterling, Delhi, 1981.

———, Healthcare Administration Levels and Aspects, Sterling, Delhi, 1981.

Goel, S.L., Healthcare Administration Ecology, Principles and Modern Trends, Sterling, Delhi, 1981.

———, Family Planning Programme and Beyond, New Delhi, Deep & Deep Publications Pvt. Ltd., New Delhi, 1990.

———, International Administration: WHO, South-East Asia Regional Office, Sterling, New Delhi, 1977.

———, Modern Management Techniques, Deep & Deep Publications Pvt. Ltd., New Delhi, 1987.

———, Public Health Administration, Sterline, New Delhi, 1984.

———, Public Personnel Administration, Sterling, New Delhi, 1984.

———, Hospital Administration and Management, Deep & Deep Publications Pvt. Ltd., New Delhi, 1903.

———, Distance Education in 21st Century, Deep & Deep Publications Pvt. Ltd., New Delhi, 2000.

Hanlon, John, Principles of Public Health Administration, C.V. Mobsy, Sthouis, 1969.

ICSSR & ICMR, Health for All-an Alternative Strategy—Report of a Study Group set-up Jointly by ICSSR & ICMR, Pune, Indian Institute of Education, 1981.

Govt. of India, Annual Reports of the Ministry of Health and Family Welfare, Delhi.

———, Committee on Multi-purpose Workers under Health and Family Welfare Programme (Kartar Singh Report), Delhi, Ministry of Health and Family Welfare, Delhi, 1973.

———, Govt. of India, Health in Independent India (G. Borkar Report), Delhi, 1961.

———, Health Survey and Development Committee (Bhore Committee), Delhi, 1946.

———, Lok Sabha Secretariat, Estimates Committees and Public Accounts Committees Reports.

———, Planning Commission, Five Year Plans, New Delhi.

———, Report of Health Survey and Planning Committee, (Mudaliar Committee) Ministry of Health, August-October, 1961.

———, Ministry of Information and Broadcasting, India, 1999, A Refresher Manual, New Delhi, 1999.

———, Initiatives and Best Practices of Government of India for Effective and Responsive Administration, New Delhi, Ministry of Personnel, Public Grievances, and Pensions, 1997.

———, Deptt. of Family Welfare, Reproductive and Child Health (World Bank Component), Vols. I and II, New Delhi, 1997.

———, Report of the Working Group on Health for All by 2000 A.D., New Delhi Ministry of Health and Welfare, 1981.

Gunaratne Herat, V.T., Challenges and Response Health in South-East Asia Region, New Delhi, McGraw Hill, 1977.

Hardon, A., et. al., Monitoring Family Planning and Reproductive Rights, A Manual for Empowerment, London, Zed Books, 1997.

Indian Society of Health Administrators, Bangalore.

Annual Conference Reports

Health for all by 2000 (AD 1980).
The Role of Hospitals in Healthcare (1981).
Health Manpower Requirements for 2000 (1982).
Role of the Health Administrator in India (1983).
On Growing Needs of Urban Health Management (1985).
Cost Reduction in Hospitals and Healthcare (1986).
Health of the High Risk Groups Mothers, Children and Elderly (1985).
Health of Women and Children for Development (1988).
Healthcare for the Villages and Urban Slums (1989-90).
Health of the Youth and the Female Child.
Role of Voluntary Organizations in Healthcare in India (1992).

Books

Stress and Health of Executives and Professionals.
Hospital and Health Administration.
Modern Technology for Hospitals and Healthcare.
Management for Nursing Administrators.
Community Participation in Health and Family Welfare-Indian Experiences.
Health of the Metropolis-Bangalore-A Guide to Health Planning and Development of Urban Cities in India.
Leadership and Human Resources Development for Healthcare.
Managerial Effectiveness for Organizational Excellence.
Computer Applications to Hospitals, Healthcare and Medical Education.
Health and Development of the Tribal People in India-A Guide for Professionals and Administrators.
Retirement Planning, Adjustment and Health.
Janovsky, K., Health Policy and Systems Development on Agenda for Research, WHO/SHS/NHP/96.1, Geneva, 1996.
Jesani, Amar & Ganguly, Shilpi, Some Issues in Community Participation in Health Services, FRCH, Mumbai, 1993.
Khandewale, Shreekant V., Health Administration and the Weaker Sections in an Indian Metropolis, Devika Publications, Delhi, 1996.
Klinoboul Krienkrai, Health and Family Welfare Administration in Thailand—A Case Study of Lampang Province (Doctoral Thesis).
Kumar, R., Child Development in India, Ashish, New Delhi, 1988.
———, Environment Pollution and Health Hazards in India, Ashish, New Delhi (Year not mentioned).
———, Youth Health, Problem, Planning and Development, Deep and Deep Publications Pvt. Ltd., New Delhi, 1986.
Lane, S.D., From Population Control to Reproductive Health: An Emerging Policy Agenda, Social Science and Medicine, 1994.
Lush, L., Integrating Services, from Rhetroic to Action, Development Research Insights, 1997.
Mattoo, P.K., Project Formulation in Developing Countries, Macmillan, Delhi, 1978.

Meher, C. Nanavaty and P.D. Kulkarni, NGO's in the Changing Scenario, New Delhi, Uppal, 1998.

Miller, George E. and Tamas Fulop, Educational Strategies for the Health Professionals, Geneva, WHO, 1974.

Mishra, R.P., Medical Geography of India, NBT, Delhi, 1970.

Murray, C.J.L., Lopez, A.D., The Global Burden of Diseases, WHO, Geneva, Switzerland, 1996.

Myrdal Gunnar, Asian Drama, An Enquiry into the Poverty of Nations, Vol. III, Penguis, London, 1968.

Naik, J.P., An Alternative System of Healthcare Service in India Some Proposals, Allied, Bombay, 1988.

National Institute of Health and Family Welfare, New Delhi

Management Training Modules for District Health Offices.

Management Training Modules for Health Offices.

Management Training Modules for Health Assistants (Male and Female).

Management Training Modules for Health Workers (Male and Female).

Management Training Modules for TBA.

Management Training Modules for Health Guide.

Park, J.E. and K. Park (1990), Textbook on Preventive and Social Medicine, Banarasidas Bhanot Publishers, Jabalpur.

Pai Panadiker, V.A., et. al., Organizational Policy for Family Planning, New Delhi, Uppal, 1983.

Pathak, Shankar, Social Welfare, Health and Family Planning in India, Marwah Publications, Delhi, 1979.

Rao, C. Hayavandana, Mysore Gazetteer, Vol. IV, B.R. Publishing Corporation, Delhi, 1984.

Ramanathan, S. (ed.), Landmarks in Karnataka Administration, New Delhi, Uppal, 1998 (Published for Indian Institute of Public Administration, Karnataka, Regional Branch, Bangalore).

Rafei, Dr. Uton M., Primary Healthcare in Changing World South-East Asia Regional Perspectives, WHO Regional Office for South-East Asia, Delhi, India, 1993.

Ranga, R.K., Admn. of Family Planning Programmes in India—A Case Study of Haryana (Doctoral Thesis, Panjab University, 1998).

Rao, V.K.R.V., Food, Nutrition and Poverty in India, Vikas, New Delhi, 1982.

Rifikin, S.B., Health Planning and Community Participation, Crown Helm, London, 1985.

Sahni, Ashok, The Third Force in Healthcare—Voluntary Sector, Bangalore Indian Society of Health Administrators (1992).

Scott-Samuel A., Total Participation, Total Health, Scottish Academic Press, 1990.

Sarjivi, K.S., Planning India's Health, Orient Longman, Delhi, 1971. Shenoi, P.V. (ed.), Contours of Social and Economic Development Political Issues, Concept, New Delhi, 1997.

Sharma, R.D., Advanced Public Administration, New Delhi, H.K. Publishers, 1994.

Singh, Sarabjit, Management Information System in a Hospital—A Case Study of General Hospital, Chandigarh (Doctoral Thesis, Panjab University, 1991).

Taori, Kamal, People's Participation in Sustainable Human Development (A Unified Approach), New Delhi, Concept, 1998.

Vaeth, R.M., A Theory of Medical Ethics, New York, Basic Books, 1981.

Vettivel, S.K., People's Participation in Social Development, Role of NGO, New Delhi, Vetri Publishers, 1992.

World, Health Organisation Alma Ata Revisited, WHO/SHS/CC/ 94.2, WHO, Geneva, 1994.

Werner, D., Where there is no Doctor?, The Voluntary Health Association of India, Delhi, 1984.

World Bank Financing of Health Services in Developing Countries, Washington, 1987.

World Bank, Development Report, 1993, New York, Oxford University Press.

World Bank, World Development Report, 1997, New York, Oxford University Press, 1997.

World Health Organisation, Annual Report of South-East Asia Regional Office, Delhi, 1997.

———, Bulletin of Regional Health Information, Regional Office for South-East Asia, Delhi, 1980, 1981, 1982, 1983, 1984-85, 1986-87, 1988-90, and 1991-93.

World Health Organization, Collaboration in Health Development in South-East Asia, 1948-88, Fortieth Anniversary Volume (Revised), Delhi, 1992.

———, Community Action for Health, SEA/HSD/185, Regional Office for South-East Asia, Delhi, 1993.

———, Development of Indicator for Monitoring Progress Towards Health for all by the Year 2000, Geneva, 1981.

———, Eighth General Programme of Work—Covering the Period 1990-95, Geneva, 1987.

———, Evaluation of the Strategy for Health for All by the year 2000, Regional Office for South-East Asia, Delhi, 1986.

———, Formulating Strategies for Health for all by the year 2000, Geneva, 1979.

———, Global Strategy for Health for all by the year 2000, Geneva, 1981.

———, Health in Development—Prospects for 21st Century, WHO! DGH/ 94.5, Geneva, 1994.

World Health Organization, Health Situation in the South-East Asia Region, 1991-93, Regional Office for South-East Asia, Delhi, 1995.

———, Implementation of the Global Strategy for Health for All by the year 2000, Second Evaluation, Regional Office for South-East Asia, Delhi, 1993.

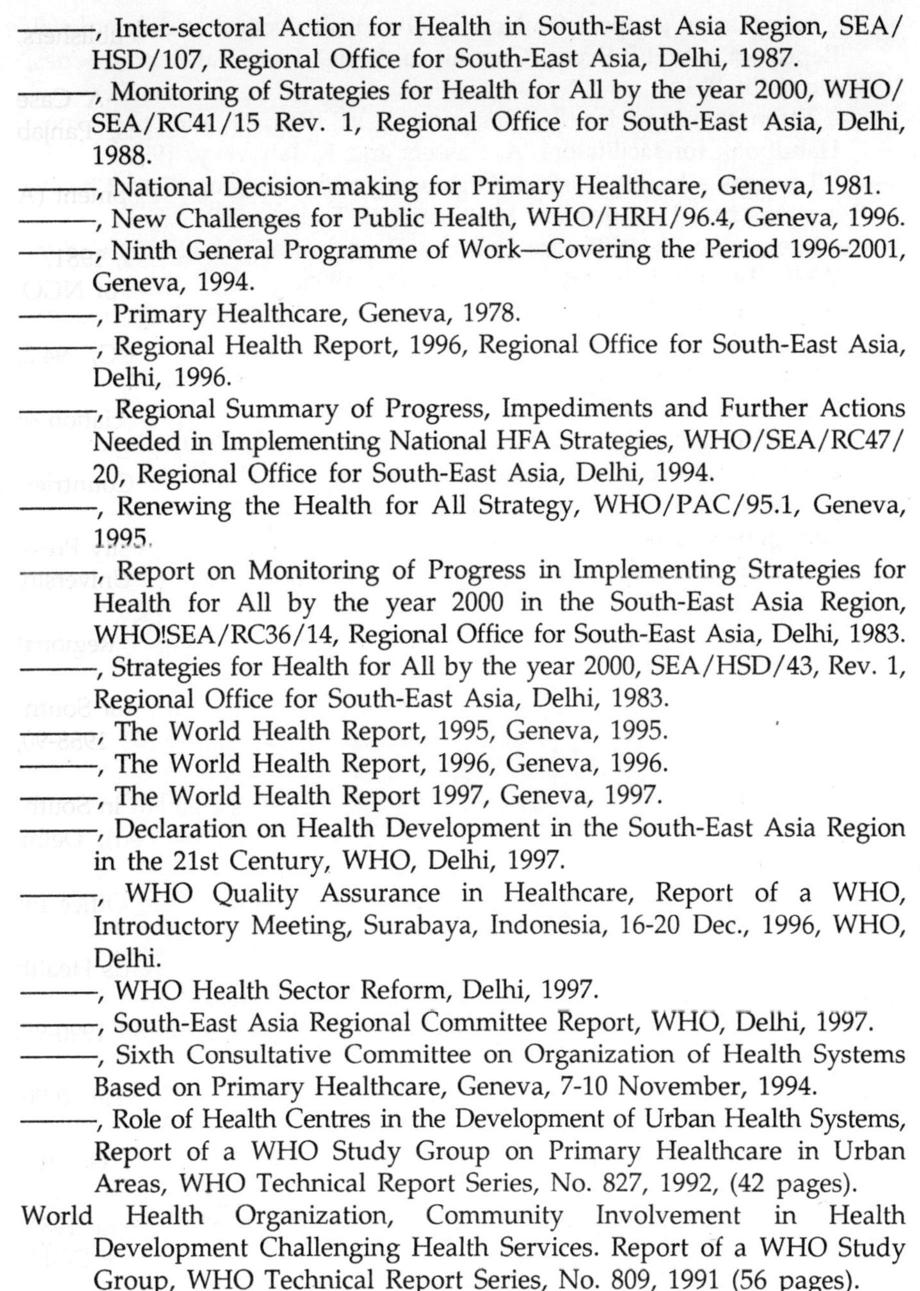

———, Inter-sectoral Action for Health in South-East Asia Region, SEA/HSD/107, Regional Office for South-East Asia, Delhi, 1987.

———, Monitoring of Strategies for Health for All by the year 2000, WHO/SEA/RC41/15 Rev. 1, Regional Office for South-East Asia, Delhi, 1988.

———, National Decision-making for Primary Healthcare, Geneva, 1981.

———, New Challenges for Public Health, WHO/HRH/96.4, Geneva, 1996.

———, Ninth General Programme of Work—Covering the Period 1996-2001, Geneva, 1994.

———, Primary Healthcare, Geneva, 1978.

———, Regional Health Report, 1996, Regional Office for South-East Asia, Delhi, 1996.

———, Regional Summary of Progress, Impediments and Further Actions Needed in Implementing National HFA Strategies, WHO/SEA/RC47/20, Regional Office for South-East Asia, Delhi, 1994.

———, Renewing the Health for All Strategy, WHO/PAC/95.1, Geneva, 1995.

———, Report on Monitoring of Progress in Implementing Strategies for Health for All by the year 2000 in the South-East Asia Region, WHO!SEA/RC36/14, Regional Office for South-East Asia, Delhi, 1983.

———, Strategies for Health for All by the year 2000, SEA/HSD/43, Rev. 1, Regional Office for South-East Asia, Delhi, 1983.

———, The World Health Report, 1995, Geneva, 1995.

———, The World Health Report, 1996, Geneva, 1996.

———, The World Health Report 1997, Geneva, 1997.

———, Declaration on Health Development in the South-East Asia Region in the 21st Century, WHO, Delhi, 1997.

———, WHO Quality Assurance in Healthcare, Report of a WHO, Introductory Meeting, Surabaya, Indonesia, 16-20 Dec., 1996, WHO, Delhi.

———, WHO Health Sector Reform, Delhi, 1997.

———, South-East Asia Regional Committee Report, WHO, Delhi, 1997.

———, Sixth Consultative Committee on Organization of Health Systems Based on Primary Healthcare, Geneva, 7-10 November, 1994.

———, Role of Health Centres in the Development of Urban Health Systems, Report of a WHO Study Group on Primary Healthcare in Urban Areas, WHO Technical Report Series, No. 827, 1992, (42 pages).

World Health Organization, Community Involvement in Health Development Challenging Health Services. Report of a WHO Study Group, WHO Technical Report Series, No. 809, 1991 (56 pages).

World Health Organization, Coordinated Health and Human Resources Development. Report of a WHO Study Group, WHO Technical Report Series, No. 801, 1990.

———, Health System Decentralization. Concept, Issues and Country Experience, A. Mills, J.P. Vaughan, D.L. Smith, I. Tabibzadehg, eds., 1990.

———, Information support for New Public Health action at district-level, Report of a WHO Expert Committee, WHO Technical Report Series, No. 845, 1994.

———, Strengthening Health Management in districts and provisions. Handbook for facilitators, A. Cassels and K. Janovsky, 1991.

———, Towards a healthy district, Organizing and managing district health systems based on primary healthcare, E. Tarimo, 1991.

———, Integration of Healthcare Delivery, Report of a WHO Study Group, WHO Technical Report Series, No. 861, 1996.

———, Primary Healthcare Reviews, Guidance and Methods, A. El Bindari-Hammad and D.L. Smith, 1992.

———, Health Promotion and Community Action for Health in Developing Countries, H.S. Dhillon and L. Philip, 1994.

———, Achieving Health for All by the year 2000, Midway Reports of Country Experiences, E. Tarimo, A. Creese, eds., (1990).

Young, Paul V., Scientific Social Surveys and Research, Englewood Cliffs, New Jersey, 1966.

Index